AF449256

CT and MRI
of the Genitourinary Tract

Contemporary Issues in Computed Tomography
Volume 13

SERIES EDITOR

Elliot K. Fishman, M.D.
Associate Professor, The Russell H. Morgan Department of Radiology and Radiologic Science, The Johns Hopkins University School of Medicine; Director, Division of Computed Body Tomography, Department of Radiology, The Johns Hopkins Hospital, Baltimore, Maryland

Volumes Already Published

Forthcoming Volumes in the Series

CT and MRI of the Genitourinary Tract

Edited by

Stanford M. Goldman, M.D., F.A.C.P.

Professor, Departments of Radiology and Urology
The Johns Hopkins University School of Medicine
Radiologist-in-Chief
Department of Radiology
Francis Scott Key Medical Center
Baltimore, Maryland

Olga M. B. Gatewood, M.D.

Associate Professor, Departments of Radiology and Urology
The Johns Hopkins University School of Medicine
Director, Section of Uroradiology
Department of Radiology
The Johns Hopkins Medical Institutions
· Baltimore, Maryland

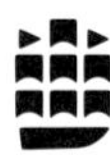

CHURCHILL LIVINGSTONE
NEW YORK, EDINBURGH, LONDON, MELBOURNE

RC
874
.C7
1990

Library of Congress Cataloging-in-Publication Data

CT and MRI of the genitourinary tract/edited by Stanford M.
Goldman, Olga M. B. Gatewood.
       p. cm.—(Contemporary issues in computed tomography; v. 13)
     Companion to and extension of: Computed tomography of the
kidneys and adrenals/edited by Stanley S. Siegelman, Olga M. B.
Gatewood, Stanford M. Goldman. 1984.
   Includes bibliographical references.
   Includes index.
   ISBN 0-443-08657-5
   1. Genitourinary organs—Tomography.   2. Genitourinary organs—
Magnetic resonance imaging.   I. Goldman, Stanford M.
II. Gatewood, Olga M. B.   III. Computed tomography of the kidneys
and adrenals.   IV. Series.
   [DNLM: 1. Adrenal Gland Diseases—diagnosis.   2. Genital
Diseases, Male—diagnosis.   3. Magnetic Resonance
Imaging.   4. Tomography, X-Ray Computed.   5. Urogenital
Neoplasms—diagnosis.   6. Diseases—diagnosis.   W1 CO769MQK
v. 13/WJ 141 C959]
RC874.C7   1990
616.6'07572—dc20
DNLM/DLC
for Library of Congress   90–1940
                                                                              CIP

© **Churchill Livingstone Inc. 1990**

All rights reserved. No part of this publication may be reproduced,
stored in a retrieval system, or transmitted in any form or by any
means, electronic, mechanical, photocopying, recording, or otherwise, without prior permission of the publisher (Churchill Livingstone Inc., 1560 Broadway, New York, NY 10036).

Distributed in the United Kingdom by Churchill Livingstone, Robert
Stevenson House, 1-3 Baxter's Place, Leith Walk, Edinburgh EH1
3AF, and by associated companies, branches, and representatives
throughout the world.

Accurate indications, adverse reactions, and dosage schedules for
drugs are provided in this book, but it is possible that they may
change. The reader is urged to review the package information data
of the manufacturers of the medications mentioned.

The Publishers have made every effort to trace the copyright holders
for borrowed material. If they have inadvertently overlooked any,
they will be pleased to make the necessary arrangements at the first
opportunity.

Acquistions Editor: *Robert A. Hurley*
Copy Editor: *Bridgett Dickinson*
Production Designer: *Marci Jordan*
Production Supervisor: *Jeanine Furino*

Printed in the United States of America

First published in 1990

To my wife, Harriet, and children, Etan Boaz and Nava

Stanford M. Goldman

Contributors

Marco A. Amendola, M.D.
Professor, Department of Radiology, University of Miami School of Medicine; Chief, Section of Uroradiology, Department of Radiology, Jackson Memorial Hospital, Miami, Florida

Bruce R. Baumgartner, M.D.
Associate Professor of Radiology, Department of Medicine, Emory University School of Medicine, Atlanta, Georgia

Michael E. Bernardino, M.D.
Professor of Radiology, Department of Medicine, Emory University School of Medicine, Atlanta, Georgia

Bernard A. Birnbaum, M.D.
Assistant Professor, Department of Radiology, New York University School of Medicine, New York, New York

Morton A. Bosniak, M.D.
Professor, Department of Radiology, New York University School of Medicine, New York, New York

Charles B. Brendler, M.D.
Associate Professor, Department of Urology, The Johns Hopkins University School of Medicine, Baltimore, Maryland

Steven H. Brick, M.D.
Staff Radiologist, Department of Radiology, Washington Adventist Hospital, Takoma Park, Maryland

Judith L. Chezmar, M.D.
Assistant Professor, Department of Radiology, Emory University School of Medicine, Atlanta, Georgia

Peter L. Choyke, M.D.
Associate Professor, Department of Radiology, Georgetown University School of Medicine, Washington, D.C.; Staff Radiologist, Department of Radiology, Warren G. Magnuson Clinical Center National Institutes of Health, Bethesda, Maryland

N. Reed Dunnick, M.D.
Professor, Department of Radiology, Duke University School of Medicine; Director, Division of Imaging, Department of Radiology, Duke University Medical Center, Durham, North Carolina

Elliot K. Fishman, M.D.
Associate Professor, The Russell H. Morgan Department of Radiology and Radiologic Science, The Johns Hopkins University School of Medicine; Director, Division of Computed Body Tomography, Department of Radiology, The Johns Hopkins Hospital, Baltimore, Maryland

Arnold C. Friedman, M.D.
Professor, Department of Diagnostic Imaging, Temple University School of Medicine; Chief, Section of Abdominal Imaging, Temple University Hospital, Philadelphia, Pennsylvania

Olga M. B. Gatewood, M.D.
Associate Professor, Departments of Radiology and Urology, The Johns Hopkins University School of Medicine; Director, Section of Uroradiology, Department of Radiology, The Johns Hopkins Medical Institutions, Baltimore, Maryland

Stanford M. Goldman, M.D., F.A.C.P.
Professor, Departments of Radiology and Urology, The Johns Hopkins University School of Medicine; Radiologist-in-Chief, Department of Radiology, Francis Scott Key Medical Center, Baltimore, Maryland

Michael Hallowell, M.D.
Instructor, Department of Radiology, The Johns Hopkins University School of Medicine; Staff Radiologist, Department of Radiology, Francis Scott Key Medical Center, Baltimore, Maryland

Philip J. Kenney, M.D.
Associate Professor, Department of Radiology, Administrative Director of Magnetic Resonance Imaging, Department of Radiology, University of Alabama School of Medicine, Birmingham, Alabama

Ron Khazan, M.D.
Instructor, Department of Radiology, The Johns Hopkins University School of Medicine; Staff Radiologist, Department of Radiology, Francis Scott Key Medical Center, Baltimore, Maryland

Richard A. Leder, M.D.
Assistant Professor, Department of Radiology, Duke University School of Medicine, Durham, North Carolina

William J. Marasco, M.D.
Post-Graduate Fellow, Department of Radiology, The Johns Hopkins University School of Medicine, Baltimore, Maryland

Robert Mattrey, M.D.
Associate Professor and Director of Magnetic Resonance Research, Department of Radiology, University of California, San Diego, School of Medicine, La Jolla, California; Chief, Body Magnetic Resonance Section, Department of Radiology, Magnetic Resonance Institute, San Diego, California

Timothy J. Miller, M.D.
Radiology Resident, Department of Radiology, The Johns Hopkins University School of Medicine, Baltimore, Maryland

Steven H. Millmond, M.D.
Assistant Professor, Department of Radiology, The Johns Hopkins University School of Medicine; Staff Radiologist, Department of Radiology, Francis Scott Key Medical Center, Baltimore, Maryland

Howard M. Pollack, M.D.
Professor of Radiology and Urology, Department of Radiology, University of Pennsylvania School of Medicine; Chief, Section of Uroradiology, Department of Radiology, Hospital of the University of Pennsylvania, Philadelphia, Pennsylvania

Paul D. Radecki, M.D.
Associate Professor, Department of Diagnostic Imaging, Temple University School of Medicine; Physician, Section of Abdominal Imaging, Temple University Hospital, Philadelphia, Pennsylvania

Michael C. Soulen, M.D.
Fellow, Department of Radiology, Thomas Jefferson University Hospital, Philadelphia, Pennsylvania

Harvey V. Steinberg, M.D.
Assistant Professor of Radiology, Department of Medicine, Emory University School of Medicine, Atlanta, Georgia

Ray E. Stutzman, M.D.
Associate Professor of Urology, Department of Surgery, The Johns Hopkins University School of Medicine; Chief, Division of Urology, Francis Scott Key Medical Center, Baltimore, Maryland

John P. Volpe, M.D.
Research Assistant, Department of Radiology, Warren G. Magnuson Clinical Center National Institutes of Health, Bethesda, Maryland

Byrn Williamson, Jr., M.D.
Associate Professor, Department of Diagnostic Radiology, Mayo Medical School, Rochester, Minnesota

Andrew Yang, M.D.
Instructor of Magnetic Resonance Imaging, Department of Radiology, The Johns Hopkins University School of Medicine; Attending Radiologist, Department of Radiology, Union Memorial Hospital, Baltimore, Maryland

Shirley Yang, M.D.
Instructor, Department of Radiology, The Johns Hopkins University School of Medicine; Attending Radiologist, Department of Radiology, Union Memorial Hospital, Baltimore, Maryland

Preface

It is now six years since we edited *Computed Tomography of the Kidneys and Adrenals,* volume 3 of this series. As a companion to and an extension of volume 3 the scope of this volume and its title have been expanded to encompass the entire urinary tract. We have included magnetic resonance imaging (MRI) as a guide for the reader in understanding the appropriate utilization of MRI in the evaluation of urinary tract disease. Although there are areas where CT clearly remains the modality of choice, MRI currently has a significant role in the evaluation of the prostate, the inferior vena cava, and the adrenal gland. In addition, we have included new state-of-the-art uses of CT in the evaluation of the kidney, which have emerged since 1984.

We would like to take this opportunity to thank the authors who have contributed to this volume and to recognize the time they have devoted to writing their chapters. We also would like to thank Mr. Robert Hurley at Churchill Livingstone whose advice and direction led to the completion of this text. Finally, we wish to thank Mrs. Joyce Schreiber who kept constant tabs on its status and development. We hope and believe that our readers will find the result of these efforts useful in their clinical practice.

Stanford M. Goldman, M.D.
Olga M. B. Gatewood, M.D.

Contents

1 CT and MRI of the Adrenal Gland

RICHARD A. LEDER
N. REED DUNNICK

Adrenal lesions can be divided into those that produce clinical syndromes, in which the patient manifests signs and symptoms of hormone excess, and nonfunctional disease, in which no recognizable hormone is overproduced. The adrenal glands are also a common site of metastatic disease. Detection of disease can be accomplished by plain film, excretory urography, ultrasound, radionuclide scanning, and angiography. However, accurate delineation and characterization of adrenal pathology often require CT and MRI.

ANATOMY

The adrenal gland lies within the perirenal space along with the kidney and perirenal fat and is enclosed by Gerota's fascia. Located at the level of the eleventh or twelfth rib lateral to the vertebra, the adrenal glands rest in the superior portion of the perirenal space.[1] The right adrenal gland lies immediately posterior to the inferior vena cava and anterosuperior to the kidney. The gland has a roughly triangular shape; as one proceeds caudally, the gland has the configuration of an inverted V or an inverted Y. The apical portion of the V or the "tail" of the Y constitutes the anteromedial portion of the gland. The two posteriorly directed limbs are the lateral (hepatic) and medial (crural) limbs.[2]

Since the left kidney is usually higher than the right kidney, the left adrenal gland is lower in relation to the left kidney and lies anteromedial to the kidney's upper pole. The left gland may extend down to the left renal hilum in up to 10 percent of normal persons.[3] The gland is lateral to the aorta and posterior to the pancreas and splenic vein. Similar to the right adrenal, the gland on the left may have an inverted V or Y shape. The multiple normal appearances of the adrenal glands were appreciated even on early CT studies.[4–6] Current

"

scanners should be able to detect both adrenal glands in nearly 100 percent of cases.

Multiple small arteriae arise from three main feeding arteries to supply the adrenal glands. These major vessels are the inferior adrenal artery (arising from the renal artery), the middle adrenal artery (arising from the aorta), and the superior adrenal artery (a branch of the inferior phrenic artery).[7]

Venous drainage is via a single central vein. The right adrenal vein empties into the posterior aspect of the inferior vena cava, while the left adrenal vein empties into the inferior phrenic vein, which then enters the superior aspect of the left renal vein.

The adrenal gland is composed of cortical and medullary regions. The cortex, which is 50 percent of the adrenal gland by weight, is comprised of three zones of cells. The zona glomerulosa is the outermost layer and is formed by small columnar cells in ovoid groups. This layer produces the mineralocorticoids, in particular aldosterone. The middle layer is the zona fasciculata, which is responsible for the production of glucocorticoids (cortisol). The zona reticularis is the innermost layer and produces glucocorticoids and cortical androgens. The adrenal medulla is responsible for the production of epinephrine and norepinephrine.[8] A basic understanding of this architectural arrangement allows for better understanding of the location of particular pathologic processes.

TECHNIQUE

CT is the single best imaging modality for examining the adrenal glands. In many cases this will be the only radiographic study required. The adrenal glands are routinely examined with contiguous 5-mm sections through the entire gland. For small lesions to clarify equivocal findings, 3- or 1.5-mm sections may be obtained. Patients are scanned at end-inspiration using a large field of view. Spatial resolution is improved if a smaller medium display field of view is used. Since numerous adrenal lesions are associated with disease elsewhere in the abdomen, a full field of view is generally employed. The raw scan data are then used for subsequent target reconstruction of the adrenal glands.

Oral contrast should be provided to delineate the gastrointestinal (GI) tract. This helps avoid misinterpreting vessels, a loop of bowel, the fundus of the stomach, or a gastric diverticulum as an adrenal mass[9,10] (Fig. 1-1). Intravenous (IV) contrast material is not necessary, but is helpful in separating the adrenal gland from the kidney and in defining possible venous tumor extension.

Generally, IV contrast is not given to patients suspected of having a pheochromocytoma. Hypertensive crises induced by IV contrast material, drugs (glucagon), or physical manipulation (percutaneous biopsy) have been reported.[11] Fortunately, a high noncontrast detection rate obviates the need for IV contrast in most patients. In addition, MRI scanning and radionuclide imaging with metaiodobenzylguanidine (MIBG) provide alternative methods of diagnosis.

MRI can provide valuable information about the nature of adrenal masses.

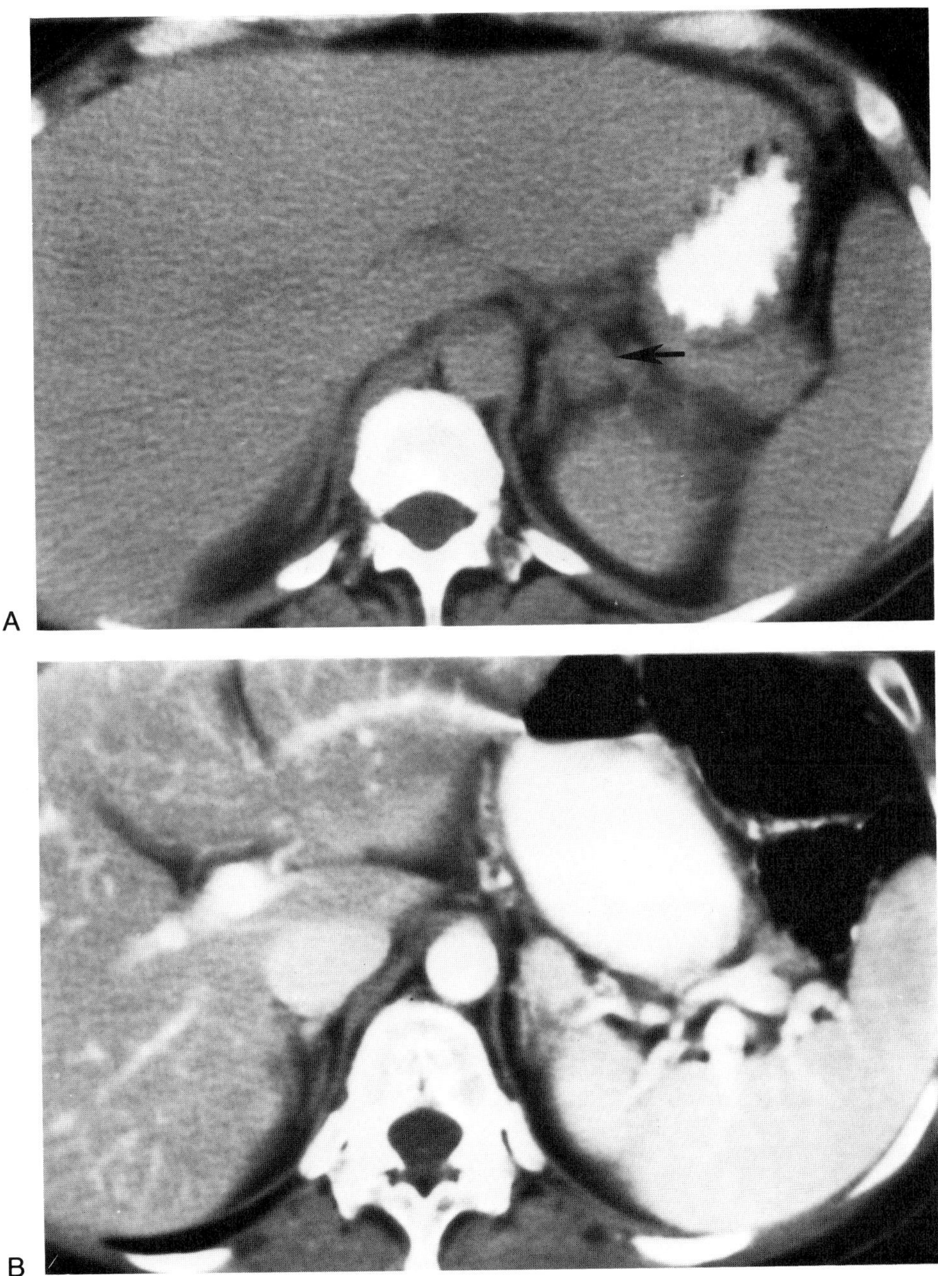

FIG. 1-1.   Pseudotumor. (A) A soft tissue mass (arrow) is seen anterior to the upper pole of the left kidney, simulating an adrenal mass. (B) Following intravenous contrast, this mass is enhanced and is seen to be a portion of the spleen.

While spatial resolution is poorer than CT, differences in proton density reflected in tissue relaxation time (T_1, T_2) can help to further characterize abnormal mass lesions.

Numerous examination protocols may be used to study the adrenal glands. Image slices are typically 5 mm thick and contiguous. Operating a magnet at 1.5 T, spin-echo pulse sequences 500/25 (TR ms/TE ms) and 2,000/25, 80 or 2,000/40, 80 are acquired. Images obtained with a 500/25 sequence are considered T_1-weighted, while 2,000/80 sequences are considered T_2-weighted images. The morphologic features of the adrenal gland are emphasized on T_1-weighted images, while T_2-weighted images provide more specific information about the nature of a mass. Body coils are used to image both glands; for small lesions and improved signal-to–noise (S/N) ratio, a surface coil may be used. Limitations to the use of surface coils include a complicated study setup and a restricted field of view. The role of paramagnetic contrast material is still under investigation. Improved image quality may be achieved using cardiac and respiratory gating.[12]

NONFUNCTIONING ADRENAL LESIONS

Frequently an adrenal lesion will be detected during imaging studies performed for tumor staging or an unrelated problem. These masses do not produce a recognizable hormone, and no symptoms relative to the adrenal mass are evident. Numerous congenital, developmental, traumatic, inflammatory, and neoplastic masses may occur in the adrenal gland.

Adenoma

At autopsy, nonfunctioning adenomas of the adrenal glands are found in approximately 2 to 9 percent of adult patients.[13] Adrenal adenomas are usually single and encapsulated. CT cannot differentiate between functioning and nonfunctioning adenomas. In addition, adenomas must be distinguished from metastases. In patients without biochemical evidence of adrenal hyperfunction and without a known primary malignancy, these masses are almost always nonfunctioning adrenal adenomas or focal nodular hyperplasia.[14]

CT findings in adrenal adenoma include a smooth, round, or oval mass. These lesions have a well-delineated margin, and no growth is demonstrated on serial CT studies. Follow-up scanning in 2 to 3 months, followed by 6 months and then 1 year, has been advocated to exclude malignant disease.[15] Lesions that are stable at 1 year should be considered benign, and no further follow-up is required. Percutaneous fine-needle biopsy, MRI or radionuclide examination with a cortical labeling agent have all been advocated to further define these masses.

Most adenomas are less than 5 cm in diameter. Larger lesions should be viewed with suspicion. Adenomas may arise in any portion of either adrenal gland. The lesion is of variable density, but more than one-half have soft tissue

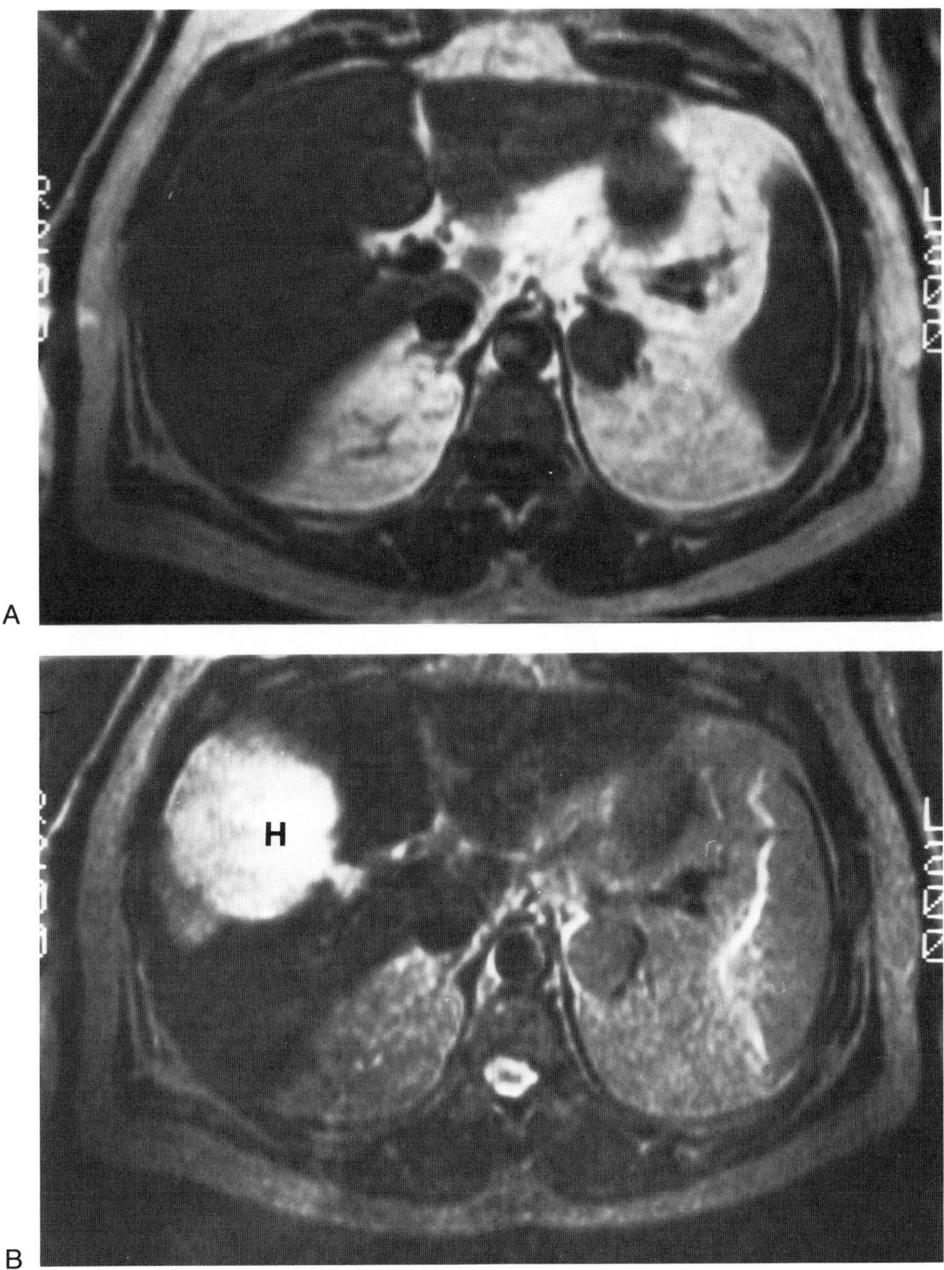

FIG. 1-2.   Nonfunctioning adenoma. (A) A 4-cm left adrenal mass is seen on this T_1-weighted image (TR 500/TE 25). (B) The signal intensity is minimally prolonged on T_2-weighted images (TR 2,500/TE 80). Incidental note is made of a high-signal cavernous hemangioma (H) of the liver.

density similar to the rest of the normal gland. Some lesions may demonstrate decreased attenuation due to high lipid content. Hyalinization or necrosis within adenomas may also cause areas of decreased attenuation.[15]

MRI studies reveal a generally homogeneous adrenal mass. Nonhyperfunctioning adenomas have T_1 and T_2 relaxation times similar to those of the normal gland. On T_1-weighted images, they appear slightly hypointense or isointense compared with the liver. Isointensity or slight hyperintensity is found in nonhyperfunctioning adenomas on T_2-weighted pulse sequences[16] (Fig. 1-2). Overlap may occur with metastatic adrenal lesions. Difficulties arise when hemorrhage occurs into benign adrenal adenomas.

Adrenal adenomas may occur in adrenal glands that contain other mass lesions. For example, combined adrenal adenoma and myelolipoma has been reported.[17] Furthermore, adrenal adenomas have been associated with renal cell carcinoma. Adrenal adenomas occur in 12 to 15 percent of patients with renal cell carcinoma as compared with 2 to 3 percent of the general population.[18] Adrenal mass lesions in patients with renal cell carcinoma may be misdiagnosed as metastases. In this setting MRI scanning should be performed to further clarify this situation.

Myelolipoma

Adrenal myelolipomas are rare benign tumors of the adrenal gland. The tumor is composed of varying portions of fat and bone marrow elements. Reported autopsy incidence ranges from 0.08 to 0.2 percent.[19,20] Most cases are discovered in the fourth to sixth decades (age range 17 to 93 years). Males and females are equally affected. Although typically asymptomatic, pain may occur as a result of hemorrhage, necrosis, or pressure on adjacent structures. These lesions have no significant malignant potential and are nonfunctioning.[21]

CT diagnosis depends on the identification of fatty tissue within the lesion. The demonstration of a fatty component that is slightly less dense than normal fat but more lucent than water or soft tissue is sought. Most lesions are unilateral. Focal or diffusely increased density may be caused by calcification, hemorrhage, or a relatively greater amount of myeloid tissue. These tumors appear as well-defined, discrete masses that may have a pseudocapsule. Myelolipomas range from microscopic to more than 8 cm in size[22] (Fig. 1-3). Myelolipomas may coexist with nonfunctional and functional adrenal adenomas.[17,23]

MRI reveals a mass with signal intensity equal to that of subcutaneous or retroperitoneal fat. This holds true for all pulse sequences. As with CT, MRI may reveal heterogeneous features based on the particular elements composing the mass. The simplicity and accuracy of CT scanning of myelolipoma makes this modality sufficent for assessing these masses. Other fatty suprarenal masses exist, including lipomas, lymphangiomas, angiomyolipomas, retroperitoneal teratomas, and liposarcomas. If a retroperitoneal fatty mass can be localized to the adrenal gland, myelolipoma is highly likely.[21]

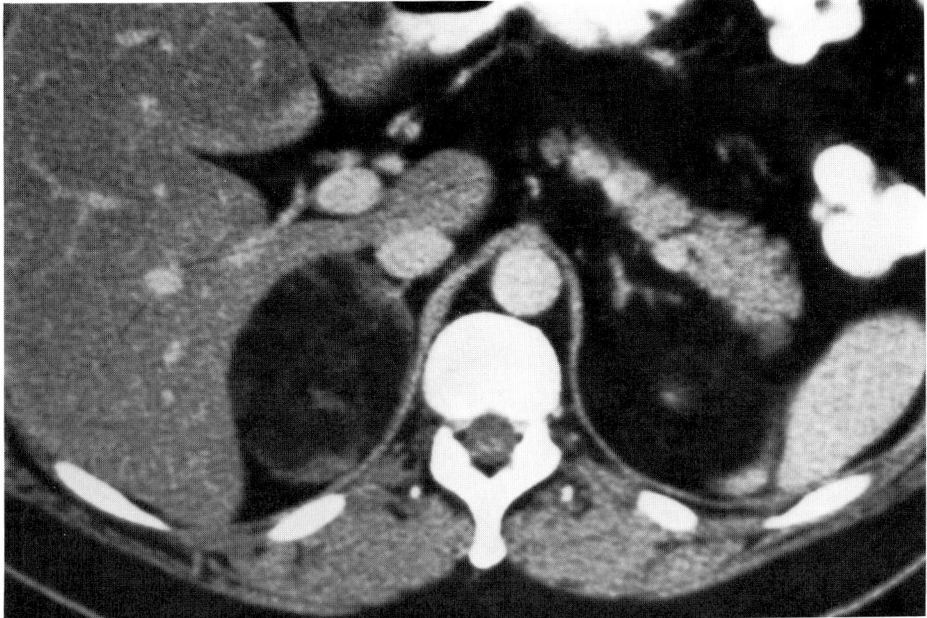

FIG. 1-3.   Myelolipoma. The fatty density of this 6-cm right adrenal mass indicates a myelolipoma.

Cyst

Adrenal cysts are usually incidentally discovered during evaluation of abnormalities of the genitourinary system. The prevalence of an adrenal cyst at autopsy is less than 0.1 percent. Cysts occur with equal frequency in the right and left adrenal glands. Bilateral cysts may occur, but are rare. Women are affected more often than men (2 to 1). Large cysts may cause abdominal pain or GI symptoms or may result in a palpable mass. Endothelial cysts are most common (45 percent), followed by pseudocysts (39 percent) and epithelial cysts (9 percent). Most cysts are small and may go undiagnosed. Pseudocysts tend to be larger and occur secondary to hemorrhage into a normal or abnormal adrenal gland[24] (Fig. 1-4).

Adrenal cysts, like cysts in other organs, appear as round, sharply marginated lesions with a thin wall. The density of these cysts is near that of water, and they lack contrast enhancement. Calcification may occur in the wall of a cyst and is more commonly seen in pseudocysts. Septae may be present in pseudocysts.[25] Areas of high attenuation within adrenal cysts may be caused by hemorrhage.[26]

Low signal intensity on T_1-weighted images with high T_2 signal are typical of adrenal cysts.[27] These cysts have signal characteristics similar to cysts of other organs, such as the liver or kidney.

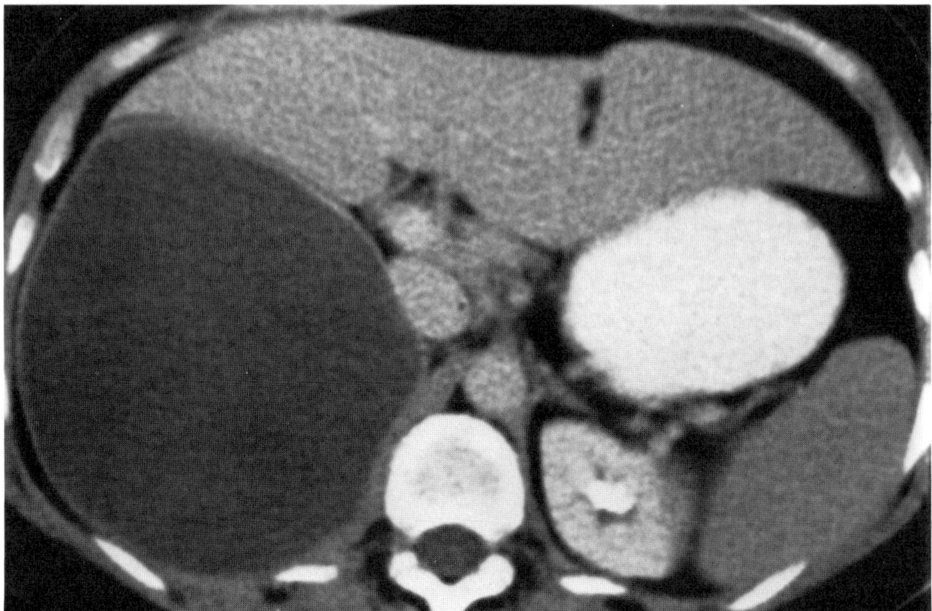

FIG. 1-4.   Pseudocyst. A 12 × 15 cm cystic mass is identified in the right adrenal bed. At surgery, a 1,650-g adrenal pseudocyst was removed.

Hemorrhage

The diagnosis of adrenal hemorrhage is frequently made at autopsy. The degree of adrenal insufficiency created by an adrenal bleed may not be great enough to produce clinical symptoms. Adrenal insufficiency does not result until approximately 90 percent of the cortex is affected.[26] Symptoms of adrenal hemorrhage, such as abdominal or flank pain, may mimic acute myocardial infarction or an acute surgical abdomen. Nausea, vomiting, and diaphoresis may also occur. If adrenal insufficiency does result from adrenal hemorrhage, the symptoms of lethargy, hypotension, tachycardia, and fever may be incorrectly attributed to sepsis.[28]

The etiology of adrenal hemorrhage includes the postoperative and postpartum setting, congestive heart failure, pulmonary embolic disease, myocardial infarction, sepsis, and commonly thrombocytopenia and use of anticoagulant therapy. Anticoagulant-related adrenal hemorrhage is noted to occur during the initial 3 weeks of treatment.[29] Neonatal adrenal hemorrhage is common and is best diagnosed by ultrasound. Classic laboratory abnormalities in patients with adrenal hemorrhage include hyponatremia, hyperkalemia, and hypoglycemia; however, this is not universally found.[30]

Bilateral adrenal masses are frequently found in cases of adrenal hemorrhage. These masses range from 2 to 5 cm in diameter. An acute bleed will appear as homogeneously increased attenuation (50 to 80 HU). The adrenal gland will appear more dense than the kidney on noncontrast imaging. Follow-up scans in cases of hemorrhage show diminution or disappearance of areas of hemorrhage. In addition, there will be progressive diminution of attenuation, with the gland eventually becoming soft tissue or water density.[31] Unilateral adrenal hemorrhage may occur in the setting of blunt trauma, in which 85 percent of hemorrhages involve the right adrenal gland.[32]

The precise role of MRI in the evaluation of hematomas is uncertain. Acute hematomas do not have a distinctive MRI appearance and can usually be diagnosed on CT because of their high attenuation. Subacute and chronic hematomas are expected to have signal characteristics similar to those of other extracranial hematomas. Most subacute hematomas appear inhomogeneous with low-intensity centers and high signal in the periphery. This finding is best appreciated on T_1-weighted images but may also be seen on T_2-weighted images. Low signal regions of hematomas on T_1- and T_2-weighted images correspond to areas of high attenuation on CT. Low-attenuation areas have a high signal on MRI.[33] Chronic hematomas are likely to have hyperintensity both centrally and peripherally. This may be explained by the magnetic characteristics of the constituents of blood, oxyhemoglobin, deoxyhemoglobin, and methemoglobin.[34] MRI of hematomas is heavily dependent on the age of the hematoma, and the appearance will change on follow-up examinations.

Metastasis

The adrenal glands are a frequent site of metastatic disease. Adrenal metastases were found by Abrams and co-workers[35] in 27 percent of autopsied patients with malignant epithelial neoplasms. Examination of the adrenal glands by CT is included in tumor staging for a wide variety of neoplasms, particularly bronchogenic carcinoma. The most common primary tumors that produce adrenal metastases are lung, breast, stomach, colon, and renal neoplasms. This list is not complete as virtually any neoplasm may metastasize to the adrenal gland.

The incidence of adrenal metastasis in lung cancer is as high as 30 percent.[36] CT detection of adrenal metastases is high; using proper technique, lesions smaller than 1 cm may be detected. False-negative scans can occur with microinvasion, which does not distort the normal architecture of the gland. Fine-needle aspiration biopsy has detected metastases in as many as 17 percent of patients with bronchogenic carcinoma and a negative CT scan.[37] False-positive cases arise when masses are found in the adrenals that are subsequently found to be adenomas, hyperplasia, or adrenal cysts. The detection of an adrenal mass (particularly if bilateral) in a patient with a known malignancy is highly suggestive of metastatic disease. The presence of liver metastasis or adenopathy, both of which can be detected by CT, further increases the likelihood that an adrenal mass is attributable to metastatic disease. If an adrenal mass is the only evidence of disease, however, confirmation is needed, and may be achieved with percutaneous aspiration biopsy.[38,39]

The detection of an adrenal metastasis frequently occurs during the course of CT scanning for tumor staging. These patients are frequently asymptomatic, although abdominal or back pain may occur. Adrenal insufficiency is unusual as a high percentage of the adrenal cortex must be replaced before insufficiency occurs.

The CT appearance of metastatic disease to the adrenal gland is variable. Most lesions are small, homogeneous, oval, or round masses. Most lesions are less than 6 cm in diameter. Bilaterality of lesions favors metastatic disease. Metastatic lesions can have low attenuation, in the range of water density. Larger lesions are frequently inhomogeneous because of hemorrhage or necrosis. Calcification is rare, although it may occur with metastases from primary mucin-producing tumors.[26]

Adrenal metastases usually demonstrate less signal intensity than does the liver on T_1-weighted images, with high signal intensity on T_2-weighted images. However, small metastatic deposits or metastases from a tumor with a low T_2 may not show increased signal intensity.[40] Glazer et al.[41] reported three metastatic masses in the adrenal glands that were low signal intensity on T_2 images. This finding is troublesome, since the impression would be that of a benign adenoma; therefore, further workup would not necessarily be recommended.[41] Benign lesions with high T_2 signal have also been reported. These lesions would present less of a dilemma, since biopsy or surgery would be recommended to exclude malignancy.[42]

The ability of MRI to separate metastatic disease from nonhyperfunctioning adenomas is imperfect. Many recent studies have attempted to establish criteria by which adrenal metastases can be distinguished from adrenal adenomas.[43-45] National Institutes of Health (NIH) data indicate that all adrenal lesions with lesion/liver intensity ratios less than or equal to 1.2 at SE 2,500/80 (0.5 T) were adenomas, while all lesions with an intensity ratio greater than or equal to 1.4 were malignant (ratios of 1.2 to 1.4 were indeterminate).[46] How this lesion/liver intensity ratio will work at 1.5 T is as yet undetermined, although the T_2 should not change with field strength. Other limitations of this ratio are relative to both the adrenal lesion and the liver. Signal intensity of adrenal lesions will be affected by size, blood flow, necrosis, active inflammation, and hemorrhage (Fig. 1-5). Liver pathology will also contribute to misinterpretation of the ratio. Hepatic T_1 and T_2 signal intensity can be affected by hepatitis, fatty infiltration, and iron deposition.[42] Until further prospective data are available, a conservative approach is recommended. In equivocal or indeterminate cases, biopsy is warranted.

Lymphoma

Adrenal involvement in lymphoma is unusual. Most patients show evidence of other extranodal abdominal disease.[47] The response to chemotherapy is similar to that of other lymphomatous masses. CT density and mass margination are variable, although a solid homogeneous mass is most common.[48]

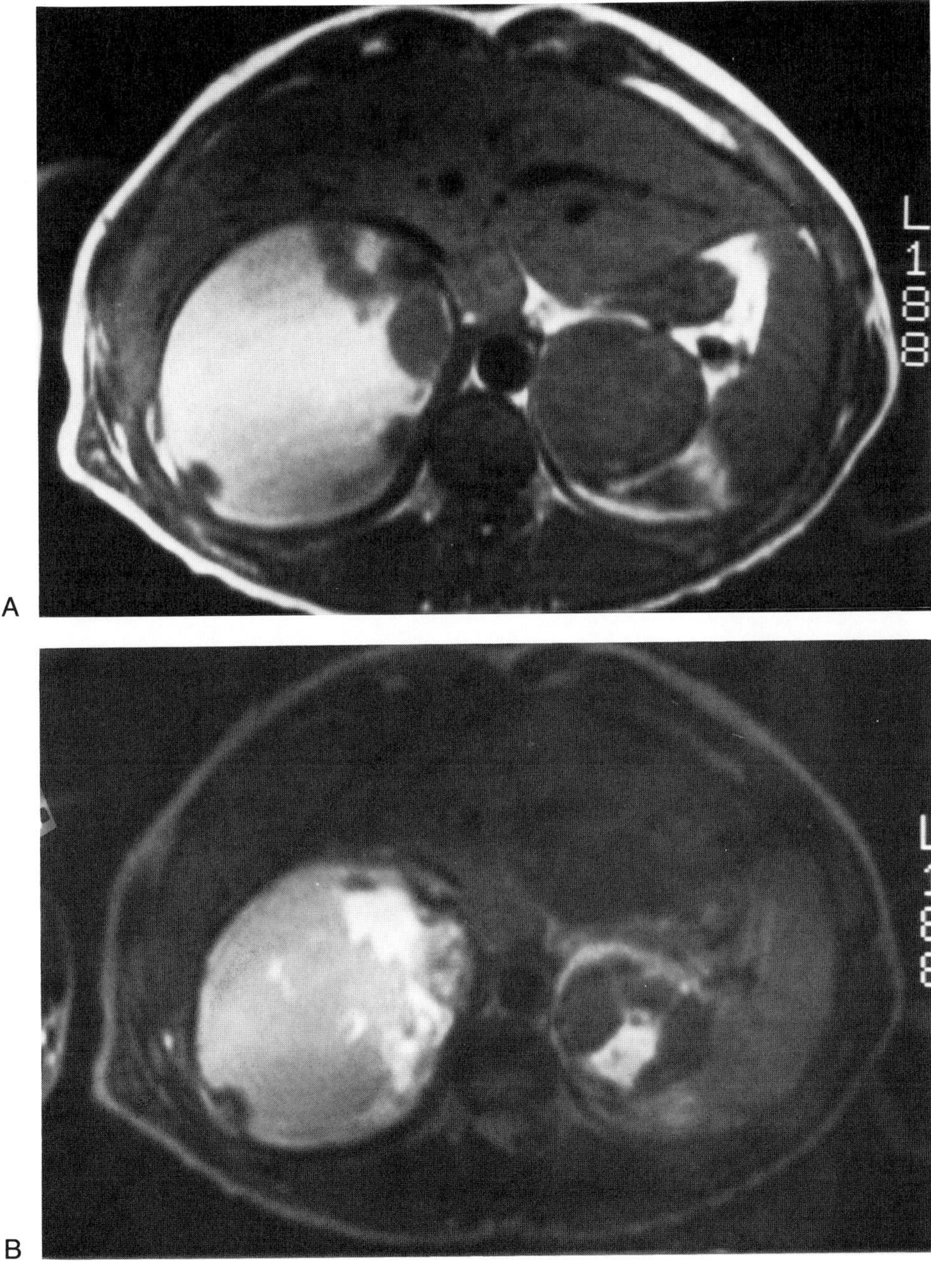

FIG. 1-5.   Metastasis. (A) A 14-cm mass is seen in the right adrenal gland. The high signal on this T_1-weighted image is due to methemoglobin and is consistent with subacute hemorrhage. A low-signal 6-cm left adrenal metastasis is also present in this patient with malignant melanoma. (B) High signal on T_2-weighted image confirms subacute hemorrhage; necrosis is seen in the left adrenal metastasis.

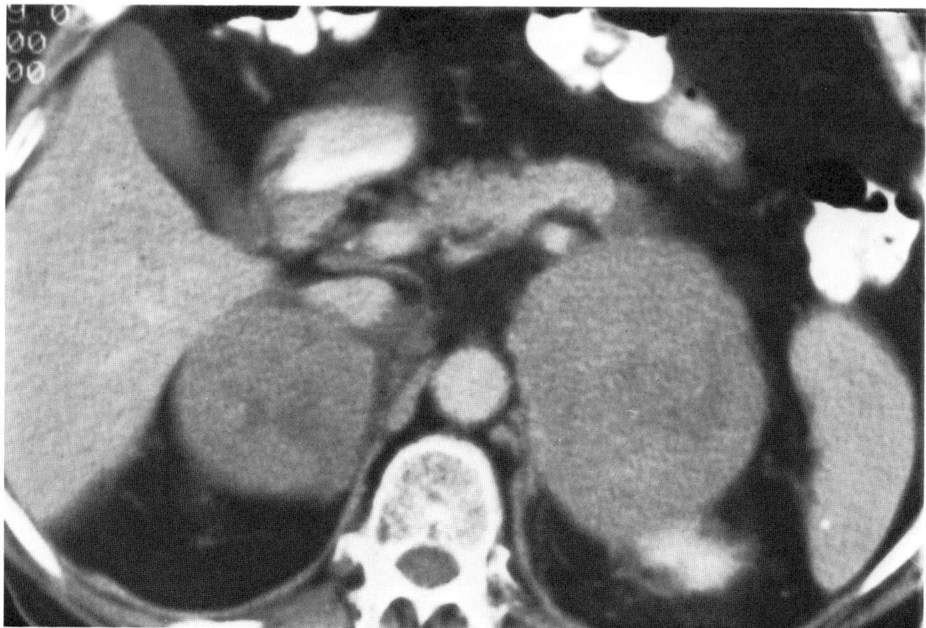

FIG. 1-6.   Lymphoma. Large bilateral solid masses are seen in this patient with non-Hodgkin's lymphoma.

Necrosis may cause inhomogeneity of lymphomatous masses. In up to one-half of cases, the adrenal masses will be bilateral (Fig. 1-6). Lymphomatous involvement of the adrenal is more common in non-Hodgkin's lymphoma than in Hodgkin's lymphoma.

Inflammatory Disease

Granulomatous infection of the adrenal gland is caused primarily by *Mycobacterium tuberculosis* and by *Histoplasma capsulatum,* less frequently by *Blastomyces* and *Cryptococcus.* Tuberculosis and histoplasmosis are responsible for most of the adrenal calcifications seen in the adult population. Many affected patients may also show evidence of disease in the chest or in other extra-adrenal sites.[49,50]

CT findings in inflammatory disease are usually bilateral and symmetric. With active disease, the gland is enlarged but maintains its normal shape. Regions of inhomogeneity within the gland are generally of low attenuation and suggest foci of necrosis.[51] With treatment, the adrenals may revert to normal size or have an atrophic appearance.[52] Improvement may occur slowly over months to years. Calcification is a sequela of healed disease. Calcification can be minimal or dense, unilateral or bilateral. Symptomatic adrenal insufficiency may occur in the setting of adrenal infection.[53] If the diagnosis is uncertain, fine-needle aspiration biopsy may be performed.

FUNCTIONING ADRENAL LESIONS

The diagnosis of the nonfunctional adrenal mass depends primarily on its imaging characteristics. Without appropriate history, the finding of an adrenal soft tissue mass is nonspecific. Clinical data are crucial in imaging the functional adrenal lesions. Diagnosing these tumors requires high-quality imaging combined with pertinent clinical history.

Aldosteronoma

Primary hyperaldosteronism, or Conn's syndrome, is characterized by sodium and fluid retention resulting in hypertension, metabolic alkalemia, and hypokalemia. Increased production of aldosterone causes retention of sodium and fluid in the collecting tubules of the kidney, with concomitant loss of potassium. Hypokalemia may manifest as weakness, cardiac arrhythmia, carbohydrate intolerance, or nephrogenic diabetes insipidus.

Less than 1 percent of patients with hypertension have an aldosteronoma. Clinical and laboratory testing demonstrate elevated plasma and urinary aldosterone levels, as well as suppressed plasma-renin activity.[54] When primary aldosteronism has been confirmed biochemically, the role of radiology is the identification and localization of the adrenal tumor.

Primary aldosteronism may be caused by an adrenal adenoma, bilateral adrenal hyperplasia and rarely adrenal carcinoma. Almost 80 percent of cases are caused by an adrenal adenoma, and approximately 70 percent of patients are female. Diffuse or nodular adrenal hyperplasia accounts for more than 20 percent of cases, with males and females equally affected.[55] Treatment will depend on which type of lesion is present; therefore, imaging is critical.

Because of the small size of these adrenal tumors, the CT examination should be performed with narrow 5-mm collimation. The adrenocortical adenomas responsible for Conn's syndrome typically range in size from 0.5 to 3.5 cm in diameter. These appear as small, round masses that may be isodense or slightly less dense than the remainder of the gland. Low-attenuation areas are attributed to a high lipid content.[56] IV contrast may be used to enhance the normal adrenal tissue, which may allow for improved detection of the adenoma. While the CT detection rate for aldosteronomas is above 70 percent, approximately one-fourth to one-third of aldosteronomas will not be detected. In these cases, adrenal venous sampling may be employed.[57] Adrenal venous sampling localized 96 percent of 23 adenomas, as reported by Geisinger et al.[58]

Adrenal hyperplasia may also cause hyperaldosteronism. In these cases, CT will detect 40 percent of glands as visibly enlarged, while 60 percent of glands will appear normal. Hyperplastic glands may be unilaterally or bilaterally enlarged; they may appear nodular or normal.[59] The presence of multiple or bilateral nodules in the setting of hyperaldosteronism is compatible with nodular hyperplasia, since adenomas are rarely multiple.[16]

Most aldosteronomas are isointense to slightly hypointense relative to the liver on T_1-weighted images. Falke et al.[60] suggested that the MRI signal of aldosteronomas was higher than for nonhyperfunctioning adenomas on T_2-weighted imaging.[60] However, the ability to discriminate between functional and nonfunctional adenomas by MRI is unproven. Given the superiority of CT in the detection of both adenomas and hyperplasia, this is advocated as the primary modality in the workup of primary aldosteronism.

Accurate detection and localization allows for adequate treatment of affected patients. In patients with hypertension caused by adenomas, surgical removal should result in cure. Bilateral adrenalectomy in patients with hyperplasia results in a low cure rate and subjects the patient to lifelong steroid replacement. Thus medical therapy is employed for hyperplasia.[61]

Cushing's Syndrome

The diagnosis and management of hypercortisolism remains a complex problem. Cushing's syndrome is caused by an excess production of glucocorticoids, primarily cortisol. Clinical features of this syndrome include truncal obesity, hirsutism, acne, moon facies, facial plethora, muscle wasting, easy bruising, purple striae, fatigue, weakness, psychological impairment, hypertension, edema, impaired glucose tolerance, atherosclerosis, amenorrhea, and osteopenia. Cushing's syndrome most commonly afflicts patients in the third and fourth decades of life, with women affected four times more frequently than men.

Excess cortisol has multiple potential causes. Exogenous glucocorticoids prescribed for many medical conditions are the most common cause. A complex internal mechanism serves to regulate the body's cortisol level. Cortisol releasing factor secreted by the hypothalamus stimulates the anterior portion of the pituitary gland to secrete adrenocorticotropic hormone (ACTH). This hormone acts on the adrenal cortex to increase production of cortisol. A negative feedback mechanism will turn off further production. Thus, disease in any of the regulatory organs or in the end organ can result in excess glucocorticoid production. Pituitary overstimulation of the adrenal gland is responsible for 70 percent of cases of Cushing's syndrome. Adrenal adenomas are found in 20 percent of patients; less frequent causes include adrenocortical carcinoma in 10 percent[62] and ectopic ACTH production in 1 percent.

The largest group of patients will have adrenal hyperplasia secondary to ACTH stimulation from either pituitary or hypothalamic disease. Provocative biochemical testing as well as pituitary CT can be performed to determine whether this is the cause of excess cortisol production. Abdominal CT scanning is performed to visualize the effect on the adrenal gland of excess stimulation. The excess fat induced by this syndrome will aid in visualizing the gland. In most patients, the adrenal glands will appear normal, while in others there will be diffuse, uniform thickening of both limbs.[63]

Occasionally, hyperplastic glands may become nodular or lumpy. Nodular hyperplasia can at times be massive. Only a minority of cases show this macronodular hyperplasia. The macroscopic cortical nodules measure 0.6 to 7.0 cm in diameter.[64] In severe long-standing macronodular hyperplasia, autonomous function may develop. One must be careful not to mistake a dominant macronodule for an adenoma. Careful inspection of the ipsilateral and contralateral gland for nodular and hyperplastic change should permit one to differentiate these entities.

Ectopic ACTH production may also cause adrenal hyperplasia and glucocorticoid excess. The syndrome of ectopic ACTH production is associated with various neoplasms, including small cell carcinoma of the lung, thymoma, pancreatic islet cell tumor, carcinoid, medullary carcinoma of the thyroid, pheochromocytoma, paraganglioma, and chemodectoma.[65]

Adrenal adenomas make up the second largest group of lesions causing hypercortisolism. Most adenomas are 2 to 5 cm in diameter. The detection of masses less than 1 cm in size is rarely necessary. Excess cortisol production sufficient to cause syndromal effects occurs in larger masses.[66] Since there is abundant retroperitoneal fat, CT is highly successful in identifying these tumors (Fig. 1-7). The adenomas are well marginated, round, or oval masses.

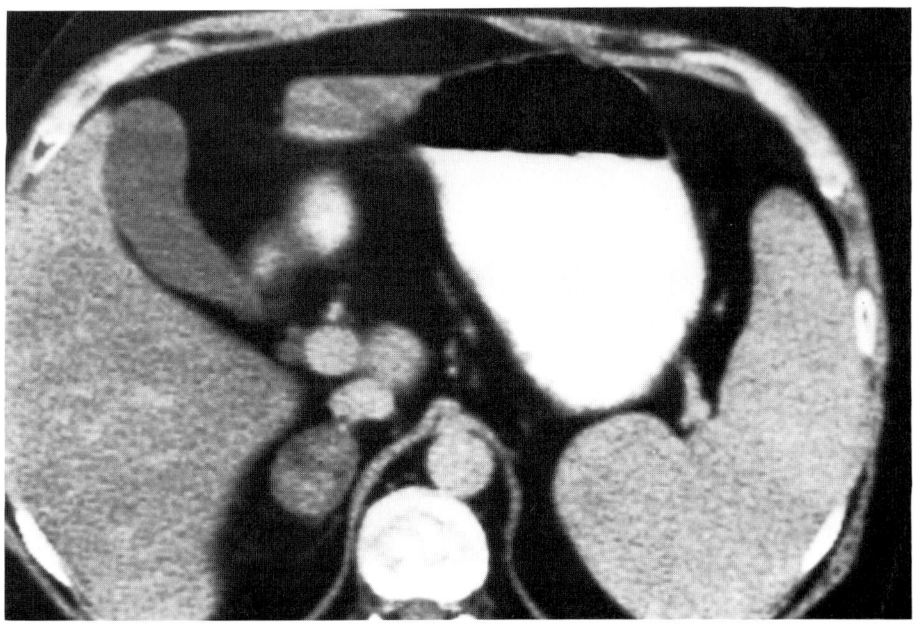

FIG. 1-7.   Functional adenoma causing Cushing's syndrome. The right adrenal mass is smoothly marginated.

Lesions are usually homogeneous, but low-attenuation areas may be present due to necrosis or hemorrhage. Uniform low attenuation may result from high fat content of the adenoma. Atrophy of the contralateral gland is a helpful adjunctive finding, but is difficult to detect. Associated CT findings in Cushing's syndrome include increased retroperitoneal, mediastinal, and subcutaneous fat, as well as fatty infiltration of the liver.

The MRI features of adrenal adenomas causing Cushing's syndrome appear to be similar to those of other functioning adenomas. However, further work is necessary to separate functional from nonfunctional adenomas, as well as aldosteronomas (Conn's syndrome) from the adenomas of Cushing's syndrome.

Adrenal carcinomas may be hormonally active and therefore may also cause hypercortisolism. There are both radiographic and biochemical differences between these masses and adenomas. Carcinomas are large masses that frequently have areas of hemorrhage and necrosis. Carcinomas produce mixed hormonal products, while the adenomas of Cushing's syndrome produce only cortisol. Specific biochemical tests can help make this distinction.

Pheochromocytoma

Pheochromocytomas are catecholamine-secreting neoplasms that arise from the chromaffin cells of the sympathetic nervous system. Ninety percent of pheochromocytomas lie in the adrenal medulla, while 10 percent reside in extra-adrenal locations. The most common extra-adrenal sites are the paravertebral nerves or plexuses (including the organ of Zuckerkandl), which lie adjacent to the aorta or the inferior vena cava. Other abdominal sites include the urinary bladder, spermatic cord, vagina, and anus. Two percent of pheochromocytomas are extra-abdominal, with sites including the chest, neck, and skull base.[67]

Clinically, patients suffer from hypertension caused by the excess secretion of the catecholamines epinephrine and norepinephrine. Increased blood pressure may be either sustained or paroxysmal and may be accompanied by palpitations, perspiration, and headaches. Other symptoms include facial pallor, chest or abdominal pain, paresthesias, nausea, and vomiting. Biochemical testing is necessary to establish the diagnosis of pheochromocytoma. Elevated urinary metanephrine and vanillylmandelic acid (VMA) is sought.

Although pheochromocytomas usually are isolated tumors, they may occur as part of other disease entities. Pheochromocytomas, often bilateral, occur in patients with von Hippel-Lindau syndrome, multiple endocrine neoplasia (MEN) Type II and Type III, and familial pheochromocytoma. Briefly reviewed, MEN II (Sipple's syndrome) consists of medullary carcinoma of the thyroid, as well as hyperparathyroidism and pheochromocytoma (in 75 percent of patients). Bilaterality is sufficiently common that both adrenal glands may be removed in cases in which only a unilateral mass is discovered preoperatively. MEN III (multiple mucosal neuroma syndrome) is a variant of MEN II in which patients have multiple mucosal neuromas and intestinal ganglioneuromatosis instead of parathyroid adenomas. Patients with von Hippel-Lindau syndrome suffer from retinal angiomatosis, hemangioblastomas of the cerebellum and medulla or spine, and renal cell carcinoma. Familial pheochromocytomas are rare, accounting for only 10 percent of all pheochromocytomas.[68]

Because of the various locations that may harbor a pheochromocytoma, CT scanning must include not only the adrenal glands, but other areas of the abdomen and pelvis. Thin-section imaging should be performed through the adrenal glands; if unrevealing, scanning should continue through the remainder of the abdomen and pelvis.[69] Scanning the chest is seldom helpful if the chest radiograph is normal.

Initially, scanning should be performed without IV contrast, as it may elevate plasma catecholamine levels and could precipitate a hypertensive crisis in patients with pheochromocytoma. If IV contrast is to be used, adequate α-adrenergic blockade is advocated.[70]

The CT appearance of a pheochromocytoma is that of a round, homogeneous soft tissue mass. Most lesions are greater than 3 cm in size. Approximately 7 percent contain calcifications. The density of these tumors is frequently similar to that of the renal parenchyma. In these cases, it may be difficult to distinguish the pheochromocytoma from the upper pole of the adjacent kidney.[71] If necessary, contrast may be used to separate the enhanced parenchyma of the kidney from a suprarenal pheochromocytoma. The various scan planes offered by MRI should also help in this respect. Areas of low attenuation in pheochromocytomas may be found; they represent regions of hemorrhage, necrosis, or cyst formation.

Approximately 20 percent of pheochromocytomas are malignant, and there is a high female predominance in these patients. Extension of tumor into the capsule, invasion of the peripheral venous sinuses, or pulmonary metastases may occur. The diagnosis of malignancy can also be established by lymph node invasion, tumor recurrence, or liver metastases.[72]

MRI provides multiplanar imaging capability. Large anatomic areas can be scanned, thus improving detection of extra-adrenal (and extra-abdominal) lesions. Coronal and sagittal scans permit assessment of the cephalic and caudal margins of a lesion, as well as the interface between the abnormal mass and adjacent organs. On T_1-weighted images, pheochromocytomas are isointense or hypointense to the liver. T_2-weighted images reveal a hyperintense homogeneous or heterogeneous mass (Fig. 1-8). As with other adrenal lesions, signal intensity will vary with necrosis and hemorrhage. Metastatic lesions to the retroperitoneum, liver, and chest may be identified on MRI and will display signal intensities similar to that of the primary tumor.[73] The presence of surgical clips limits the ability of CT to detect recurrent tumor. MRI does not suffer from metallic streak artifact and is likely to improve detection of recurrent tumors. Furthermore, MRI does not require IV or intra-arterial contrast, thereby avoiding potential adverse reactions. Localization of ectopic pheochromocytomas is also likely to be improved with MRI as opposed to CT scanning.[74]

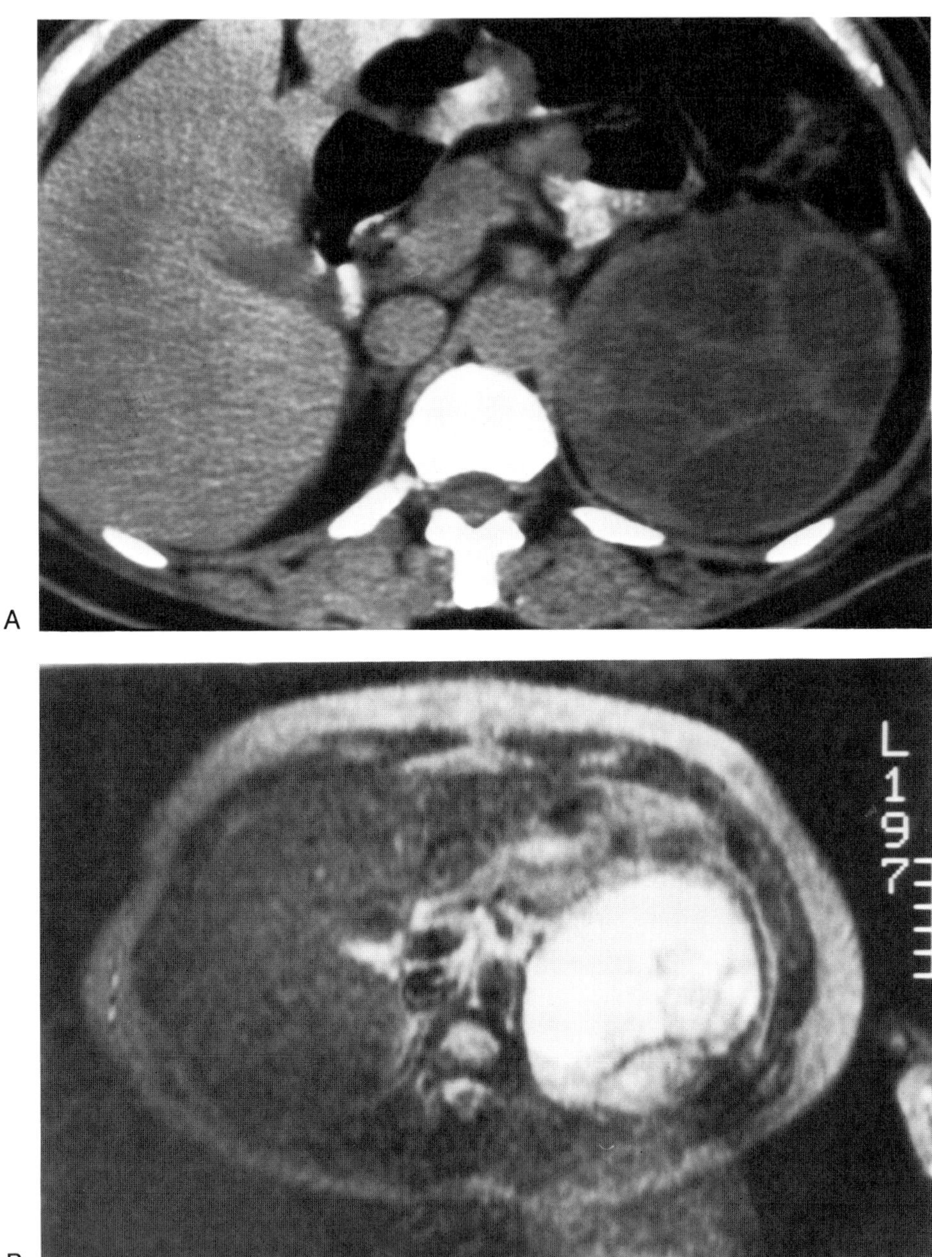

FIG. 1-8. Pheochromocytoma. (A) Adrenal pheochromocytomas are readily detected with CT. (B) The high signal intensity on T_2-weighted images (TR 2,500/TE 80) is consistent with a pheochromocytoma.

Carcinoma

Carcinoma of the adrenal gland is included with the functional lesions, since many are hormonally active.[75] Functioning adrenocortical neoplasms may manifest as Cushing's syndrome, adrenogenital syndrome, or precocious puberty. Virilization after birth in a prepubertal girl, Cushing's syndrome in a child, and combined Cushing's syndrome and virilization suggest an adrenal carcinoma. Feminization in adult men is suggestive of an estrogen-producing malignant adrenal tumor.

Nonfunctioning adrenal carcinomas are usually discovered when large, or they present with metastases. Hemorrhage and necrosis may cause pain, backache, or fever. Weight loss, anorexia, and muscle weakness may also be present. Adrenocortical neoplasms occur in both sexes; however, there is a female predominance in patients with functional neoplasms. Masses may be found in either the right or left adrenal gland, without definite predilection. In patients with functional disease, determination of plasma and urinary steroid levels is necessary. Although nonfunctional adrenocortical carcinomas do not produce an excess of active hormone, they are capable of forming excess amounts of precursor steroids. Increased urinary excretion of metabolic precursors may be found.[76]

Most adrenal carcinomas are large (greater than 6 cm in diameter), round, or lobular inhomogeneous masses. Central necrotic regions and hemorrhage are often present. Enhancement is irregular within the solid portions of the tumor.[77] The identification of local invasion, venous extension into the adrenal or renal veins, as well as metastatic lesions to the lungs, liver, or lymph nodes allow for more certain diagnosis of malignancy (Fig. 1-9). Fishman et al.[78] reported a thin, enhancing, capsulelike rind surrounding adrenocortical neoplasms.[78] These capsules were continuous, smooth, and not adherent to adjacent structures. Following injection of IV contrast material, all capsules are enhanced, suggesting that they represent well-vascularized portions of the tumor. On CT scanning, difficulty may arise in accurately determining the tissue of origin when masses are large. Multiplanar MRI can aid in establishing intra-abdominal anatomic relationships.

The differentiation of malignant from benign adrenal masses is of obvious importance. The typical features of cortical carcinoma are large size, central necrosis, and irregular enhancement. Since some of these features are seen in benign adrenal disease, other features are sought to aid in differentiation. Hussain et al.[79] reported a 0.31 probability of malignancy in a 5-cm adrenal mass without enhancement. A mass of the same size that demonstrated enhancement had a 0.68 probability of being malignant.[79]

T_1-weighted MRI scans of adrenal carcinoma reveal a low-signal adrenal mass. Depending on the degree of necrosis present, these masses may be homogeneous or inhomogeneous. Cystic necrotic areas appear as regions of higher signal on T_1 images. On T_2-weighted images, adrenal carcinomas are hyperintense (Fig. 1-10). Liver metastases appear similar to the primary tumor and display increased intensity on T_2-weighted images. MRI provides the

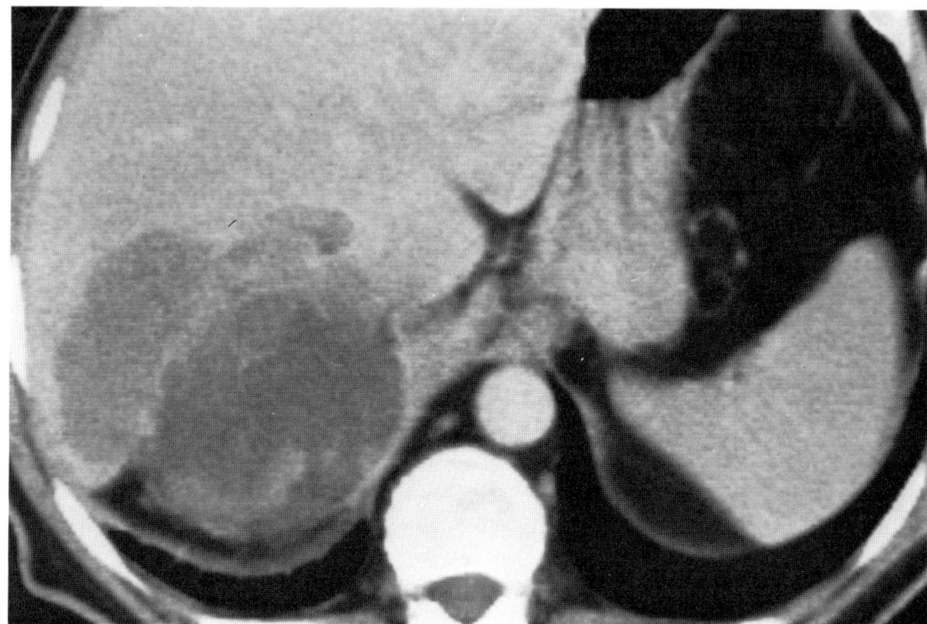

FIG. 1-9.   Carcinoma. A large mixed attenuation mass is seen in the right adrenal gland. Extension to the liver confirms the malignant nature of this adrenal mass.

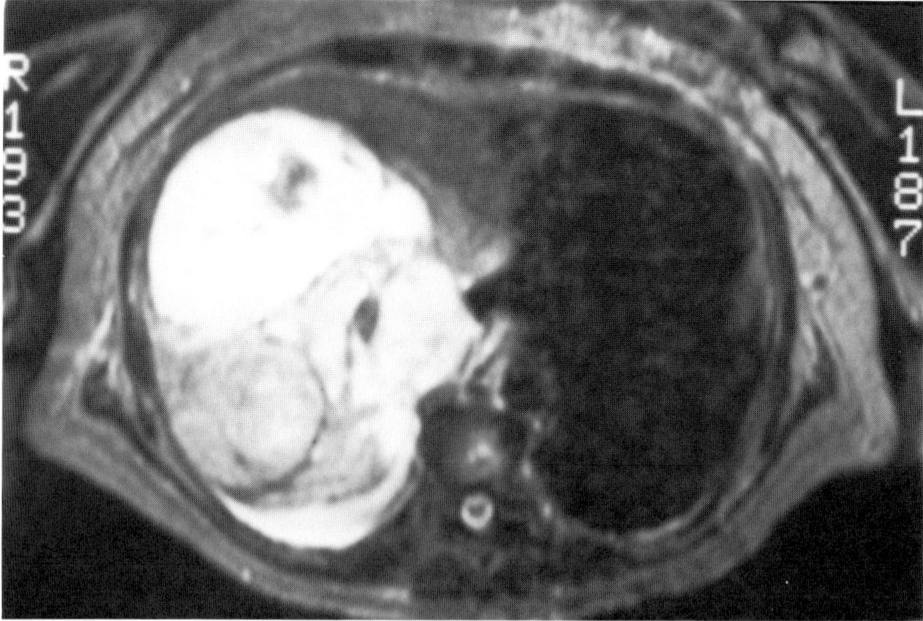

FIG. 1-10.   Carcinoma. This high-signal intensity (T_2-weighted) right adrenal mass is typical of adrenocortical carcinoma.

added benefit of being able to characterize intraluminal pathology. MRI is capable of distinguishing signal intensity secondary to slow flow and signal intensity indicative of intraluminal thrombus. Furthermore, signal intensity of intravascular thrombus similar to that of the primary tumor may permit differentiation of tumor from nontumor thrombus. This has been demonstrated in the case of venous extension of adrenocortical carcinoma.[80]

CHOICE OF MODALITY

CT remains the primary tool for evaluating adrenal masses. Contiguous images (5 mm) through the adrenal glands will detect the vast majority of adrenal lesions. If a high index of suspicion exists for an adrenal mass, 3-mm or even 1.5-mm images may be obtained. The density of some adrenal lesions permits a specific diagnosis. Numerous other lesions have nonspecific soft tissue density. MRI may be used to help differentiate metastatic lesions from adenomas. The accuracy with which MRI can differentiate metastatic disease from adenomas and functional and nonfunctional adenomas is still being investigated. Any "typical" adrenal mass can assume an atypical appearance when complicated by either necrosis or hemorrhage. This will affect both its CT and MRI appearance. Diagnoses rest on not only imaging characteristics but also clinical data. History of functional activity will be critical to determine which of the adrenal lesions is being imaged. Further work with MRI using surface coils, contrast agents, fast acquisition techniques, and dynamic imaging will help improve the imaging of adrenal masses.

REFERENCES

1. Mitty HA: Embryology, anatomy, and anomalies of the adrenal gland. Semin Roentgenol 23:271, 1988
2. Siegelman SS, Fishman EK, Gatewood OMB, et al: CT of the adrenal gland. p. 223. In Siegelman SS, Gatewood OMB, Goldman SM (eds): Computed Tomography of the Kidneys and Adrenals. Churchill Livingstone, New York, 1984
3. Brownlie K, Kreel L: Computer assisted tomography of normal suprarenal glands. J Comput Assist Tomogr 2:1, 1978
4. Karstaedt N, Sagel SS, Stanley RJ, et al: Computed tomography of the adrenal gland. Radiology 129:723, 1978
5. Montagne JP, Kressel HY, Korobkin M: Computed tomography of the normal adrenal glands: AJR 130:963, 1978
6. Wilms G, Baert A, Marchal G, et al: Computed tomography of the normal adrenal glands: Correlative study with autopsy specimens. J Comput Assist Tomogr 3:467, 1979
7. Kadir S: Diagnostic Angiography. WB Saunders, Philadelphia, 1986
8. Bloom W, Fawcett DW: A Textbook of Histology. 10th Ed. WB Saunders, Philadelphia, 1975
9. Berliner L, Bosniak MA, Megibow A: Adrenal pseudotumors on computed tomography. J Comput Assist Tomogr 6:285, 1982
10. Mitty HA, Cohen BA, Sprayregen S, et al: Adrenal pseudotumors on CT due to dilated portosystemic veins. AJR 141:727, 1983
11. Casola G, Nicolet V, van Sonnenberg E: Unsuspected pheochromocytoma: Risk of blood-pressure alterations during percutaneous adrenal biopsy. Radiology 159:733, 1986

12. Falke THM, te Strake L, Sandler MP, et al: Magnetic resonance imaging of the adrenal glands. Radiographics 7:343, 1987

13. Commons RR, Callaway CP: Adenomas of the adrenal cortex. Arch Intern Med 81:37, 1948

14. Glazer HS, Weyman PJ, Sagel SS, et al: Nonfunctioning adrenal masses: Incidental discovery on computed tomography. AJR 139:81, 1982

15. Mitnick JS, Bosniak MA, Megibow AJ, et al: Nonfunctioning adrenal adenomas discovered incidentally on computed tomography. Radiology 143:495, 1983

16. Glazer GM, Francis IR, Quint LE: Imaging of the adrenal glands. Invest Radiol 23:3, 1988

17. Weiner SN, Bernstein RG, Lowy S, et al: Combined adrenal adenoma and myelolipoma. J Comput Assist Tomogr 5:440, 1981

18. Ambos MA, Bosniak MA, Lefleur RS, et al: Adrenal adenoma associated with renal cell carcinoma. AJR 136:81, 1981

19. Olsson CA, Krane RJ, Klugo RC, et al: Adrenal adenoma. Surgery 73:665, 1973

20. McDonnell WY: Myelolipoma of adrenal. Arch Pathol 61:416, 1956

21. Vick CW, Zeman RK, Mannes E, et al: Adrenal myelolipoma: CT and ultrasound findings. Urol Radiol 6:7, 1984

22. Leibman R, Srikantaswamy S: Adrenal myelolipoma demonstrated by computed tomography. J Comput Assist Tomogr 5:262, 1981

23. Whaley D, Becker S, Presbrey T, et al: Adrenal myelolipoma associated with Conn syndrome: CT evaluation. J Comput Assist Tomogr 9:959, 1985

24. Kearney GP, Mahoney EM: Adrenal cysts. Urol Clin North Am 4:273, 1977

25. Johnson CD, Baker ME, Dunnick NR: CT demonstration of an adrenal pseudocyst. J Comput Assist Tomogr 9:817, 1985

26. Moulton JS, Moulton JS: CT of the adrenal glands. Semin Roentgenol 23:288, 1988

27. Pastakia B, Miller I, Wolfman M, et al: MR imaging of a large adrenal cyst. J Comput Assist Tomogr 10:710, 1986

28. Ling D, Korobkin M, Silverman PM, et al: CT demonstration of bilateral adrenal hemorrhage. AJR 141:307, 1983

29. O'Connell TX, Aston SJ: Acute adrenal hemorrhage complicating anticoagulant therapy. Surg Gynecol Obstet 139:355, 1974

30. Albert SG, Wolverson MK, Johnson FE: Bilateral adrenal hemorrhage in an adult. JAMA 247:1737, 1982

31. Wolverson MK, Kannegiesser H: CT of bilateral adrenal hemorrhage with acute adrenal insufficiency in the adult. AJR 142:311, 1984

32. Wilms G, Marchal G, Baert A, et al: CT and ultrasound features of post-traumatic adrenal hemorrhage. J Comput Assist Tomogr 11:112, 1987

33. Unger EC, Glazer HS, Lee JKT, et al: MR of extracranial hematomas: Preliminary observations. AJR 146:403, 1986

34. Grossman RI, Gomori JM, Goldberg HI, et al: MR imaging of hemorrhagic conditions of the head and neck. Radiographics 8:441, 1988

35. Abrams HL, Spiro R, Goldstein N: Metastases in carcinoma. Cancer 3:74, 1950

36. Anderson EE: Nonfunctioning tumors of the adrenal gland. Urol Clin North Am 4:263, 1977

37. Pagani JJ: Normal adrenal glands in small cell lung carcinoma: CT-guided biopsy. AJR 140:949, 1983

38. Nielsen ME, Heaston DK, Dunnick NR, et al: Preoperative CT evaluation of adrenal glands in nonsmall cell bronchogenic carcinoma. AJR 139:317, 1982

39. Pagani JJ: Non-small cell lung carcinoma adrenal metastases. Cancer 53:1058, 1984

40. Reinig JW, Doppman JL, Dwyer AJ, et al: Distinction between adrenal adenomas and metastases using MR imaging. J Comput Assist Tomogr 9:898, 1985

41. Glazer GM: MR imaging of the liver, kidneys and adrenal glands. Radiology 166:303, 1988

42. Baker ME, Spritzer C, Blinder R, et al: Benign adrenal lesions mimicking malignancy on MR imaging: Report of two cases. Radiology 163:669, 1987

43. Glazer GM, Woolsey EJ, Borrello J, et al: Adrenal tissue characterization using MR imaging. Radiology 158:73, 1986

44. Reinig JW, Doppman JL, Dwyer AJ, et al: Adrenal masses differentiated by MR. Radiology 158:81, 1986

45. Chang A, Glazer HS, Lee JKT, et al: Adrenal gland: MR imaging. Radiology 163:123, 1987

46. Reinig JW, Doppman JL, Dwyer AJ, et al: MRI of indeterminate adrenal masses. AJR 147:493, 1986

47. Jafri SZH, Francis IR, Glazer GM, et al: CT detection of adrenal lymphoma. J Comput Assist Tomogr 7:254, 1983

48. Paling MR, Williamson BRJ: Adrenal involvement in non-Hodgkin lymphoma. AJR 141:303, 1983

49. Wilson DA, Muchmore HG, Tisdal RG, et al: Histoplasmosis of the adrenal glands studied by CT. Radiology 150:779, 1984

50. Wilms GE, Baert AL, Kint EJ, et al: Computed tomographic findings in bilateral adrenal tuberculosis. Radiology 146:729, 1983

51. Doppman JL, Gill JR Jr, Nienhuis AW, et al: CT findings in Addison's disease. J Comput Assist Tomogr 6:757, 1982

52. McMurry JF Jr, Long D, McClure R, et al: Addison's disease with adrenal enlargement on computed tomographic scanning. Am J Med 77:365, 1984

53. Shah B, Taylor HC, Pillay I, et al: Adrenal insufficiency due to cryptococcus. JAMA 256:3247, 1986

54. Weinberger MH, Grim CE, Hollifield JW, et al: Primary aldosteronism. Ann Intern Med 90:386, 1979

55. Williams TC: Functional disorders of the adrenal glands: An overview. Semin Roentgenol 23:304, 1988

56. Kenney PJ, Berlow ME, Ellis DA: Current imaging of adrenal masses. Radiographics 4:743, 1984

57. Dunnick NR, Doppman JL, Gill JR Jr, et al: Localization of functional adrenal tumors by computed tomography and venous sampling. Radiology 142:429, 1982

58. Geisinger MA, Zelch MG, Bravo EL, et al: Primary hyperaldosteronism: Comparison of CT, adrenal venography and venous sampling. AJR 141:299, 1983

59. Roberts L Jr, Dunnick NR, Thompson WM, et al: Primary aldosteronism due to bilateral nodular hyperplasia: CT demonstration. J Comput Assist Tomogr 9:1125, 1985

60. Falke THM, te Strake L, Shaff MI, et al: MR imaging of the adrenals: Correlation with computed tomography. J Comput Assist Tomogr 10:242, 1986

61. Auda SP, Brennan MF, Gill JR Jr: Evolution of the surgical management of primary aldosteronism. Ann Surg 191:1, 1980

62. Ling D, Lee JKT: The adrenals. p. 827. In Lee JKT, Sagel SS, Stanley RJ (eds): Computed Tomography of the Body with MRI Correlation. 2nd Ed. Raven Press, New York 1989

63. Eghrari M, McLoughlin MJ, Rosen IE, et al: The role of computed tomography in assessment of tumoral pathology of the adrenal glands. J Comput Assist Tomogr 4:71, 1980

64. Doppman JL, Miller DL, Dwyer AJ, et al: Macronodular adrenal hyperplasia in Cushing disease. Radiology 166:347, 1988

65. Johnson CM, Sheedy PF, Welch TJ, et al: CT of the adrenal cortex. Semin US CT MR 6:241, 1985

66. Carpenter PC: Cushing's syndrome: Update of diagnosis and management. Mayo Clin Proc 61:49, 1986

67. Thomas JL, Bernardino ME, Samaan NA, et al: CT of pheochromocytoma. AJR 135:477, 1980

68. Glownaik JV, Shapiro B, Sisson JC, et al: Familial extra-adrenal pheochromocytoma. Arch Intern Med 145:257, 1985

69. Francis IR, Glazer GM, Shapiro B, et al: Complementary roles of CT and ^{131}I-MIBG scintigraphy in diagnosing pheochromocytoma. AJR 141:719, 1983

70. Raisanen J, Shapiro B, Glazer GM, et al: Plasma catecholamines in pheochromocytoma: Effect of urographic contrast media. AJR 143:43, 1984

71. Radin DR, Ralls PW, Boswell WD Jr, et al: Pheochromocytoma: Detection by unenhanced CT. AJR 146:741, 1986

72. Mahoney EM, Harrison JH: Malignant pheochromocytoma: Clinical course and treatment. J Urol 118:225, 1977

73. Fink IJ, Reinig JW, Dwyer AJ, et al: MR imaging of pheochromocytomas. J Comput Assist Tomogr 9:454, 1985

74. Schmedtje JF Jr, Sax S, Pool JL, et al: Localization of ectopic pheochromocytomas by magnetic resonance imaging. Am J Med 83:770, 1987

75. Nader S, Hickey RC, Sellin RV, et al: Adrenal cortical carcinoma: A study of 77 cases. Cancer 52:707, 1983

76. Richie JP, Gittes RF: Carcinoma of the adrenal cortex. Cancer 45:1957, 1980

77. Dunnick NR, Heaston D, Halvorsen R, et al: CT appearance of adrenal cortical carcinoma. J Assist Comput Tomogr 6:978, 1982

78. Fishman EK, Deutch BM, Hartman DS: Primary adrenocortical carcinoma: CT evaluation with clinical correlation. AJR 148:531, 1987

79. Hussain S, Belldegrun A, Seltzer SE, et al: Differentiation of malignant from benign adrenal masses: Predictive indices on computed tomography. AJR 144:61, 1985

80. Falke THM, Peetoom JJ, de Roos A, et al: Gadolinium-DTPA enhanced MR imaging of intravenous extension of adrenocortical carcinoma. J Comput Assist Tomogr 12:331, 1988

2 CT and MRI of Renal Cell Carcinoma

BERNARD A. BIRNBAUM
MORTON A. BOSNIAK

Renal neoplasms represent approximately 2 percent of all adult malignancies. The vast majority are composed of renal cell carcinomas (RCC) (80 to 85 percent), with transitional cell carcinoma, nephroblastoma (Wilms' tumor), and miscellaneous sarcomas occurring much less frequently.[1] RCC tends to occur in patients over age 40, the peak incidence noted in the sixth and seventh decades of life. It has been reported with a male preponderance in the ratio of almost 2:1. While its etiology remains uncertain, epidemiologic studies demonstrate an increased incidence in tobacco users and possibly those exposed to long-term doses of phenacetin. Genetics also plays a role, as patients with the autosomal-dominant disorder of von Hippel-Lindau syndrome (cerebelloretinal hemangioblastomatosis) have been noted to have an increased risk of developing RCC (10 to 25 percent). Familial cases need not be associated with this syndrome and, unlike nonfamilial cases, it has been shown that RCC ascribed to genetic factors are more likely to be bilateral, multifocal, and to have an earlier age of onset.[2]

The presenting signs and symptoms of RCC are quite variable and include hematuria, flank pain or mass, fatigability, weight loss, fever, and varicoceles. The classic triad of gross hematuria, flank pain, and palpable abdominal mass is encountered in less than 10 percent of cases. Furthermore, patients may present with a variety of hematologic disturbances and paraneoplastic syndromes that has led this tumor to be dubbed the "internist's tumor," as it may produce a diversity of symptoms unrelated to the kidney.

Over the past 10 years, there has been a significant change in the presentation of these tumors. While previously 25 to 33 percent of patients with RCC presented with metastatic disease at the time of diagnosis, a greater percentage of these tumors are now being serendipitously discovered when they are smaller and before they have become symptomatic or metastasized. This has occurred because the kidneys are now routinely imaged in a larger proportion of the population due to the widespread use of CT and ultrasound. The earlier discovery of these masses should lead to an improvement in the overall cure rate of this neoplasm.[3]

Originally termed *hypernephromas*, the yellow-gray color of these fleshy tumors initially led to the erroneous belief that they arose from "adrenal rests." It is now known that RCCs are parenchymal neoplasms that originate in the renal tubular epithelial cells. While they do not possess a true capsule, they may appear well encapsulated by virtue of a pseudocapsule composed of compressed renal parenchyma and fibrous tissue, which may be associated with peripheral inflammatory changes. Characteristically, these tumors are frequently associated with regions of necrosis, cystic degeneration, hemorrhage, calcification, and fibrosis. As a result, the radiographic manifestations of RCC may be quite diverse.

CT

Examination Technique

CT, by virtue of its ability to assess the tissue density and vascularity of renal masses, is extremely accurate in the detection and characterization of renal neoplasms. CT may be used both as a *screening* examination, in which case the study is usually performed with intravenous (IV) contrast enhancement, or as a *diagnostic* examination, in which case the study is performed both with and without contrast enhancement. Thus, if a renal lesion is detected on an ultrasound study or urogram and needs further evaluation, this should be accomplished by performing a CT study as a *diagnostic* examination; that is, the study is performed both before and after IV contrast, and thin (5-mm) sections can be performed as needed.

In clinical practice, a large number of renal masses are discovered on *screening* CT examinations (contrast only), usually as an incidental finding in the evaluation of another abdominal complaint. In this setting, the examination of the kidneys may not be complete or diagnostic, and a repeat *diagnostic* CT scan may be needed.

The following describes the workup of patients in which a renal mass is detected on a screening CT scan (i.e., contrast only scan):

1. If the mass has the characteristics of a classic renal cyst, the diagnosis is established and no further study is needed. This is a common finding.
2. If the mass is a clearly malignant lesion, no further study is needed unless staging is unclear; if so, a repeat CT scan is done as a *diagnostic* study or MRI is performed.
3. If the lesion clearly contains fat, this finding is diagnostic of angiomyolipoma, and no further study is needed.
4. If the lesion is indeterminate:
   a. but is probably a cyst, ultrasound should be performed. If the lesion is a cyst, no further study is needed; otherwise a *diagnostic* CT should be performed.

   b. but is a possible malignant lesion, a *diagnostic* CT examination should be performed.

   c. such as a questionable angiomyolipoma, renal anomaly, or renal pseudotumor (i.e. hematoma), a *diagnostic* CT should be obtained.

The method of administration of IV contrast for a renal CT examination is open to a difference of opinion as to whether contrast enhanced scans should be performed with bolus, bolus-infusion, or pure infusion technique. As a general rule, the kidneys should be scanned when a high and prolonged iodine concentration exists within the bloodstream and renal parenchyma as contrast is being concentrated and excreted after the injection. This is usually best achieved by using either pure bolus or bolus-infusion types of contrast administration, which also permits dynamic incremental scanning through the level of the renal vasculature, if so desired.[4]

At our institution, a *diagnostic* renal CT scan of a suspected renal lesion generally begins with non-IV contrast enhanced scans consisting of contiguous 10-mm-thick slices (10s at 10s) obtained through both kidneys. In those cases in which the lesion is small or in which a particular area of a larger mass needs further attention, contiguous 5-mm-thick sections (5s at 5s) are then taken. These initial noncontrast images are critical, allowing one to detect enhancement later as well as to identify regions of calcification, fat, or hemorrhage, which may sometimes be obscured by contrast media. The patient is then rescanned, using identical exposure factors, after the administration of IV contrast with both slice thickness and positioning remaining unchanged so as to match ideally with the precontrast images. Contrast (200 ml of Conray-43, 40.4 g of iodine) is administered via a 50-ml bolus followed by a 150-ml infusion and is best delivered by a power injector, if available, to ensure rapid and constant elevation of serum iodine levels. At a minimum, the scan should span the region from the retrocrural nodes extending to the inferior aspect of the kidneys if the remainder of the abdomen and pelvis are not to be imaged. If a renal neoplasm is diagnosed, a careful search for metastases should be performed.

Once the images are reconstructed, CT Hounsfield numbers are measured and compared over the regions of interest (ROIs) on the pre- and postcontrast studies to evaluate for vascular enhancement. Often, this will involve ROIs not only of the renal mass, but also of the renal parenchyma, and such structures as the gallbladder or simple cysts (if present) which may be used as measurement controls. Dynamic or axial scanning can be performed.

Findings of Renal Cell Carcinoma

Renal cell carcinoma has many varied appearances on CT. Generally speaking, any renal mass that enhances with IV contrast should be considered an RCC until proven otherwise. The goal of the radiologist is to separate RCC from all other renal masses so that the diagnosis of RCC can be made with total confidence. This means that simple and complicated renal cysts, abscesses, hematomas, infarcts, and localized inflammatory pseudotumors, angiomyolipomas, lymphoma, and metastatic cancer should be identified and differentiated from RCC if possible. The combination of clinical history and CT findings is generally able to make the differentiation.

Most RCCs appear as heterogeneous, solid masses that may be easily distinguished from simple renal cysts. Applying strict CT criteria, simple cysts possess thin, smooth, well-marginated walls with sharp interfaces with adjacent renal parenchyma. The cyst contents should be of homogeneous water density and, most importantly, there should be no enhancement either in the density of the cyst wall or in the cyst contents following IV contrast infusion.[5] On the other hand, most RCCs tend to have thick, irregular walls with asymmetric, lobulated contours. A thickened pseudocapsule may be seen. The density of the tumor is greater than water density in at least some portions of the mass. On non-IV enhanced scans, tumor attenuation may be similar to or higher than that of normal renal tissue. Frequently, areas of necrosis are

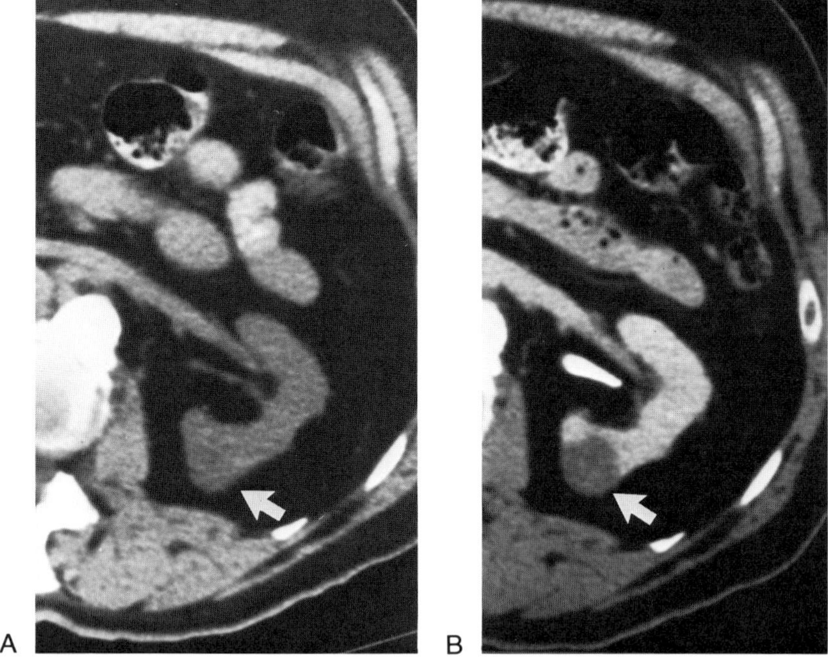

FIG. 2-1.   Small renal cell carcinoma. A 71-year-old man had lower urinary tract symptoms. A diagnostic CT scan was performed to evaluate a left renal mass detected by sonography. Nonenhanced CT scan (A) reveals a small, 2.3-cm, round, well-circumscribed solid lesion (arrow). The mass measured 25 HU. Contrast-enhanced CT scan (B) clearly depicts the mass, which now measured 43 HU. This vascular enhancement confirms the neoplastic nature of this lesion. A partial nephrectomy was performed. Pathologic diagnosis was renal cell carcinoma.

seen as regions of decreased attenuation, close to fluid density, within the mass. Following the administration of IV contrast, the neovascularity of the tumor is reflected by enhancement of the lesion, which appears different from normal enhancing renal parenchyma (Fig. 2-1). The degree of enhancement is often quite variable, depending both on tumor vascularity as well as the rate and volume of contrast administered.

At times, cystic-type renal neoplasms (e.g., cystic necrotic tumors, cystadenocarcinomas, and tumors based within a cyst) may be difficult to differentiate from benign complicated cysts. This differentiation is based on evaluation of a number of radiologic findings, which include the following:

1. *Calcification.* While the appearance of stippled or irregular calcification is always suggestive of possible malignancy, CT is useful in evaluating the pattern and amount of calcification present (Fig. 2-2). If all the CT and ultrasound criteria for a cyst are met, yet a small amount of calcium or a thin, fine area of calcification is identified in the wall or a septa of

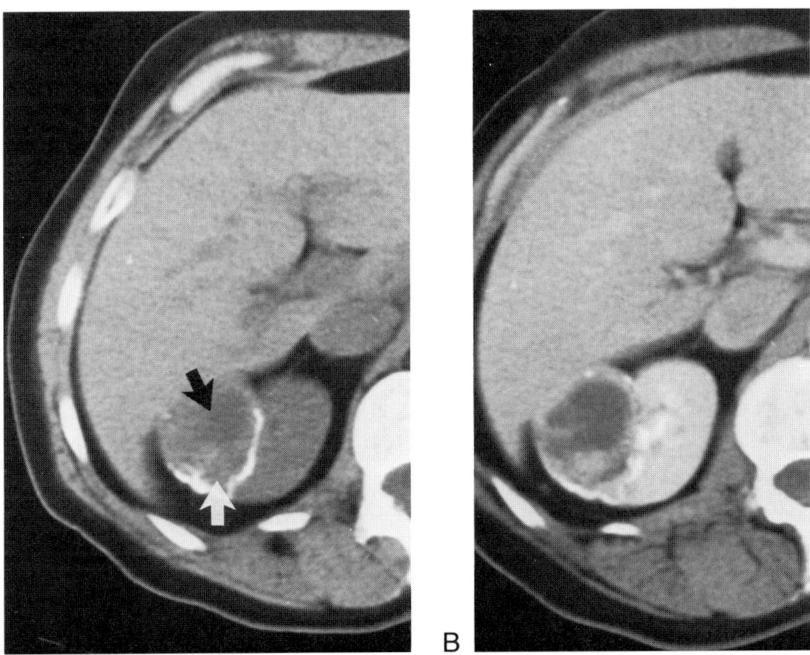

FIG. 2-2.   Calcified cystic renal cell carcinoma. A 49-year-old woman had lower urinary tract symptoms, and a calcified mass was detected at the upper pole of the right kidney by IV urography. Nonenhanced CT scan (A) reveals a complex renal mass containing an incomplete peripheral rim of calcification with solid and fluid components. The cyst fluid (black arrow) measured 19 HU, while the peripheral soft tissue region (white arrow) measured 43 HU. Contrast-enhanced CT scan (B) reveals enhancement of the soft tissue elements to 99 HU. No enhancement of the cystic region was noted. A right nephrectomy was performed for a cystic renal cell carcinoma.

a cystic lesion, the mass may be regarded as a complicated benign cyst, and not a neoplasm, if there is no evidence of associated soft tissue density or contrast enhancement.[6] More extensive calcification within a renal mass, especially if thick and irregular, may occasionally be seen with benign masses; however, surgical exploration is usually indicated in these instances to exclude a neoplasm.

2. *Contour of the mass and thickness of the wall.* Contour irregularity and poor margination of a cystic mass are always highly suggestive of malignancy, as is an irregular, thickened enhancing wall. Benign lesions have thin walls with sharp, smooth margination.

3. *Number and thickness of septations.* Many benign complicated cysts contain septations. As a rule of thumb, benign cysts may be associated with thin septations (1 mm or less) that are smooth and that attach to the cyst walls without associated thickened soft tissue elements. However, the presence of irregular or thickened enhancing septa (often associated with solid elements) indicates probable neoplasia, for which surgical exploration is necessary[6] (Fig. 2-3).

4. *Density of the fluid within a cyst.* Fluid within a renal cyst generally measures 20 HU or lower. Cyst fluid occasionally measures higher than 20 to 40 HU because of the presence of protein or blood breakdown products. Nevertheless, the diagnosis of a benign cyst can usually be made if all other CT criteria suggest the diagnosis of a cyst and if there is *no* enhancement of the lesion following IV contrast. Correlation with sonography can also be helpful in such lesions.[6]

A common finding is the hyperdense renal cyst, a renal cyst (usually containing old hemorrhage) that has greater attenuation than that of adjacent renal parenchyma on a non-contrast-enhanced CT scan.[7,8] Often detected as an incidental small mass (less than 3 cm in diameter) arising from the periphery of the cortex, hyperdense cysts usually measure approximately 60 to 70 HU, in a range of about 40 to 100 HU. On contrast-enhanced examination, these masses become either hypodense or isodense with respect to the renal parenchyma. They may be diagnosed as nonsurgical lesions only if they appear homogeneous and *do not enhance* following administration of IV contrast, and if all other strict CT criteria for a simple cyst are met. At least a portion of the mass must protrude from the kidney so that wall thickness can be evaluated. Lack of enhancement is a critical finding in these lesions because at times the other CT criteria for a cyst may be difficult to evaluate. Therefore, 5-mm sections are necessary in the study of these cases to show that *no portion* of the lesion enhances with contrast. Further confidence for the benign nature of these masses is afforded if sonography confirms the characteristics of a cyst. However, larger lesions measuring greater than 3 cm, totally intrarenal lesions, and those lesions not appearing cystic by sonography have to be handled by either surgical exploration or follow-up studies depending on the individual case. Other fluid-filled masses that may be difficult to distinguish from RCC include proteinacious or infected cysts as well as centrally placed chronic abscesses. Their diagnosis may be aided by history and cyst puncture.

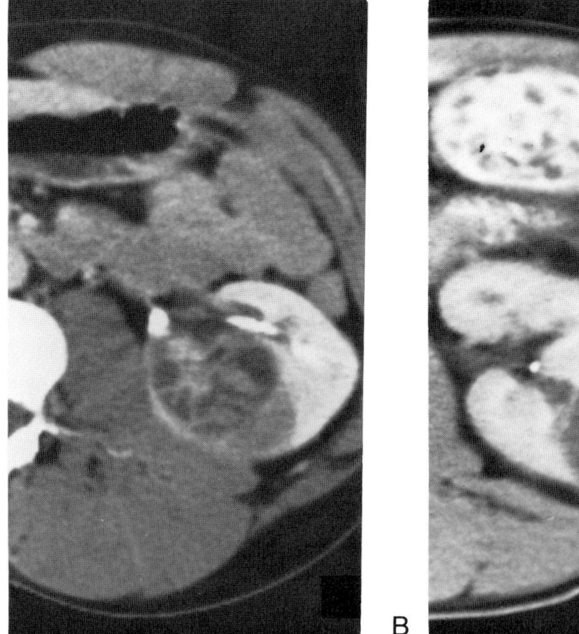

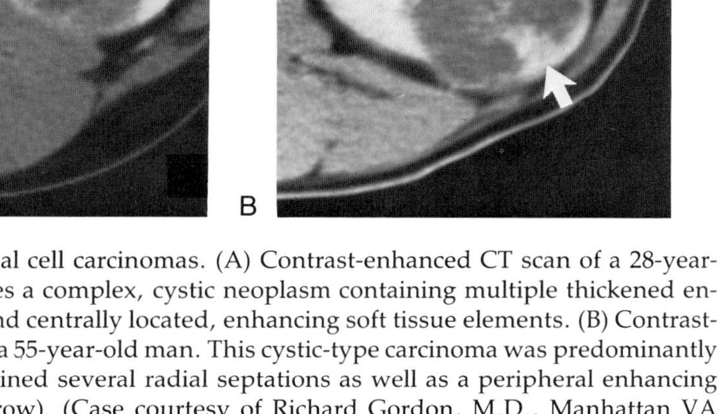

FIG. 2-3.   Cystic renal cell carcinomas. (A) Contrast-enhanced CT scan of a 28-year-old man demonstrates a complex, cystic neoplasm containing multiple thickened enhancing septations and centrally located, enhancing soft tissue elements. (B) Contrast-enhanced CT scan of a 55-year-old man. This cystic-type carcinoma was predominantly fluid filled, yet contained several radial septations as well as a peripheral enhancing solid component (arrow). (Case courtesy of Richard Gordon, M.D., Manhattan VA Medical Center.)

A renal angiomyolipoma is a benign hamartoma of the kidney that may be differentiated from an RCC by CT if one is able to establish the presence of fat within the mass. While this is usually not a problem, occasionally only small amounts of fat are present, and this may require the use of 5-mm thin-section noncontrast images for increased spatial and density resolution.[9] On the other hand, it may be difficult for CT to distinguish an RCC from an oncocytoma, another benign renal neoplasm thought to arise from the proximal tubular epithelial cells of the kidney.[10] Further discussion of these lesions is included in Chapter 3.

MRI

Examination Technique

MRI represents an alternative and complementary imaging modality to CT for the diagnosis and staging of RCC. Its use is advocated for those patients who are unable to receive iodinated contrast agents, when prior contrast-enhanced CT examinations are suboptimal, and for select cases in which the CT findings are equivocal.

The specific MRI parameters, sequences, and imaging planes chosen for a particular examination will depend on the goals of that study. While we believe that MRI should not be used as the initial screening modality for renal tumors, the following protocol is suggested for medium-field strength systems for those cases in which both lesion detection and staging are desired. T_1-weighted images are first obtained in the axial plane as well as in an angled coronal plane along the long axis of the kidney. This latter view is important for allowing a more accurate assessment of the polar regions of the kidney. Such views may be achieved using either spin-echo (TR 300 ms, TE 20 ms) or inversion-recovery (TR 1,400 ms, TI 400 ms, TE 20 ms) pulse sequences. T_2-weighted images are then acquired in both planes using spin-echo technique (TR 2,000 ms, TE 50 and 100 ms). Slice section thickness is 1 cm, with an interslice factor of 1.1 resulting in 1-mm intersection gaps. In cases in which adjacent organ invasion is suggested, we obtain additional sagittal views as needed using similar parameters. While even-echo rephasing phenomena may be used to help distinguish slow flow from vascular thrombus, occasionally the slice sequence acquisition order may need to be altered to exclude the presence of signal generated by flow-related enhancement on entry slices of a multislice package.[11,12] Use of fast, low flip angle imaging to demonstrate suspected renal vein or LVC tumor thrombus can be used in select cases (i.e., GRASS, FLASH, etc.).

At this time, IV Gadolinium-DTPA (Gd-DTPA) has not yet been approved by the Food and Drug Administration (FDA) for routine renal imaging. Following its IV administration, this paramagnetic complex is known to cause renal parenchymal enhancement on T_1-weighted images.[13] It is hoped that such a contrast agent will prove valuable as a vascular marker for tumor enhancement. If so, it should increase the sensitivity of MRI in the detection of small RCCs and allow MRI to help distinguish complex renal cysts from enhancing neoplasms.

Findings in the Diagnosis of Renal Cell Carcinoma

Renal cell carcinomas appear as masses of variable signal intensity on T_1- and T_2-weighted images, with signal characteristics ranging from hypointense to hyperintense with respect to the normal renal parenchyma. No specific morphologic features, signal intensities, or absolute T_1 or T_2 measurements are diagnostic of these neoplasms. On T_1-weighted images, they most commonly present as lesions with signal intensities intermediate between that of the renal cortex and medulla, or similar to or greater than that of the cortex, while on T_2-weighted images they are usually hyperintense.[14,15] Areas of necrosis often demonstrate decreased signal intensity on T_1-weighted scans, while regions of hemorrhage may appear hyperintense. In general, both necrotic and hemorrhagic areas show high signal intensity on T_2-weighted images, but this too is variable, since the signal generated from blood will depend to a great extent on the concentrations of paramagnetic hemoglobin breakdown products present and the particular TR and TE chosen.

MRI is not sensitive for the detection of intratumoral calcification. Furthermore, because this modality presently lacks the spatial resolution possessed by CT, MRI is not able to characterize fully a complicated benign renal cyst as such and may not be able to distinguish complex renal cystic disease from cystic neoplasm. MRI is less sensitive than CT in demonstrating solid lesions smaller than 3 cm in diameter. If poor tissue contrast exists between the neoplasm and the surrounding normal parenchyma on both T_1- and T_2-weighted spin-echo images, the mass will not be detected by MRI unless it deforms the renal contour[16] (Fig. 2-4). On the other hand, MRI is the complementary procedure of choice in evaluating large tumors in which the tumor origin may be difficult to define with CT. The multiplanar imaging capabilities of MRI facilitate distinguishing a polar renal neoplasm from an adjacent tumor of adrenal or retroperitoneal origin.

MRI may differentiate an RCC from an angiomyolipoma if enough fat exists within the lesion. Because of the short T_1 and moderately long T_2 of fatty tissue, the hamartoma should demonstrate high signal intensity on both T_1-

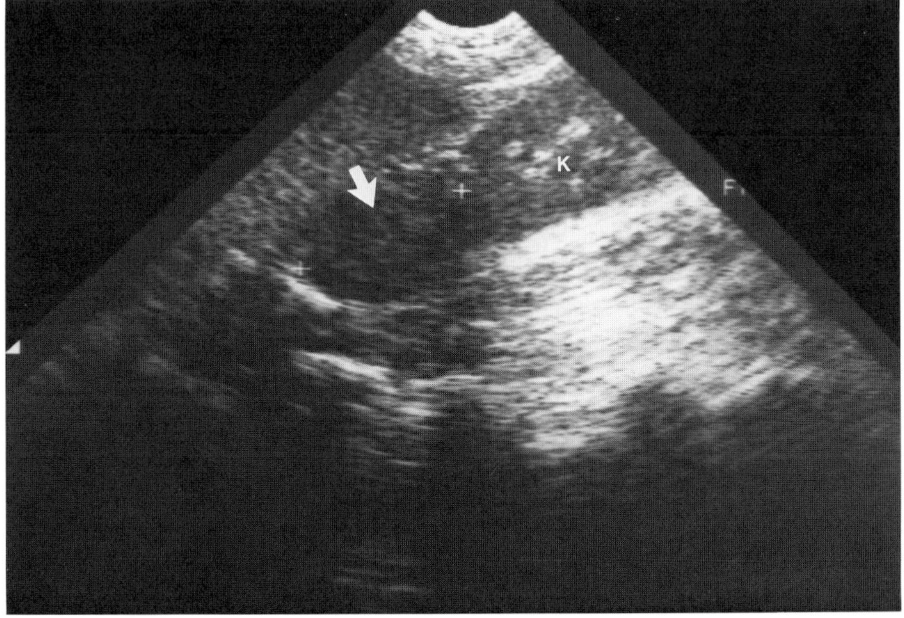

A

FIG. 2-4.   Renal cell carcinoma. A 73-year-old man presented with hematuria. Because of a known allergic history to IV contrast, the patient was initially studied by sonography and then further evaluated with MRI. (A) Sonogram demonstrates a mass (arrow) arising from the superior aspect of the right kidney (K). The mass contains multiple low-level echoes with no through-transmission, indicative of a solid tumor. (*Figure continues.*)

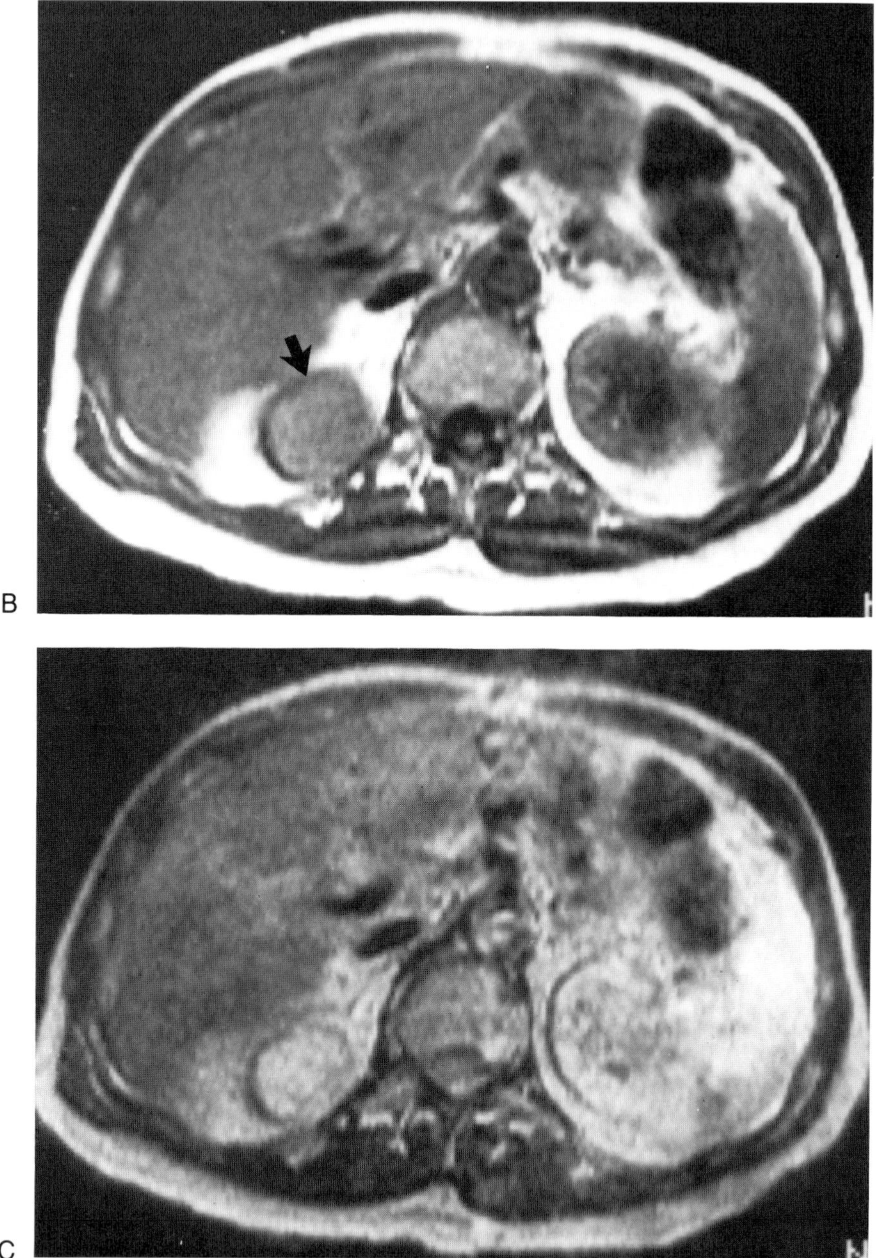

FIG. 2–4 (*Continued*). (B) Short TR, short TE (525 ms/32 ms) axial MRI scan taken through the tumor (arrow) reveals homogeneous signal intensity similar to that of normal renal cortex in the contralateral normal kidney. (C) T_2-weighted scan (TR 2,000 ms, TE 60 ms) confirms that lesion signal intensity increases, tracking with that of normal renal parenchyma. Small lesions with similar signal characteristics may be difficult to detect using MRI.

and T_2-weighted images. MRI lacks the capability of distinguishing RCCs from most other solid renal lesions, whether benign or malignant.

STAGING OF RENAL CELL CARCINOMA: COMPARISON OF CT AND MRI

The accurate staging of RCC is essential for proper patient management. While surgical-pathologic staging offers the most accurate prognosis, preoperative radiologic staging guides the therapeutic approach and aids the surgeon in operative planning. The current staging system used in clinical practice, according to Robson et al.,[17] is presented in Table 2-1.

Until recently, the staging of renal neoplasms was performed predominantly by CT, which has demonstrated overall accuracy rates of greater than 90 percent in distinguishing between surgical stages I and III.[18-20] MRI is now being increasingly used for staging, with recent series revealing overall accuracy rates ranging from 74 to 96 percent.[15,16,21] However, direct comparison of such overall accuracy rates may be misleading, as different studies did not necessarily attempt to detect tumor microinvasion through the renal capsule or to subclassify stage III lesions. It is best, then, to compare these two modalities on a stage-by-stage basis.

The differentiation of stages I and II from stages III and IV is significant because of the different surgical approaches taken for the lower-stage lesions and the different survival rates for these two groups. The primary treatment for RCC is radical nephrectomy, consisting of resection of Gerota's fascia and its contents as well as para-aortic lymph nodes in left-sided tumors, or paracaval nodes in right-sided neoplasms. While much has been made of attempting to distinguish preoperatively between stage I and II lesions, this has limited clinical significance, since both stages are usually treated by radical nephrectomy. As more patients undergo partial nephrectomies in the treatment of localized small tumors, this distinction may assume greater impor-

TABLE 2-1   Staging of renal cell carcinoma

Stage	Tumor Involvement
I	Confined to the renal capsule
II	Extension into perinephric fat but confined by perirenal fascia; ipsilateral adrenal involvement possible
IIIA	Extension into the renal vein and/or inferior vena cava
IIIB	Extension into adjacent regional lymph nodes
IIIC	Involvement of both venous and lymphatic structures
IVA	Extension into adjacent organs outside perirenal fascia
IVB	Distant metastases

tance. Nevertheless, both CT and MRI have difficulty in this area, as neither modality is able to detect microinvasion through the renal capsule, and false-positive diagnoses leading to upstaging are often made.[15,16,18]

Whereas MRI and CT show similar degrees of accuracy in evaluating lower-stage lesions, MRI appears more advantageous in characterizing stage III RCCs. This is because MRI is more sensitive and specific than CT in detecting venous tumor extension into both the renal vein and vena cava,[16] although CT may visualize tumor thrombus in most instances (Fig. 2-5). False-positive CT diagnoses may be made if enlargement of the renal vein or vena cava is identified without visualizing definite thrombus within the vessel. Vascular enlargement is a nonspecific finding, seen in both hypervascular neoplasms as well as in unrelated conditions such as right-sided heart failure. MRI clearly demonstrates tumor thrombus without the use of IV contrast and multiplanar imaging permits precise evaluation of cranial extension to aid operative management (Fig. 2-6). In addition, the need for preoperative inferior vena cavography is obviated because MRI has both a positive predictive value as well as negative predictive value of 100 percent for tumor extension into the distal renal vein and inferior vena cava[16] (Fig. 2-7).

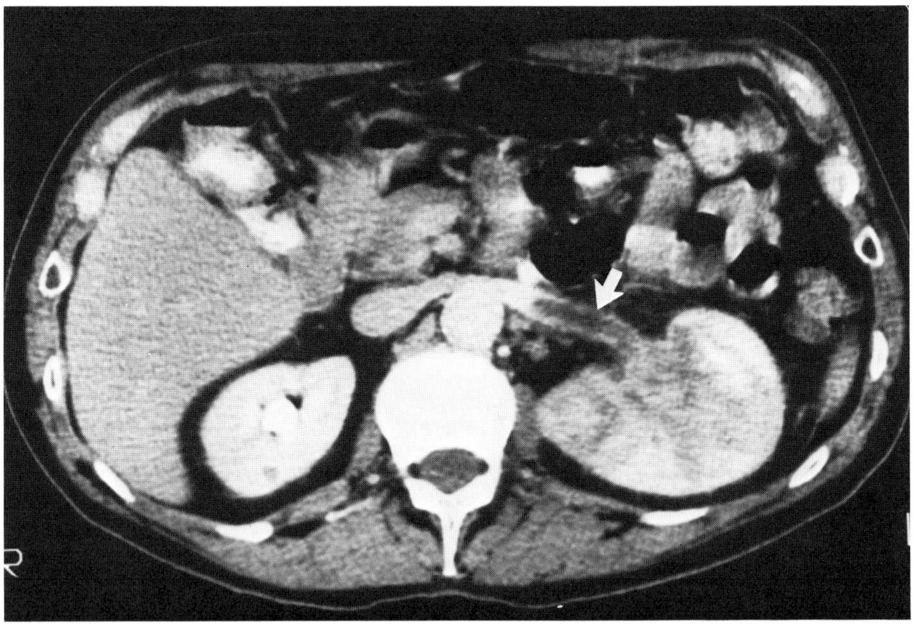

FIG. 2-5.   Renal cell carcinoma, Stage IIIA. A 59-year-old man was evaluated for hematuria. Contrast-enhanced CT scan reveals an ill-defined, infiltrating neoplasm growing throughout the posteromedial aspect of the left kidney. Tumor thrombus is seen to extend into a slightly enlarged left renal vein (arrow). At surgery, a poorly differentiated grade III renal cell carcinoma was resected with confirmed vascular invasion. Patient returned 1 year later with recurrent tumor in renal bed.

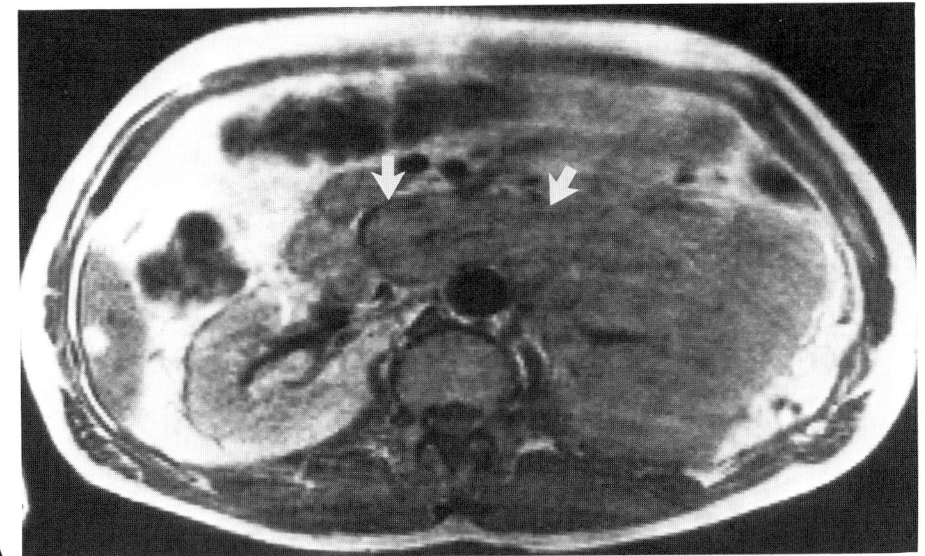

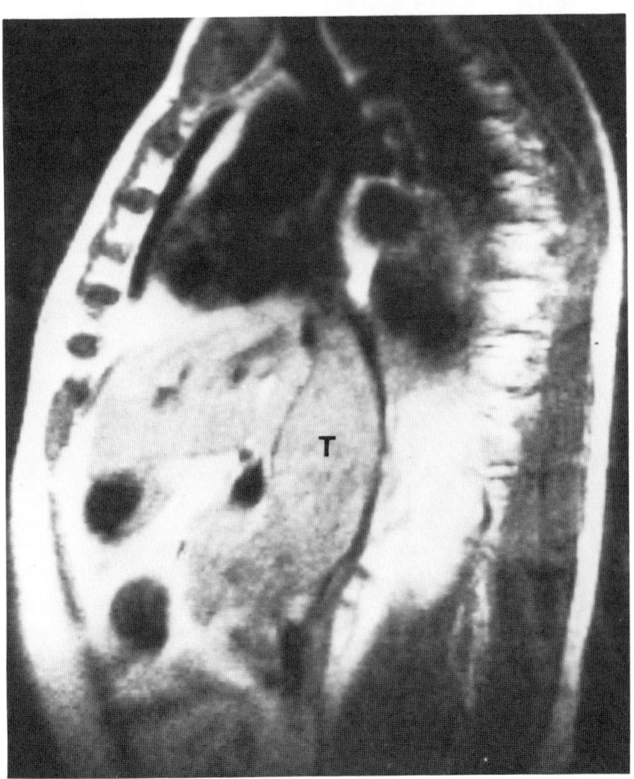

FIG. 2-6.   Renal cell carcinoma, stage IIIA. A 59-year-old man with a left renal cell carcinoma diagnosed by CT. MRI performed to evaluate the extent of vascular invasion. (A) Axial MRI scan (TR 2,000 ms, TE 30 ms) through the level of the renal hilum reveals a large left sided renal neoplasm extending into an enlarged left renal vein and inferior vena cava (arrows). Incidentally seen is a high-intensity hepatic cyst within the right lobe of the liver. (B) Sagittal MRI scan (TR 500 ms, TE 30 ms) demonstrates that tumor thrombus extends to the level of the diaphragm within a greatly enlarged inferior vena cava (T). (Case courtesy of Jeffrey C. Weinreb, M.D., New York University Medical Center.)

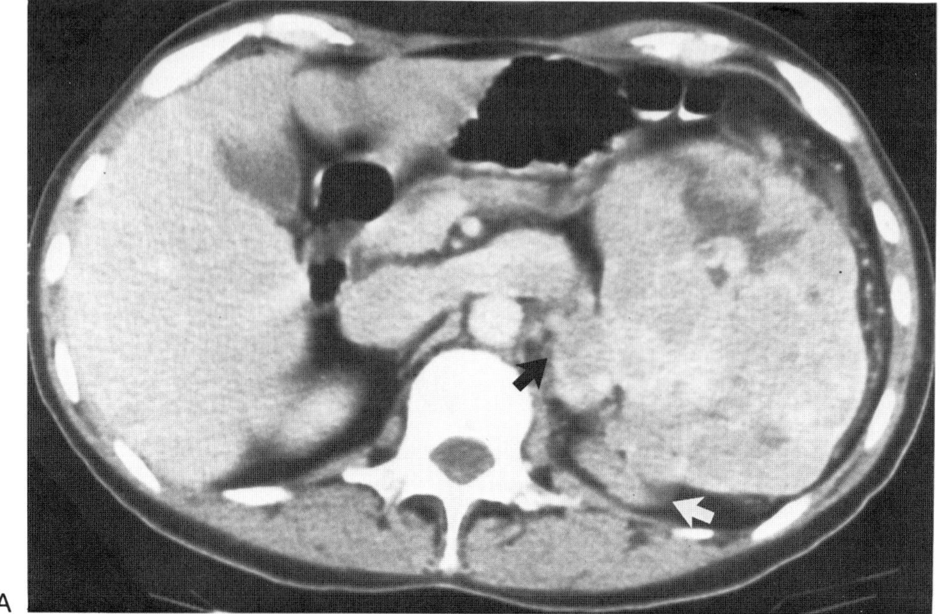

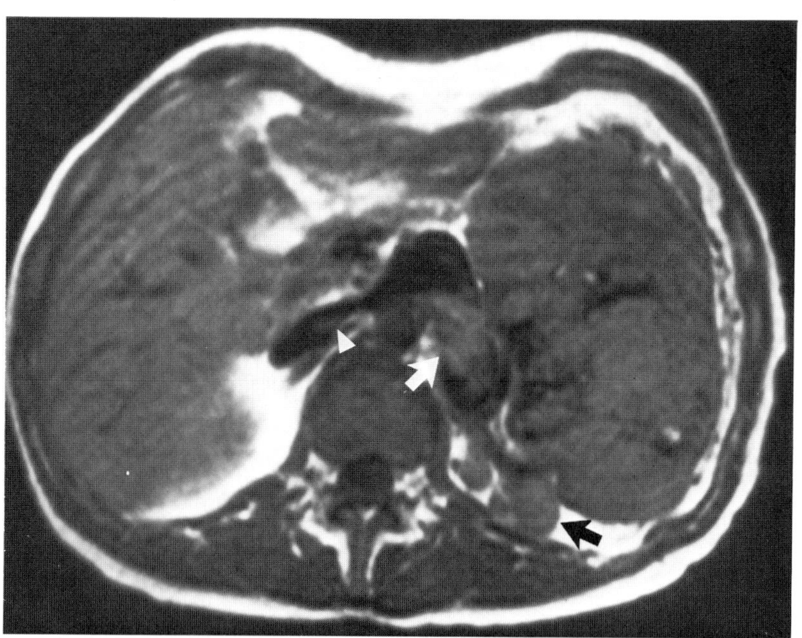

FIG. 2-7.   Renal cell carcinoma, stage IIIC. A 51-year-old man with left flank pain and a left renal mass. (A) Contrast-enhanced CT scan reveals a large, heterogeneous left renal neoplastic mass with extension into an enlarged left renal vein (black arrow) and local adenopathy (white arrow). (B) Axial T_1-weighted MRI scan (TR 300 ms, TE 30 ms, at a level comparable to Fig. A) reveals a predominantly homogeneous signal intensity renal mass with extension into the left renal vein (white arrow) with a small focus of tumor seen within the inferior vena cava (arrowhead) and local retroperitoneal nodes (black arrow). (*Figure continues.*)

38

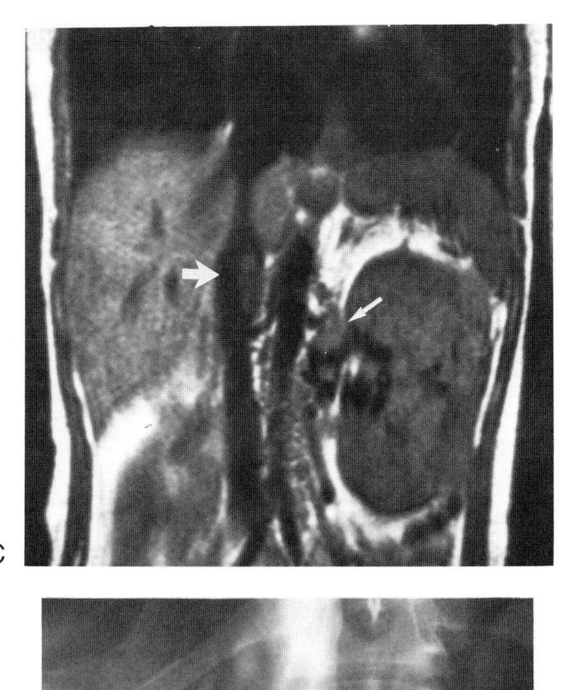

C

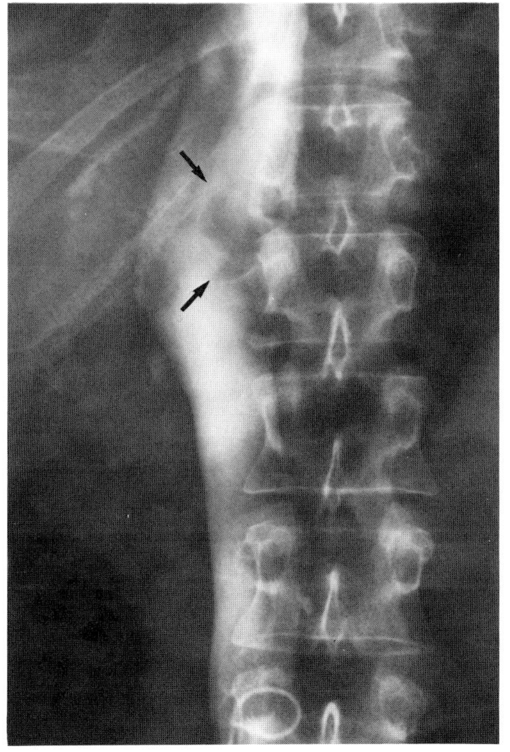

D

FIG. 2-7. (*Continued*).   (C) Coronal T$_1$-weighted MRI scan (TR 300 ms, TE 30 ms) not only demonstrates the renal carcinoma and local hilar nodes (small white arrow), but clearly depicts a short segment of non-obstructing tumor thrombus within the inferior vena cava (large white arrow). (D) Inferior venacavogram confirms the presence of tumor extension into the cava (black arrows) and correlates nicely with the MRI scan. Note unopacified blood flowing into the cava from the right renal vein.

While both CT and MRI are successful in identifying nodal size and location, neither modality is able to differentiate between normal hyperplastic nodes and metastatic adenopathy.[16,18] MRI appears to be more sensitive in nodal detection compared with CT (96 percent versus 83 percent), and MRI distinguishes adenopathy more clearly from dilated capsular or collateral veins that may not be clearly opacified on suboptimal bolus-CT studies.[15,16,18]

The demonstration of extensive metastatic disease often precludes even palliative radical surgery. Disseminated hematogenous metastases are well depicted by both CT and MRI. Because of multiplanar imaging capability, MRI has recently been shown to be more sensitive in detecting adjacent organ invasion, although both modalities have similar specificity and accuracy rates when strict criteria are applied.[16,18] Identification of a fat plane between the tumor and adjacent organs excludes direct invasion, but absence of this finding does not always indicate local invasion. For this to be reliably detected, CT must depict enlargement and/or a density change in the adjacent organ, while MRI should demonstrate disruption of tissue boundaries associated with alteration of normal signal intensities.

THE SMALL RENAL CELL CARCINOMA

The serendipitous or incidental detection of RCC by various imaging modalities is well described.[22–24] It has been estimated that in 0.3 percent of the population referred for an abdominal CT scan an occult RCC will be detected.[25] Because of the widespread application of both CT and ultrasound, as well as their improved spatial resolution and diagnostic capabilities, a significantly increased percentage of small RCCs is now being detected. These masses are being discovered earlier when they are small in size (less than 3 cm), well circumscribed, and usually stage I lesions[3] (Fig. 2-1). As a result, these patients may be offered "curative" surgery, and renal function may be preserved by performing either a partial nephrectomy or "tumorectomy" if surgically possible. The earlier diagnosis and treatment of these small carcinomas should improve the cure rate of this neoplasm. In fact, in one series, 31 of such incidentally detected lesions have been surgically resected; with follow-up ranging from 2.5 to 10 years, none has demonstrated either recurrence or evidence of metastatic disease.[3]

THE RECURRENT TUMOR

CT has proved useful for the evaluation of recurrent RCC. Following surgical resection, operative changes are allowed to subside; patients should undergo a baseline postoperative examination, particularly in cases in which there is a higher likelihood of recurrence based on operative findings. The periodicity of follow-up examinations will vary depending on the stage of the initial lesion and on the desire of both clinician and patient. The scans are carefully evaluated for local recurrence within the operative bed, as well as for evidence of either hematogenous or lymphatic metastases. Because late recurrence occurring 10 years or more after nephrectomy has been reported in approximately 11 percent of patients, patients require long-term clinical follow-up.[26]

CONCLUSION AND OVERALL ASSESSMENT

CT is extremely accurate in both the detection and characterization of complex renal mass lesions, and as such, is ideally suited as the initial screening and primary imaging modality for the evaluation of renal cell carcinoma. Properly performed contrast-enhanced CT studies are also quite accurate in the preoperative staging of these neoplasms. Because MRI lacks the capability of detecting small solid renal lesions and is unable to discriminate between complex renal masses, it presently has limited use as a screening modality. However, MRI is a promising technique that is complementary to CT. Its use is recommended when CT results are equivocal, when intravenous contrast is to be avoided, as well as to aid in the staging of renal cancer.

REFERENCES

1. Bennington JL, Beckwith JB: Tumors of the kidney, renal pelvis and ureter. p. 27. In Firminger HI (ed): Atlas of Tumor Pathology. Armed Forces Institute of Pathology, Washington, DC, 1975
2. Lynch HT, Walzak MP: Genetics in Urologic Cancer. Urol Clin North Am 7:815, 1980
3. Smith SJ, Bosniak MA, Megibow AJ, et al: Renal cell carcinoma: Earlier discovery and increased detection. Radiology 170:699, 1989
4. Zeman RK, Cronan JJ, Rosenfield AT, et al: Renal cell carcinoma: Dynamic thin section CT assessment of vascular invasion and tumor vascularity. Radiology 167:393, 1988
5. McClennan BL, Stanley RJ, Melson GL, et al: CT of renal cyst. Is cyst aspiration necessary? AJR 133:671, 1979
6. Bosniak MA: The current radiological approach to renal cysts. Radiology 158:1, 1986
7. Sussman S, Cochran ST, Pajani JJ, et al: Hyperdense renal masses: A CT manifestation of hemorrhagic renal cysts. Radiology 150:207, 1984
8. Dunnick NR, Korobkin M, Silverman PM, Foster WL Jr: Computed tomography of high density renal cysts. J Comput Assist Tomogr 8:458, 1984
9. Bosniak MA, Megibow AJ, Hulnick DH, et al: CT diagnosis of renal angiomyolipoma: The importance of detecting small amounts of fat. AJR 151:497, 1988
10. Quinn MJ, Hartman DS, Friedman AC, et al: Renal oncocytomas: New observations. Radiology 153:49, 1984
11. Bradley WG, Waluch V: Blood flow: Magnetic resonance imaging. Radiology 154:443, 1985
12. Waluch V, Bradley WG: NMR even echo rephasing in slow laminar flow. J Comput Assist Tomogr 8:594, 1984
13. Brasch RC, Weinmann H, Wesbey GE: Contrast-enhanced NMR imaging: Animal studies using Gadolinium-DTPA complex. AJR 142:625, 1984
14. Hricak H, Williams RD, Moon KL, et al: Nuclear magnetic resonance imaging of the kidney: Renal masses. Radiology 147:765, 1983
15. Fein AB, Lee JKT, Balfe DM, et al: Diagnosis and staging of renal cell carcinoma: A comparison of MR imaging and CT. AJR 148:749, 1987

16. Hricak H, Thoeni RF, Carroll PR, et al: Detection and staging of renal neoplasms: A reassessment of MR imaging. Radiology 166:643, 1988
17. Robson CJ, Churchill BM, Anderson W: The results of radical nephrectomy of renal cell carcinoma. J Urol 101:297, 1969
18. Johnson CJ, Dunnick NR, Cohan RH, Illescas FF: Renal adenocarcinoma: CT staging of 100 tumors. AJR 148:59, 1987
19. Love L, Churchill R, Reynes C: Computed tomography staging of renal carcinoma. Urol Radiol 1:3, 1979
20. Land EK: Angio-computed tomography and dynamic computed tomography in staging of renal cell carcinoma. Radiology 151:149, 1984
21. Hricak H, Demas BE, Williams RD, et al: Magnetic resonance imaging in the diagnosis and staging of renal and perirenal neoplasm. Radiology 154:708, 1985
22. Siegelman SS, Sprayregan S, Bosniak MA, Freed SZ: Serendipity in the diagnosis of renal carcinoma. J Can Assoc Radiol 23:251, 1972
23. Amendola MA, Bree BL, Pollack HM, et al: Small renal cell carcinomas: Resolving a diagnostic dilemma. Radiology 166:637, 1988
24. Curry NS, Schabel SI, Betsill WL Jr: Small renal neoplasms: Diagnostic imaging, pathologic features and clinical course. Radiology 158:113, 1986
25. Raval B, Lamki N: Computed tomography in detection of occult hypernephroma. CT 7:199, 1983
26. McNichols DW, Segura JW, Deweerd JH: Renal cell carcinoma in long-term survival and late recurrence. J Urol 126:17, 1981

3 CT and MRI of Benign Renal Neoplasms

BYRN WILLIAMSON, Jr.

Although benign renal tumors are not uncommon findings at autopsy,[1] most of these tumors are too small to cause symptoms or be detected by current imaging techniques. On the other hand, when such tumors are detected during life, they attain considerable clinical importance, primarily because they may simulate renal cell carcinoma. In recent years, advances in CT and other imaging techniques have allowed more of these masses to be discovered during life and have increased our ability to determine the nature of some of these benign masses. This chapter reviews the CT findings in renal angiomyolipoma, adenoma, oncocytoma, and multilocular cystic nephroma. MRI of angiomyolipoma and oncocytoma is also discussed.

ANGIOMYOLIPOMA

Angiomyolipoma is a tumor composed of vascular elements, smooth muscle, and adipose tissue. Because smooth muscle and fat normally do not occur in renal parenchyma, these tumors are considered heterotopic lesions rather than true neoplasms.[2] For this reason, the commonly used term *hamartoma* is misleading, because this term denotes a tumor consisting of a mixture of tissues that normally occur in the organ of origin. Renal angiomyolipoma may occur as an isolated finding or may be associated with tuberous sclerosis.

Pathologic Features

Although vascular, smooth muscle, and fatty elements may vary in their proportion in a given angiomyolipoma, all three elements are invariably present.[2] The gross and microscopic appearances are determined by the composition of the tumor. Tumors containing a large amount of fat often present a yellow appearance on cut section, while those predominantly containing smooth muscle tissue are gray. Tumors may arise in the cortex or the medulla and may be solitary or multiple, unilateral or bilateral. Angiomyolipomas located in the periphery of the kidney may elevate the renal capsule or may extend into perinephric tissues. Grossly recognizable areas of fat may be present on cut section as well as areas of recent or old hemorrhage, calcification, necrosis, or cystic degeneration.

On histologic examination the tumor is composed of tortuous, thick-walled blood vessels, sheets and collarettes of smooth muscle, and mature fat cells.[2] Angiomyolipomas have sometimes been incorrectly diagnosed as malignant because the smooth muscle component may exhibit mitotic figures, giant cells, and pleomorphic nuclei. Furthermore, multicentric tumors are not uncommon, and involvement of regional lymph nodes has been described.[3]

Clinical Features

Most angiomyolipomas are clinically silent and remain undiscovered during life or are discovered incidentally during radiologic examination of the kidneys. Larger angiomyolipomas are more likely to be evident clinically, and symptoms are usually due to hemorrhage resulting from the vascular nature of these tumors. Flank pain, either acute or chronic, is the most common symptom of angiomyolipoma. Other symptoms include palpable flank mass, hematuria, and hypertension. Massive hemorrhage from angiomyolipoma may occur and present clinically as hemorrhagic shock.

Angiomyolipomas may appear as isolated lesions or in association with tuberous sclerosis. Angiomyolipomas occurring in the absence of tuberous sclerosis tend to occur in patients beyond the age of 40 years and are more frequently discovered in women than in men. Such lesions tend to be unilateral, although they may be multiple.

Angiomyolipomas associated with tuberous sclerosis are usually multiple and bilateral. Because of aggressive radiologic evaluation of patients with tuberous sclerosis, renal angiomyolipomas in such patients are often discovered at a younger age than those in patients without evidence of tuberous sclerosis. Such lesions are frequently asymptomatic when discovered. About 20 percent of patients with angiomyolipomas have tuberous sclerosis, while 80 percent of patients with tuberous sclerosis have angiomyolipomas.

Renal angiomyolipomas also may occur in patients with lymphangiomyomatosis. This rare disease of young women may represent a "forme fruste" of tuberous sclerosis. The basic pathologic lesion in this disease is hamartomatous proliferation of smooth muscle along the lymphatic system.[4]

Radiologic Features

The radiologic diagnosis of angiomyolipoma depends on the demonstration of fat within the lesion. Angiomyolipomas that contain a large amount of fat may occasionally be diagnosed by plain radiographs of the kidneys, particularly if tomograms are obtained. After injection of contrast material for an excretory urogram, the detection of fat within a lesion is unreliable, and an angiomyolipoma presents the appearance of a indeterminate renal mass. Multiple bilateral angiomyolipomas, such as those found in patients with tuberous sclerosis, may simulate polycystic renal disease on excretory urography. The presence of fat within an angiomyolipoma gives rise to an intensely echogenic appearance on diagnostic ultrasound evaluation. Although this appearance is highly suggestive of angiomyolipoma, a small number of renal cell carcinomas can also produce a hyperechoic appearance on ultrasound.[5,6]

The angiographic appearance of angiomyolipoma is determined by the characteristics of the vascular component of the tumor. Most angiomyolipomas are hypervascular,[7] and the abnormal vessels may simulate those of renal cell carcinoma. The angiographic differentiation of angiomyolipoma from renal cell carcinoma remains a controversial subject[8]; fortunately, CT offers a reliable and less invasive means of distinguishing these entities.[9–14]

CT diagnosis of angiomyolipoma is dependent on the detection of fat within the tumor (Fig. 3-1). Thus, the rare angiomyolipoma that contains no macroscopic areas of fatty tissue will not be distinguishable from renal cell carcinoma by CT. Most angiomyolipomas, however, will contain areas of fat discernible on CT scan. The identification of fat within an angiomyolipoma on CT is facilitated by thin-section images obtained before the injection of contrast medium; this is true even in extremely small lesions.[14] Vascular and smooth muscle components of the tumor will appear as solid tissue. The typical CT findings of hemorrhage may also be detected in tumors that have bled

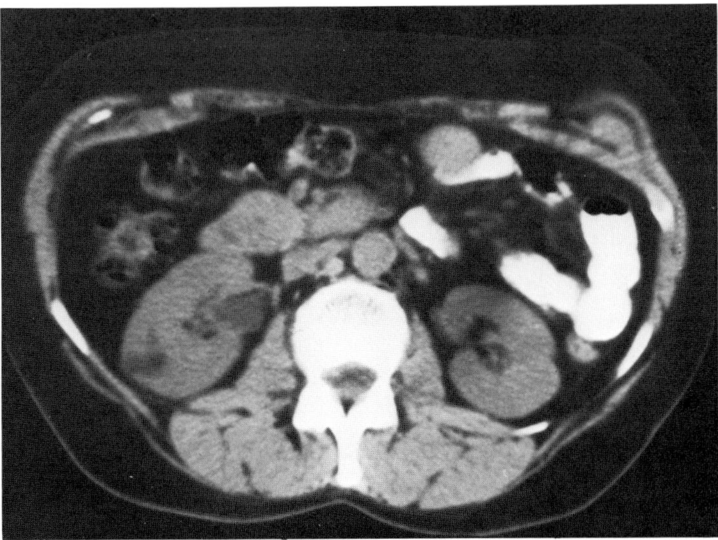

FIG. 3-1.   Angiomyolipoma. Unenhanced CT scan shows a low-attenuation mass in the lateral aspect of the right kidney. The presence of fat within this lesion allows a diagnosis of angiomyolipoma.

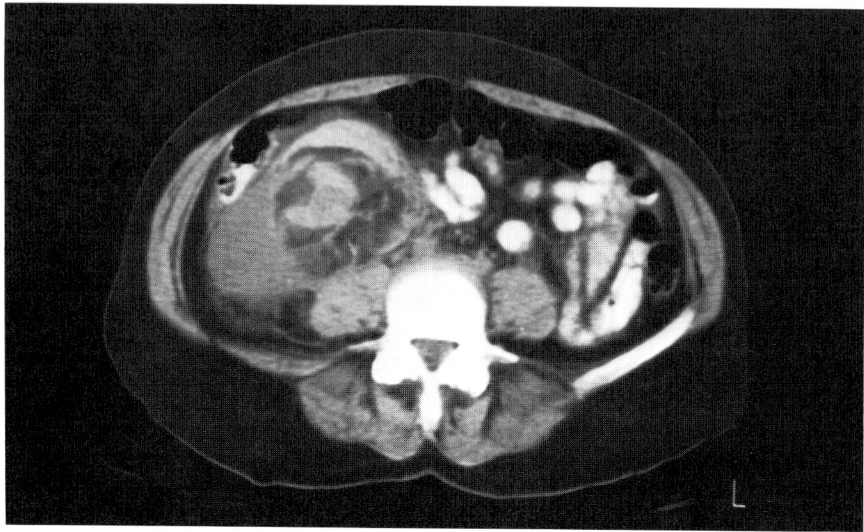

FIG. 3-2.   Hemorrhagic angiomyolipoma. Unenhanced CT scan shows a large, fat-containing mass at the lower pole of the right kidney. The crescentic high-attenuation area at the anterior aspect of the lesion and the high-attenuation area within the lesion represent areas of recent hemorrhage.

(Fig. 3-2). Massive hemorrhage from an angiomyolipoma may obscure the presence of fatty elements and prevent an accurate CT diagnosis. Although fat may be present in Wilms' tumors,[15] the presence of fat within a renal tumor in an adult is considered to be reliable evidence that the tumor represents an angiomyolipoma.

MRI may also detect fat within an angiomyolipoma and thus provide a definitive diagnosis[16,17] (Fig. 3-3). Optimal demonstration of fat can be obtained by a spin-echo technique incorporating axial T_1-weighted (TR 500 ms, TE 20 ms) and T_2-weighted (TR 2000 ms, TE 60 ms) images. Coronal imaging is usually not necessary, but may be helpful in some cases. MRI does not currently provide increased diagnostic capabilities compared with CT, so the greater expense of MRI evaluation mitigates against its use in evaluation of suspected angiomyolipoma.

Management

Because angiomyolipomas containing a significant amount of fat can be diagnosed reliably by CT, most asymptomatic lesions do not require surgery. Follow-up examinations may be helpful in evaluating growth of the lesion or episodes of recurrent hemorrhage. When clinical symptoms warrant or when kidney function is threatened, surgery may be required. In such cases, CT or angiography may be helpful in planning the surgical approach to allow pres-

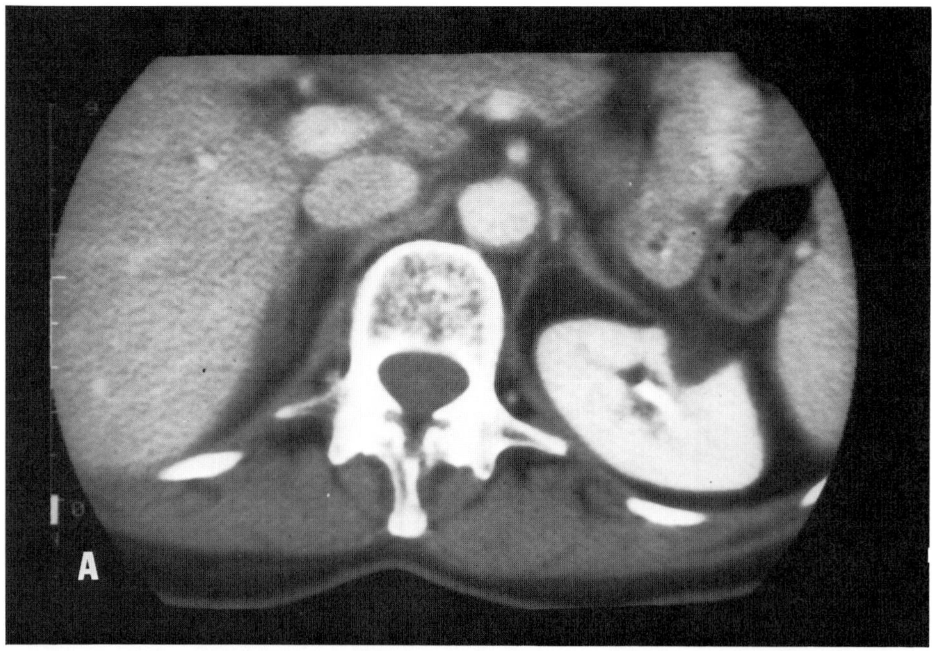

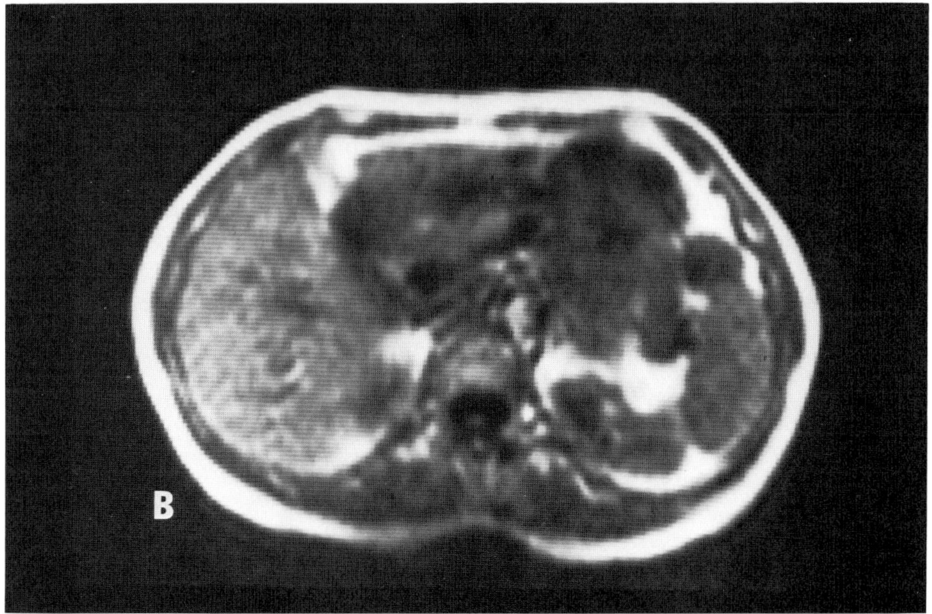

FIG. 3-3.   Angiomyolipoma. (A) Enhanced CT scan shows low-density mass in the anterior aspect of the left kidney typical of angiomyolipoma. (B) Axial T_1-weighted image (inversion recovery, TI 500 ms, TR 2,000 ms, Picker 0.15 T) of the kidneys demonstrates the left renal mass with increased signal intensity, similar to surrounding perirenal fat. An angiomyolipoma was found at surgery.

ervation of normal renal tissue. Conservation of renal tissue is particularly important in patients with multiple lesions.

ONCOCYTOMA

Oncocytic tumors may occur in the thyroid, parathyroid, adrenal, and salivary glands, as well as the kidney. Renal oncocytoma has been diagnosed with increased frequency since Klein and Valensi[18] reported 13 cases of this entity in 1976. Before the widespread recognition of this entity, most of these lesions were diagnosed as renal cell carcinomas.[19,20] Because many oncocytomas exhibit benign behavior, preoperative diagnosis may permit conservative surgery in some cases.

Pathologic Features

On gross examination, an oncocytoma exhibits a mahogany brown color and a well-developed capsule. On cut section, a central fibrous scar may be apparent, particularly if the tumor is large. Histologically, the tumor is composed of large epithelial cells containing granular eosinophilic cytoplasm. The distinctive appearance of the cytoplasm is due to the presence of a large number of mitochondria.

Some confusion exists regarding the pathologic classification of oncocytomas. Oncocytes are present in some renal cell carcinomas, and some tumors composed of oncocytes exhibit malignant characteristics. If the term *oncocytoma* is reserved for histologically benign tumors composed of oncocytes, such tumors can be expected to behave in a benign manner. Such tumors should be composed of large granular eosinophilic cells with small regular nuclei without nuclear anaplasia or mitotic activity. The tumor should not contain evidence of necrosis. A study of 90 well-differentiated oncocytic renal neoplasms at the Mayo Clinic found no metastases in 62 patients with histologically grade 1 tumors, but 4 of 28 patients with grade 2 tumors died of metastatic disease.[21]

Clinical Features

Most oncocytomas are asymptomatic and are discovered incidentally on radiographic examination.[22] In patients who are symptomatic, flank pain or gross hematuria may occur. Occasionally, a palpable flank mass or hypertension may be present. The peak incidence of oncocytoma occurs between the ages of 50 and 70, and the tumor occurs more frequently in males than in females.

Radiologic Features

Plain films and excretory urography may reveal a mass if the oncocytoma is of significant size, but oncocytoma cannot be distinguished from other solid masses by such studies. Ultrasound evaluation typically reveals a well-defined homogeneous mass with smooth contours. Ultrasound depicts a central scar in approximately 25 percent of cases; it may be either hyperechoic or hypo-echoic.[23]

Angiography may depict a hypovascular mass or, more commonly, a hypervascular mass, often containing "spoke wheel" vascularity. Such a mass exhibits well-defined margins. Vascular puddling and venous shunting are absent. Although the angiographic findings may be suggestive, oncocytoma cannot reliably be distinguished from renal cell carcinoma by this modality.[24,25]

On CT, oncocytoma appears as a well-defined, homogeneous solid mass (Fig. 3-4), occasionally containing calcification.[26] About one-third of cases exhibit a central scar, generally with a stellate configuration. Except for the scar,

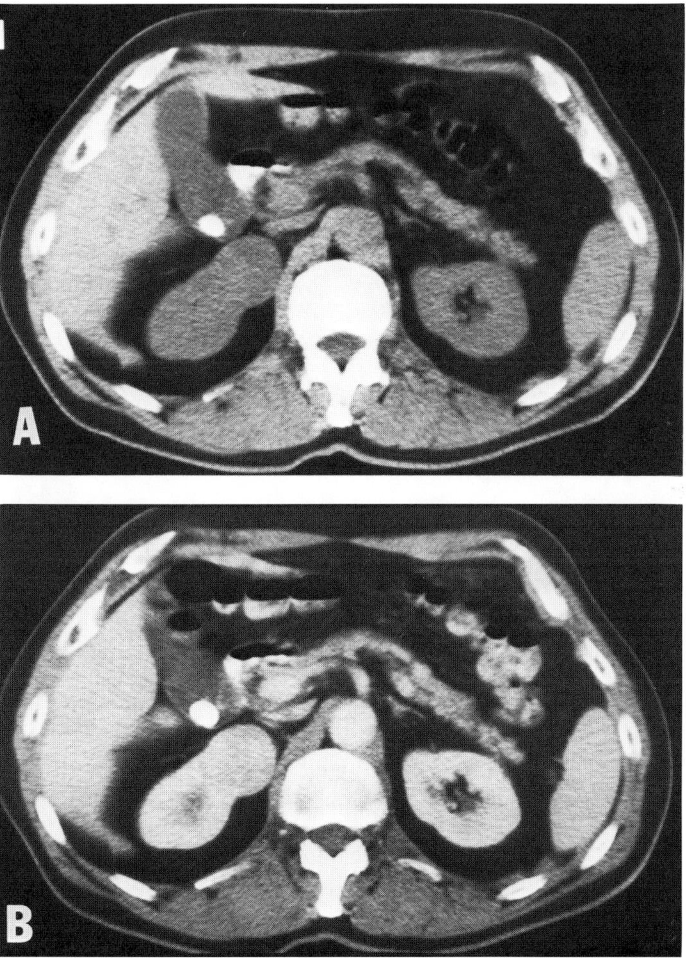

FIG. 3-4.   Oncocytoma. CT scans obtained before (A) and after (B) administration of intravenous contrast medium reveal a homogeneous mass at the medial aspect of the right kidney. This case does not demonstrate a central scar. Partial nephrectomy was performed and a renal oncocytoma was found.

the tumor enhances homogeneously following the injection of intravenous contrast material.[23]

Routine MRI of the kidneys, using spin-echo T_1-weighted (TR 500 ms, TE 20 ms) and T_2-weighted (TR 2,000 ms, TE 60 ms) axial images, can be used in the evaluation of oncocytomas. T_1-weighted coronal images can also be used to demonstrate patency of the renal veins and inferior vena cava.

MRI depicts oncocytoma as a relatively homogeneous mass[26,27] often containing a central scar (Fig. 3-5). MRI may depict a well-defined capsule. When

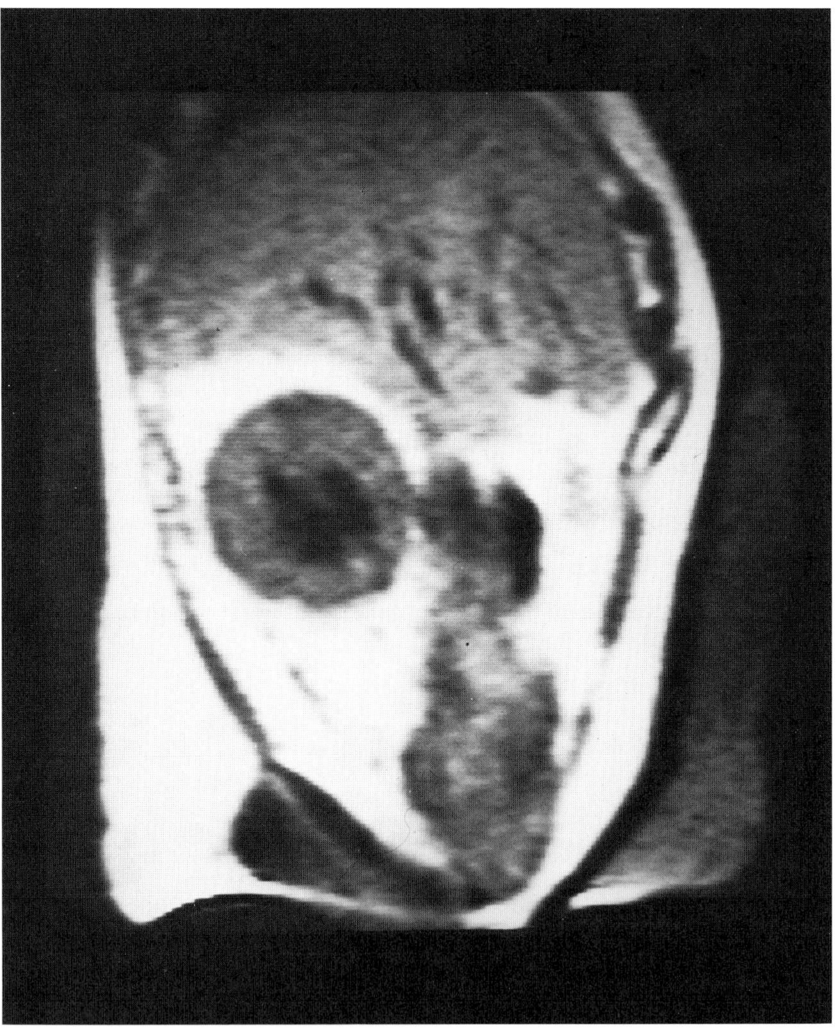

FIG. 3-5. Oncocytoma. Sagittal T_1-weighted image (inversion recovery, TI 500 ms, TR 2,083 ms, Picker 0.15 T) of the right kidney demonstrates a large renal mass with a central area of decreased signal intensity. A grade 1 renal oncocytoma was found at surgery.

present, the central scar tends to appear as an area of low intensity on inversion recovery images or an area of high intensity on spin-echo images. Although suggestive, the appearance of a scar is not pathognomonic of oncocytoma, and a similar appearance can be seen on MRI examination of renal cell carcinoma.[28]

Management

Although the diagnosis of oncocytoma can be suggested on the basis of CT or MRI, a definitive diagnosis cannot be obtained without surgery. Because renal cell carcinoma can contain areas of oncocytes, percutaneous needle biopsy may not reliably diagnose oncocytoma. Even if preoperative diagnosis of oncoctyoma were possible, the fact that some oncocytic tumors exhibit malignant behavior suggests that oncocytomas should be surgically removed. Thus, the contribution of CT and MRI is to suggest the possibility of oncocytoma so that conservative surgery can be considered.

RENAL ADENOMA

Pathologists disagree about the criteria for diagnosing renal adenomas, and some pathologists do not accept the existence of such lesions. Bennington and Beckwith[2] assert that no objective criteria exist that allow adenomas to be distinguished from carcinomas, and that all lesions thought to represent adenomas actually represent adenocarcinomas. At the other end of the spectrum, some pathologists classify all solid renal tumors measuring less than 3 cm in diameter as adenomas and consider larger tumors to represent carcinomas. The pathologists at the Mayo Clinic espouse a position between these two extremes. They classify well-differentiated tubulopapillary tumors as adenomas, even if they are larger than 3 cm in diameter. Tumors exhibiting aggressive invasive behavior, particularly with necrosis, and tumors with histologic evidence of malignancy, such as anaplasia, mitoses, or the presence of nucleoli, are considered malignant regardless of size. Similarly, all hypernephroid tumors composed of clear or lipid-laden cells in an alveolar arrangement are considered carcinomas.

Pathologic Features

Renal adenomas are generally classified histologically as papillary, tubular, or alveolar, although alveolar "adenomas" should probably be classified as adenocarcinomas as mentioned above. True adenomas may be composed of tubular elements, papillary elements, or a mixture of the two. On gross examination, these tumors may be solid or may contain cysts of variable size. In some cases, the cystic component may be the predominant feature of these tumors. Microscopic examination reveals small cells with regular nuclei arranged in either a papillary or a tubular pattern.

Clinical Features

Large adenomas may occasionally cause hematuria, flank pain,[29] or rarely may present as a palpable flank mass.[30] Hypertension rarely occurs. The vast majority of renal adenomas are asymptomatic, and most of these are not detected during life. In recent years, increasing numbers of adenomas have been detected incidentally by CT performed for unrelated causes.

Patients undergoing long-term dialysis for chronic renal failure exhibit a propensity to develop renal adenomas as well as multiple renal cysts.[31,32] In such patients, renal cysts generally appear first, often characterized by atypical cells in the cyst wall. Adenomas tend to appear later, and cases of renal cell carcinoma have been reported. Periodic evaluation of patients undergoing hemodialysis for chronic renal failure is indicated to detect the development of adenomas and carcinomas.[33,34]

Radiologic Features

A large renal adenoma may appear as a renal mass on plain radiography of the kidneys or on excretory urography.[29] Such tumors are occasionally calcified. The ultrasound appearance of an adenoma is that of a solid tumor. Although the diagnosis of adenoma is suggested by a homogeneous echo-texture and a regular distinct margin, renal cell carcinomas may also present this appearance. If the adenoma contains significant cystic areas, these may be depicted by ultrasound.

Angiography depicts a well-defined vascular mass with an orderly vascular

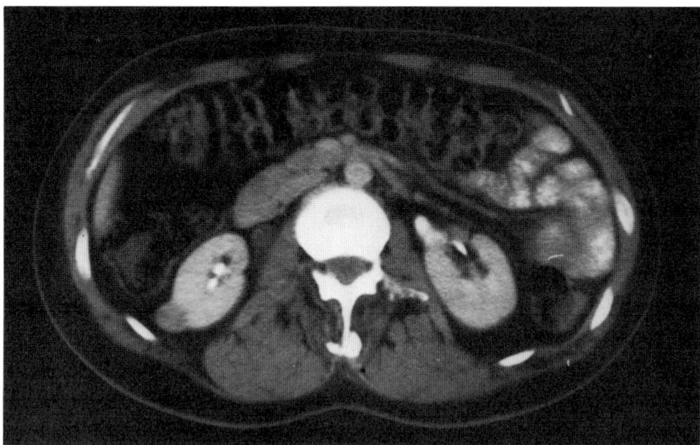

FIG. 3-6.   Cortical adenoma. Enhanced CT scan reveals a well-defined, homogeneous solid mass at the posterior aspect of the right kidney. A benign cortical adenoma was found at surgery.

pattern without venous shunting or vascular puddling.[35] Although the angiographic features may be suggestive, the possibility of renal cell carcinoma cannot be excluded on the basis of these findings alone.[36]

In common with other imaging techniques, CT of renal adenoma reveals a well-defined, homogeneous solid mass that enhances uniformly after the administration of intravenous (IV) contrast material (Fig. 3-6). Cystic components of variable size may be present. Although these findings are not sufficiently specific to allow the exclusion of renal cell carcinoma, the suggestion of the diagnosis of renal adenoma may allow conservative surgery to be performed rather than a radical nephrectomy.[37]

MULTILOCULAR CYSTIC NEPHROMA

Multilocular cystic nephroma is a benign tumor consisting of multiple noncommunicating cysts contained within a well-defined capsule. The pathogenesis of this lesion is uncertain, and the lesion has been variously considered a true neoplasm, a hamartoma, or the result of a defect in embryogenesis. The variability of pathologic findings and disagreement about the pathogenesis of the lesion have been reflected in a multiplicity of names being given to this tumor, including multilocular cyst, segmental multicystic kidney, segmental polycystic kidney, benign cystic nephroma, cystic adenoma, cystic hamartoma, and well-differentiated polycystic Wilms' tumor.[38]

Pathologic Features

Multilocular cystic nephroma is typically unilateral and solitary, although instances of bilaterality have been reported. On gross inspection, the tumor consists of multiple noncommunicating loculi with a well-defined capsule. Although the tumor may project into the renal pelvis, the loculi do not communicate with the collecting system. The individual loculi may range in size from a few millimeters to several centimeters in diameter. Multilocular cystic nephroma frequently replaces an entire pole of the kidney, although it can also occur in the midportion of the kidney or project from the surface of the kidney into perinephric tissues. Multilocular cystic nephromas have been reported as small as 2 cm in diameter and as large as 33 cm in diameter. Tumors that become clinically apparent are usually large, averaging 10 cm or more in diameter.

Microscopic examination of the collagenous capsule may reveal smooth muscle and occasionally cartilage. The loculi are lined with flattened or cuboidal epithelium, and the septa separating the loculi consist of small spindle cells with sparse cytoplasm. The intralocular septa contain no differentiated nephrons. Although the lesions are usually histologically benign, some case reports have described microscopic foci of nephroblastoma or sarcoma in the intralocular septa.

Clinical Features

Multilocular cystic nephroma is typically found in whites, only 11 cases having been reported in blacks.[39] Although the lesion affects the two sexes in equal numbers, there is marked difference in the age distribution of these lesions in the two sexes. The vast majority of multilocular cystic nephromas in males occur during the first 2 years of life, while the frequency in females is highest between the ages of 4 and 36 months and between the ages of 40 and 60 years. The right and left kidneys are involved with equal frequency.[39]

Castillo et al.[39] reported a series of 29 patients with multilocular cystic nephroma seen at the Mayo Clinic between 1976 and 1986. In 13 of these patients, the tumor was incidentally discovered during an imaging procedure performed for unrelated symptoms. In symptomatic patients, the most common clinical manifestations were abdominal pain, hematuria (either gross or microscopic), or palpable abdominal mass. Urinary tract infections have also been reported in some patients.[40] If surgery is delayed, multilocular cystic nephromas may increase in size, sometimes rapidly. The time course of development of multilocular cystic nephroma is unknown, but large tumors have been discovered only a few months following normal physical examination and as little as 2 years following a normal excretory urogram.[40]

Radiologic Features

Large multilocular cystic nephromas may appear as soft tissue masses on plain radiographs of the kidneys. Curvilinear or amorphous calcification may be visible within the mass.

Excretory urography depicts multilocular cystic nephroma as a renal mass, often protruding into the renal pelvis. If the mass causes obstruction of the collecting system, pyelocaliectasis may result. High-grade obstruction sometimes occurs with absent excretion of contrast medium in the kidney or in a portion of the kidney. If high-quality CT scans are obtained during the nephrographic phase of an excretory urogram, the septated nature of the tumor may be apparent.

The sonographic appearance of multilocular cystic nephroma depends on the size of the loculi. In a small proportion of cases, the loculi are too small to be appreciated on ultrasound examination, and the mass appears as an echogenic complex mass. More commonly, the loculi are large enough to be depicted clearly by ultrasound, and the tumor is shown to consist of numerous distinct cystic areas within a well-defined mass.[40] The septae may be several millimeters in thickness but do not display significant nodularity.

Angiography may demonstrate an avascular lesion, a hypovascular lesion, or a hypervascular mass. The nephrographic phase of the angiogram may reveal the multilocular character of the mass. Neovascularity may be present.

As with ultrasound, CT examination can fail to suggest the nature of a multilocular cystic nephroma when the cysts are quite small and the solid component predominates. In most cases, however, the cystic components of the mass are clearly visible[41] (Fig. 3-7), although not as well delineated as on ultrasound examination. The mass has a well-defined margin. The cyst fluid may be of slightly greater density than water but does not enhance after the

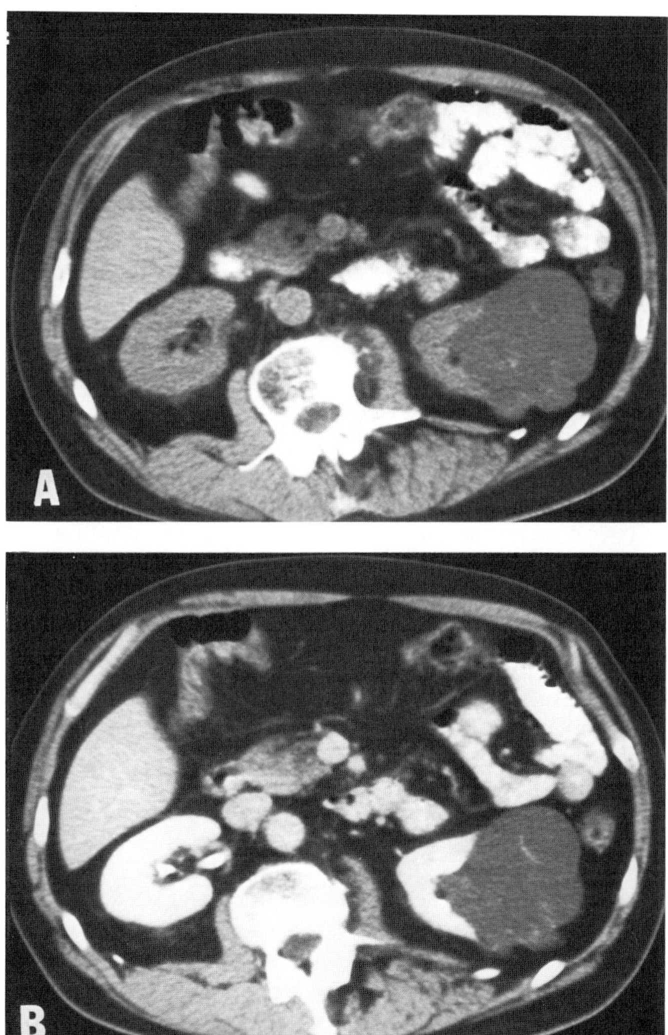

FIG. 3-7.   Multilocular cystic nephroma. (A) Unenhanced CT scan reveals a predominantly cystic mass in the lateral aspect of the left kidney. Areas of calcification are visible within the mass. (B) Enhanced CT scan confirms the cystic nature of the mass and suggests the presence of multiple loculi. The areas of calcification are located in the walls of the loculi. A 7 × 6-cm multilocular cystic nephroma was found at surgery.

administration of IV contrast material. The septae are of variable thickness and possess CT attenutation slightly less than that of renal parenchyma. Septations increase in density following administration of IV contrast material.[40]

With modern imaging techniques such as CT, MRI, and ultrasound, the diagnosis of multilocular cystic nephroma can be suggested in most cases prior to surgery, but the possibility of partially cystic renal cell carcinoma or of Wilms' tumor cannot be excluded entirely.[42–44]

Early experience with MRI of miltilocular cystic nephroma indicates that the morphologic characteristics of this tumor are well depicted by MRI. The capsule tends to be hypointense on all pulse sequences, while the fluid in the loculi may vary in intensity depending on the presence of protein or old hemorrhage. The appearance of the intralocular septae on MRI may vary depending on their cellular composition.[42]

Management

Conservative surgery can often be performed if the diagnosis of multilocular cystic nephroma is suggested by preoperative CT or ultrasound examination. Because of the presence of nephroblastoma or sarcoma cells in the septae of some multilocular cystic nephromas, some patients have undergone postoperative chemotherapy or radiation therapy. Patients with typical benign multilocular cystic nephroma require no further treatment following surgery. Incomplete excision of these tumors may result in recurrence.

REFERENCES

1. Witten DM, Myers GH, Utz DC: Emmett's Clinical Urography. Vol 3. 4th Ed. WB Saunders, Philadelphia, 1977

2. Bennington JL, Beckwith JB: Tumors of the kidney, renal pelvis, and ureter. In Firminger (ed): Atlas of Tumor Pathology. 2nd series. Part 12. Armed Forces Institute of Pathology, Washington, DC, 1975

3. Busch FM, Bark CJ, Clydine HR: Benign renal angiomyolipoma with regional lymph node involvement. J Urol 116:715, 1976

4. Rumancik WM, Bosniak MA, Rosen RJ, Hulnick D: Atypical renal and pararenal hamartomas associated with lymphangiomyomatosis. AJR 142:971, 1984

5. Hartman DS, Goldman SM, Friedman AC, et al: Angiomyolipoma: Ultrasonic-pathologic correlation. Radiology 139:451, 1981

6. Charboneau JW, Hattery RR, Ernst EC III, et al: Spectrum of sonographic findings in 125 renal masses other than benign simple cyst. AJR 140:87, 1983

7. Becker JA, Kinkhabwal AM, Pollack H, Bosniak M: Angiolipoma of the kidney: An angiographic review. Acta Radiol [Diagn] (Stockh) 14:561, 1973

8. Jander HP, Tonkin IL: Epinephrine enhanced renal angiography in the diagnosis of hamartoma (angiomyolipoma): A reevaluation. Radiology 132:61, 1979

9. Bosniak MA: Angiomyolipoma (hamartoma) of the kidney: A preoperative diagnosis is possible in virtually every case. Urol Radiol 3:135, 1981

10. Bret PM, Bretagnolle M, Gaillard D, et al: Small, asymptomatic angiomyolipomas of the kidney. Radiology 154:7, 1985

11. Raghavendra BN, Bosniak MA, Megibow AJ: Small angiomyolipoma of the kidney: Sonographic-CT evaluation. AJR 141:575, 1983

12. Sherman JL, Hartman DS, Friedman AC, et al: Angiomyolipoma: Computed tomographic-pathologic correlation of 17 cases. AJR 137:1221, 1981

13. Kolmannskog F, Kolbenstvedt A, Nakstad PH, Aakhus T: Computed tomography and angiography in renal angiomyolipoma. Acta Radiol [Diagn] (Stockh) 22:635, 1981

14. Bosniak MA, Megibow AJ, Hulnick DH, et al: CT diagnosis of renal angiomyolipoma: The importance of detecting small amounts of fat. AJR 151:497, 1988

15. Parvey LS, Warner RM, Callihan TR, Magill HL: CT demonstration of fat tissue in malignant renal neoplasms: Atypical Wilms' tumors. J Comput Assist Tomogr 5:851, 1981

16. Choyke PL, Kressel HY, Pollack HM, et al: Focal renal masses: Magnetic resonance imaging. Radiology 152:471, 1984

17. Newhouse JH, Markisz JA, Kazam E: Magnetic resonance imaging of the kidneys. Cardiovasc Intervent Radiol 8:351, 1989

18. Klein MJ, Valensi QJ: Proximal tubular adenomas of the kidney with so called oncocytic features: A clinicopathologic study of 13 cases of a rarely reported neoplasm. Cancer 38:906, 1976

19. Lieber MM: Renal oncoctyoma. p. 139. In Javadpour N (ed): Cancer of the Kidney. Thieme-Stratton, New York, 1984

20. Tessler AN, Kurusu S, Klein MJ, Valensi QJ: Proximal tubular adenoma of kidney. Urology 10:203, 1977

21. Lieber MM, Tomera KM, Farrow GM: Renal oncocytoma. J Urol 125:481, 1981

22. Merino MJ, Livolsi VA: Oncocytomas of the kidney. Cancer 50:1852, 1982

23. Quinn MJ, Hartman DS, Friedman AC, et al: Renal oncoctyoma: New observations. Radiology 153:49, 1984

24. Bonavita JA, Pollack HM, Banner MP: Renal oncocytoma: Further observations and literature review. Urol Radiol 2:229, 1981

25. Jander HP: Renal oncocytoma, a nonentity (letter to editor). Radiology 130:815, 1979

26. Sohn HK, Kim SY, Seo HS: MR imaging of a renal oncocytoma. J Comput Assist Tomogr 11:6, 1987

27. Remark RR, Berquist TH, Lieber MM, et al: Magnetic resonance imaging of renal oncocytoma. Urology 31:176, 1988

28. Ball DS, Friedman AC, Hartman DS, et al: Scar sign of renal oncocytoma: Magnetic resonance imaging appearance and lack of specificity. Urol Radiol 8:46, 1986

29. Cass AS: Large renal adenoma. J Urol 124:281, 1980

30. Weiss RM, Puchner PJ, Habif DV Jr, Tannenbaum M: Flank pain, abdominal mass, and bleeding. Urology 15:418, 1980

31. Scanlon MH, Karasick SR: Acquired renal cystic disease and neoplasia: Complications of chronic hemodialysis. Radiology 147:837, 1983

32. Hughson MD, Hennigar GR, McManus JFA: Atypical cysts, acquired renal cystic disease, and renal cell tumors in end-stage dialysis kidneys. Lab Invest 42:475, 1980

33. Kutcher R, Amodio JB, Rosenblatt R: Uremic renal cystic disease: value of sonographic screening. Radiology 147:833, 1983

34. Levine E, Grantham JJ, Slusher SL, et al: CT of acquired cystic kidney disease and renal tumors in long-term dialysis patients. AJR 142:125, 1984

35. Bruneton JN, Ballanger P, Ballanger R, Delorme G: Renal adenomas. Clin Radiol 30:343, 1979

36. Holt RG, Neiman HL, Korsower JM, Newhouser J: Angiographic features of benign renal adenoma. Urology 6:764, 1975

37. Pfannkuch F, Leistenschneider W, Nagel R: Problems of assessment in the surgery of renal adenomas. J Urol 125:95, 1981

38. Banner MP, Pollack HM, Chatten J, Witzleben C: Multilocular renal cysts: radiologic-pathologic correlation. AJR 136:239, 1981

39. Castillo OA, Boyle ET, Kramer SA, Kelalis PP: Multilocular cysts of the kidney: A study of 29 patients and review of the literature. Urology (in press)

40. Madewell JE, Goldman SM, Davis CJ Jr, et al: Multilocular cystic nephroma: A radiographic-pathologic correlation of 58 patients. Radiology 146:309, 1983

41. Parienty RA, Pradel J, Imbert MC, et al: Computed tomography of multilocular cystic nephroma. Radiology 140:135, 1981

42. Dikengil A, Benson M, Sanders L, Newhouse JH: MRI of multilocular cystic nephroma. Urol Radiol 10:95, 1988

43. Beckwith JB, Kiviat NB: Multilocular renal cysts and cystic renal tumors. (Editorial.) AJR 136:435, 1981

44. Yonezawa S, Tokunaga M, Sato E, et al: Cystic partially differentiated nephroblastoma and multilocular cyst of the kidney: Report of two cases of so-called multilocular cyst of the kidney. Acta Pathol Jpn 29:471, 1979

4 CT and MRI of Inflammatory Disease of the Kidney

STANFORD M. GOLDMAN
ELLIOT K. FISHMAN
MICHAEL C. SOULEN

Since the appearance of the excellent article by Balfé et al.[1] in Volume 3 of this series, much additional information has been accumulated about the CT appearance of renal inflammatory disease. It may well be that CT, in most cases, is now the *most* sensitive and specific method for the evaluation of the multiple renal inflammatory processes discussed in this chapter. MRI, at present, remains a secondary tool to be used in select cases and instances only.

This chapter deals with our understanding of the terminology and pathophysiology of renal infection (Table 4-1). Before dealing with individual disease patterns, certain basic concepts are reviewed in order to give the reader a true overview of the topic. With these important background concepts in hand, we then approach the various types of renal infection.

BASIC CONCEPTS

Renal Infection Is a Dynamic Process

Renal inflammation spans a continuous spectrum, from uncomplicated acute pyelonephritis through progressively worsening interstitial inflammation to frank abscess formation. It can be a multifocal process, with different parts of the kidney exhibiting different degrees of inflammation (Fig. 4-1). It is also a dynamic process that progresses and regresses over days[2] or weeks. Exact radiologic correlation with these different degrees of inflammation is difficult

TABLE 4-1   CT of inflammatory renal disease

Diffuse acute pyelonephritis (acute pyelitis, acute interstitial nephritis)

Acute bacterial nephritis (acute suppurative nephritis, severe acute pyelonephritis)

Focal acute pyelonephritis (focal lobar nephronia, focal bacterial nephritis, the preabscess state)

Emphysematous pyelonephritis

Intrarenal abscess

Pyonephrosis

Chronic pyelonephritis (chronic atrophic pyelonephritis, reflux nephropathy)

Tuberculosis

Xanthogranulomatous pyelonephritis

Echinococcosis

Aspergillosis

Pancreatitis

Renal fistula

Renal papillary necrosis

Cholesteatoma

Infected renal cyst

---

in humans because of the inability to obtain pathologic specimens in all but the most severe forms of the disease.

Current Radiologic Terminology Is At Best Confusing and At Worst May Be Incorrect

As a consequence of this lack of pathologic correlation, radiologists have spawned a confusing and conflicting medley of terms to describe the various appearances of renal infection as depicted by urography, nuclear medicine, ultrasound, CT, and/or MRI. *Focal and diffuse pyelonephritis,*[3] *focal and diffuse acute bacterial nephritis,*[4] *lobar nephronia,*[5] *pseudoabscess,*[6] *preabscess state*[7] *atrophic pyelitis,*[8] and *reflux nephropathy*[8] are but a few of the names used in the uro-radiologic literature. As might be expected when there is no definitive pathologic correlate, these terms have not been applied in any consistent fashion. For example, some authors use the terms *acute bacterial nephritis, lobar nephronia,* and *focal acute pyelonephritis* synonymously; others restrict these terms to specific disease states. To make matters worse, these terms are not always accepted by either our urologic or our pathologic colleagues. Thus, the terminology used in this chapter reflects our own bias, with the full understanding that others may not agree with some of our usage. In parentheses are found appelations used by others for the entity being described.

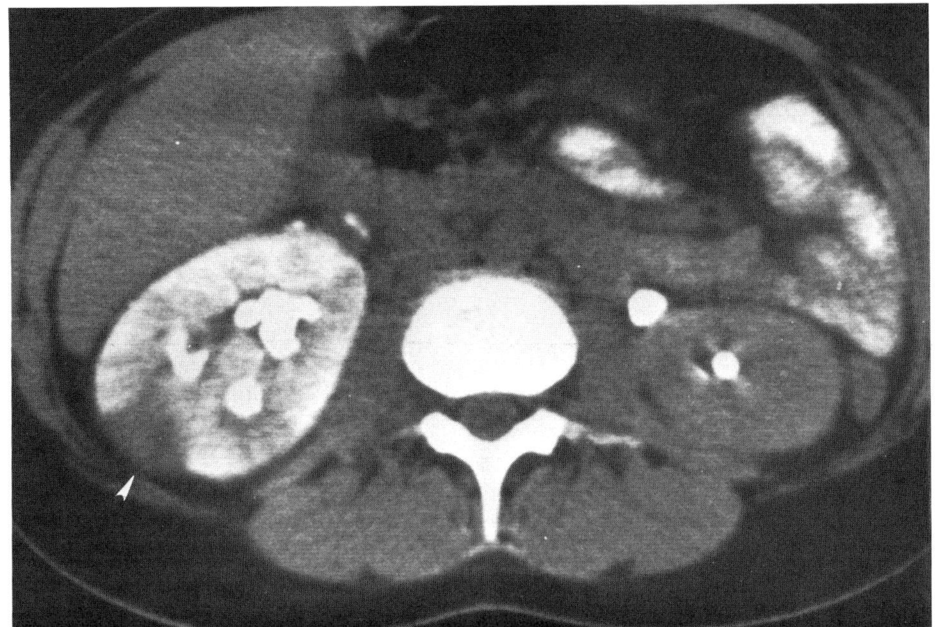

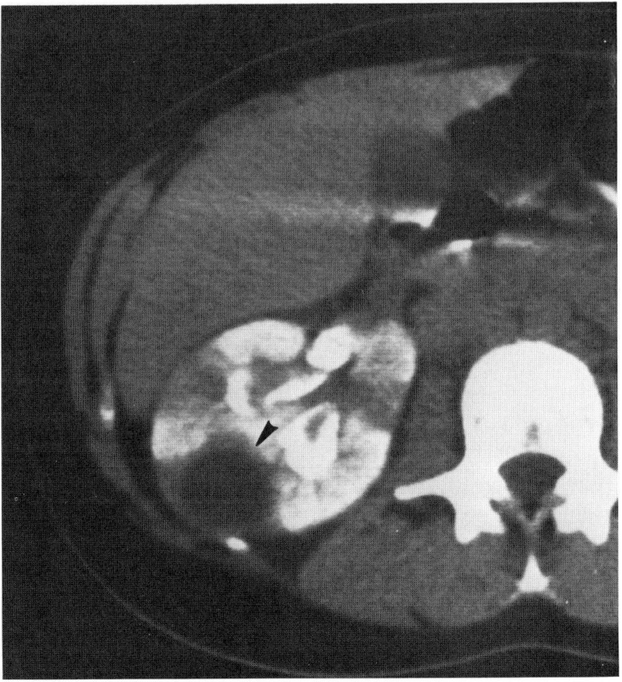

FIG. 4-1. Right renal infection demonstrating different patterns of infection in the same kidney. In (A) there is evidence of the striated pattern consistent with diffuse acute pyelonephritis (or acute bacterial nephritis) yet in the most posterior aspect of this cut there is a bulging renal lobule (white arrow) with no profusion. On another cut (B) there is a rounded area of nonperfusion (black arrow) representing either a preabscess state or more likely a true abscess. The patient responded to antibiotic therapy, making a true pathologic correlation impossible.

There Are Really Only Two Basic Defense Mechanisms Available To the Infected Kidney

In classic acute pyelonephritis, the primary defense mechanism is used; it consists of the polymorphonuclear leukocyte. In most situations, this defense (which we've termed the *star wars defense system*) is successful and no sequelae develop.

However, this primary mechanism may fail as a result of either the nature of the infecting organism or a defect in the host's primary defenses. Under these circumstances, a secondary defense mechanism (which we've termed the *fail-safe defense system*) may be activated. In this situation, the lymphocyte, histiocyte, and/or macrophage are found at the site of infection. Because this defense is often less than satisfactory, fibroblasts lay down a fibrous matrix in an attempt to isolate the infecting organism. The result is the granuloma, the primary component of all the granulomatous diseases.

TECHNIQUE OF EXAMINATION

When properly performed, CT is exquisitely sensitive to the pathologic and functional abnormalities in the kidney. Patients referred with suspected upper urinary tract infections should first be scanned without intravenous contrast administration, at contiguous 8- to 10-mm intervals through the kidneys. The unenhanced scans are done primarily to exclude calculi, which can easily be missed once the collecting systems are filled with contrast. Low-attenuation inflammatory lesions on unenhanced scans are indicative of necrosis or liquefaction. Use of an oral contrast agent is helpful since, in thin people, bowel loops can lie adjacent to the kidney and occasionally may be mistaken for a renal or perirenal mass. Intravenous contrast enhancement is critical to the detection of inflammatory lesions, and it should be performed whenever the patient's condition permits. Fifty to one hundred milliliters of 60 percent contrast should be administered intravenously as a bolus, and the entire abdomen scanned at 1-cm intervals from the diaphragms through both kidneys, then by 1.5-cm intervals through the remainder of the abdomen and pelvis until the symphysis pubis is seen. When looking for small abscesses 0.5-cm slices with overlapping scans may be needed. Occasionally, delayed scans should be performed to look for delayed enhancement or opacification in hypofunctioning or obstructed portions of the kidney.

TYPES OF RENAL INFECTION

Acute Pyelonephritis (Acute Pyelitis, Acute Interstitial Nephritis, Acute Diffuse Bacterial Nephritis)

Classically, acute pyelonephritis presents with a triad of fever, pyuria, and flank pain. A leukocytosis and a positive urine culture are often (but not invariably) present. Gram-negative bacilli are presently the most common etiologic agent. Although occasionally still seen, hematogenously spread gram-positive organisms (such as *Staphylococcus aureus*) were the most common organism in the preantibiotic era.

Uncomplicated acute pyelonephritis in the adult ordinarily does not require any imaging studies. The diagnosis is usually clinically evident, and findings on intravenous urography and renal ultrasound are normal or nonspecific. However, the diagnosis may occasionally be hindered if the specific symptoms of renal infection are occult or masked by other illness. Nonetheless, unsuspected renal infections rarely will be detected radiologically in patients referred for imaging studies for other indications, such as fever of unknown origin, cryptic illness, or immunocompromised states. The vast majority of patients referred for imaging have a known upper urinary tract infection that is unusually severe or refractory to treatment.

In our own recent review of 62 adults hospitalized with a variety of acute renal infections who had undergone one or more imaging studies of the urinary tract, two thirds were female.[9] All patients had a fever greater than 38°C for 3 to 13 days (average of 4 days) and a persistent leukocytosis despite antibiotic therapy. These persistent findings suggest the presence of a more severe upper urinary tract infection, since, for example, 95 to 99 percent of patients with uncomplicated acute pyelonephritis become afebrile within 72 hours of treatment. Urine cultures were positive in 86 percent and blood cultures were positive in 39 percent of patients. Forty percent of the positive cultures were caused by *Escherichia coli*, 40 percent by other gram-negative bacilli (*Klebsiella, Proteus, Pseudomonas,* and *Enterobacter*), and 20 percent by *S. aureus*.

Two thirds of the patients had pre-existing conditions predisposing to renal infection, including nephrolithiasis, a history of recurrent infections, and anatomic or neuropathic abnormalities of the urinary tract. Ten percent were diabetics in this series, although a prevalence of diabetes of up to 60 percent has been reported in other series of patients with severe renal infections.[10]

On gross inspection, kidneys with acute bacterial infection are diffusely enlarged owing to inflammation and edema of the parenchyma, occasionally with microabscesses ranging from 1 to 5 mm in size. Microscopic examination reveals that despte the apparent diffuse nature of the process, there are patchy and segmental areas of normal tissue. The segregation of infected and normal parenchyma is best explained by the reflux of the infecting organism into the parenchyma through individual collecting ducts, which at intervals penetrate from the papillae into the cortex.[10] Affected regions have interstitial edema and polymorphonuclear infiltration. Tubules may be obstructed by white cell casts or inflammatory debris, or by edema of the surrounding interstitium.[11] The intrarenal vasculature is narrowed by spasm and extrinsic compression, with the veins affected more than the arteries.[2] This combination of vascular and tubular abnormalities accounts for the variety of patterns seen with intravenous, contrast-enhanced studies of the kidney.

As already stated, the uncomplicated urinary tract infection in the adult requires no radiologic workup. In many instances,[12-14] the intravenous pyelogram will be normal. Even with careful technique, the distinct intravenous

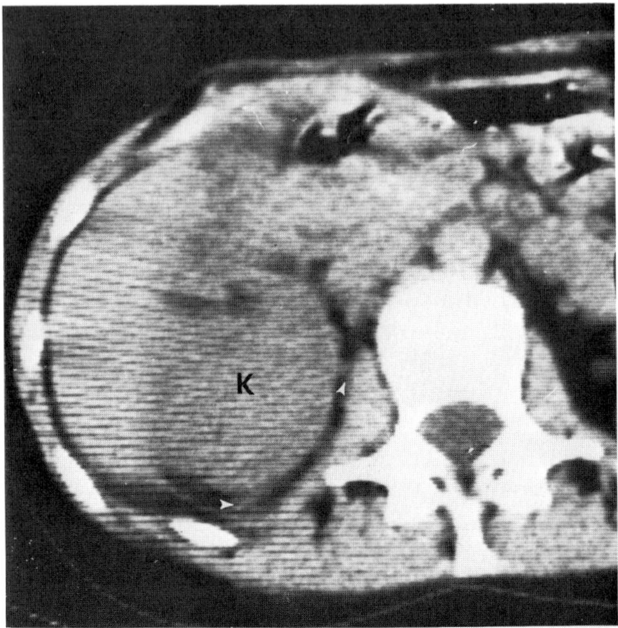

FIG. 4-2.   Unenhanced CT in acute pyelonephritis. The right kidney (K) is swollen and less dense. Small white arrows point to perinephric stranding, possibly representing infection involving the bridging septae.

pattern of acute pyelonephritis is usually identified in only 25 to 40 percent.[15] Similarly, we and others have found ultrasound[6,9] to be less sensitive than CT. Although nuclear medicine is believed to be more sensitive by some,[16,17] no large carefully controlled studies comparing these two modalities exist.

We prefer to perform CT in patients with a clinical diagnosis of acute pyelonephritis who fail to respond to antibiotics or where surgical and percutaneous intervention is being entertained because of a possible superimposed abscess.

As is to be expected, there is a spectrum of CT findings seen with acute pyelonephritis corresponding to the spectrum of pathologic findings and the severity of those findings. The most common finding on unenhanced scans is global swelling of the kidney, present in approximately 75 percent of cases (Fig. 4-2).[9,18] Occasionally, small foci of decreased attenuation are seen, reflecting microabscess formation, which may be identified with careful window setting. Abnormalities of intravenous contrast enhancement are universally present in a variety of patterns.[3,9,10] Probably the most common pattern is that of ill-defined, patchy areas of decreased and increased enhancement (Fig. 4-3).[4,9] A more classic but slightly less common pattern is that of wedged-shaped segments of striated parenchymal opacification, reflecting the distribution of the inflammatory reaction within the individual penetrating collecting ducts through which the bacteria enter the parenchyma (Fig. 4-4). The

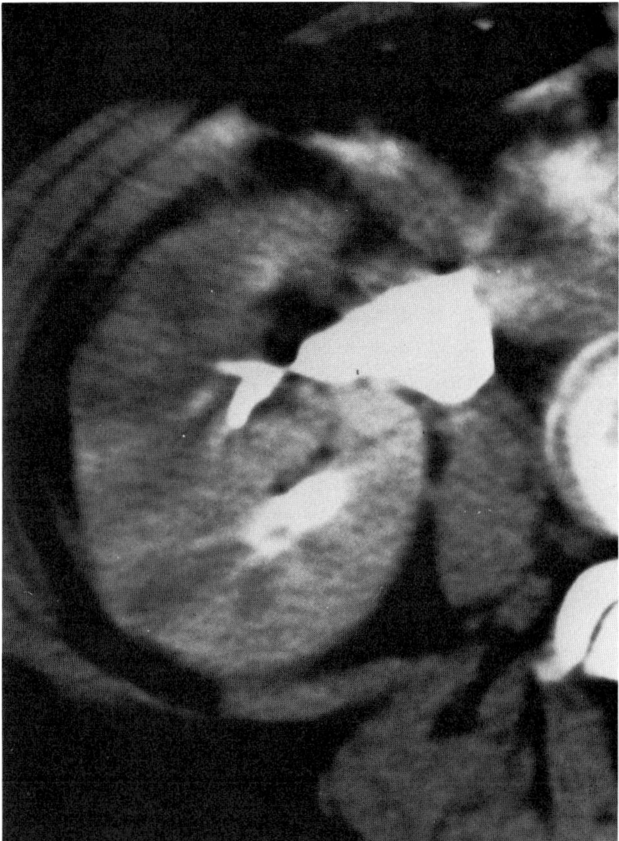

FIG. 4-3.   Acute pyelonephritis (diffuse acute bacterial nephritis) in a 53-year-old black man. In this CT pattern there are multiple areas of low attentuation. A few thickened bridging septae are seen superiorly and medially.

areas of decreased enhancement represent parenchyma that are poorly functioning or nonfunctioning owing to vasospasm, tubular obstruction, and/or interstitial edema. Abnormally increased enhancement occurs when there is slow flow or stasis of contrast within the tubules with possible increased fluid reabsorption. If delayed scans are performed, the poorly opacified areas may actually become hyperdense on occasion.[19] Although perinephric involvement is unusual in mild cases, evidence of perinephric septal and Gerota's fascia thickening will be found in more advanced cases, especially on follow-up examinations (Fig. 4-5).[9]

On MRI, loss of corticomedullary function definition is most likely the first finding in acute infection, although it is very nonspecific. T_1-weighted images will show variable degrees of low signal intensity, whereas the T_2-weighted images will demonstrate areas of high signal intensity, reflecting varying amounts of cortical or medullary edema.

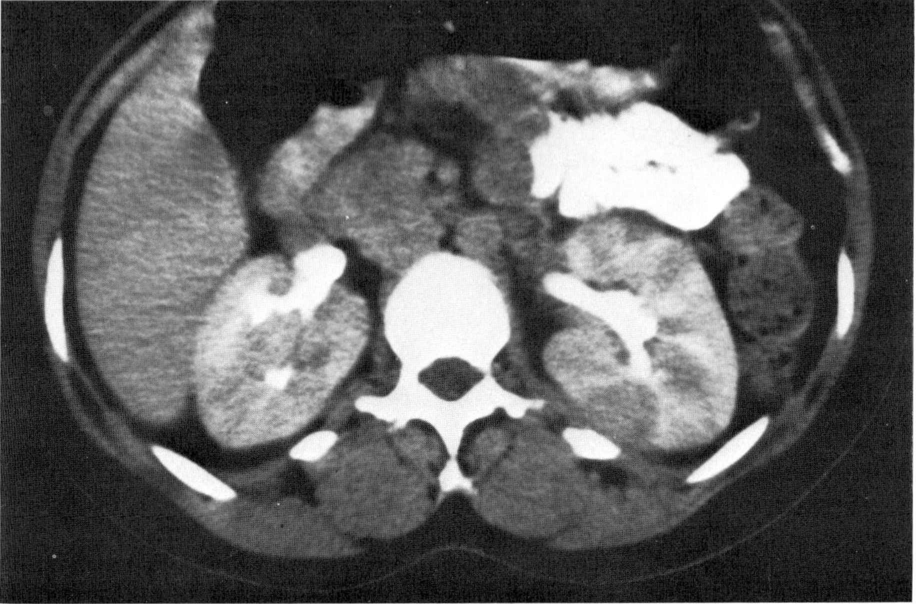

FIG. 4-4.   Diffuse bilateral acute pyelonephritis (diffuse acute bacterial nephritis). In this CT pattern, a bilateral striated pattern may be noted.

Acute Bacterial Nephritis (Acute Suppurative Nephritis, Severe Acute Pyelonephritis)

The term *acute bacterial nephritis,* which entered the literature in 1973,[20] is not recognized by pathologists. To us, this term should be reserved for the severe acute pyelonephritis most commonly seen in diabetics, immunosuppressed individuals, or patients receiving chronic steroid therapy[21] in whom there is shunting of cortical blood flow into the medulla (the Truetta phenomenon). In our estimation, most CT reports in the literature describing acute bacterial nephritis probably merely reflect the pattern of acute pyelonephritis described in the section above. The CT pattern in true cases of acute bacterial nephritis should show failure to enhance in the immediate subcortical area on initial studies secondary to the Truetta phenomenon.

Focal Acute Pyelonephritis (Focal Lobar Nephronia, Focal Bacterial Nephritis)

We use the term *focal acute pyelonephritis* when focal bacterial nephritis is found in a lobar distribution affecting only focal areas of the kidneys, most commonly the renal poles. This distribution most commonly reflects the retrograde in-

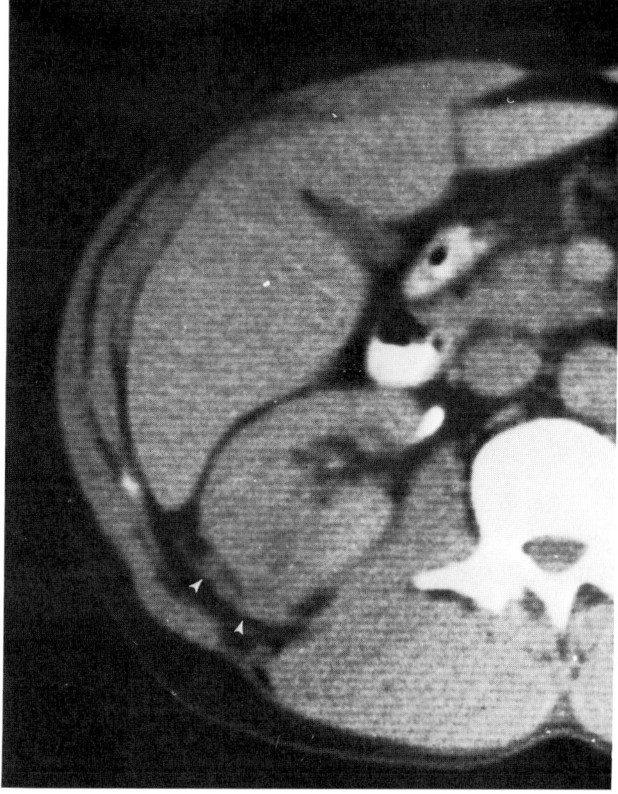

FIG. 4-5.   Acute pyelonephritis of right kidney, with evidence of thickening of Gerota's fascia. Arrows also point to thickened bridging septae and/or perinephric infection, which is the cause of the Gerota's fascia thickening.

noculation of bacteria into the renal parenchyma. No suppuration or parenchymal destruction should have occurred.

The CT correlate to the above presentation is that of one or two wedge-shaped or rounded defects seen on the enhanced scan (Fig. 4-6) or as a few wedge-shaped striated areas.[4,10,22] In rare cases, hemorrhage may occur, leading to a varying pattern of uniformly increased, mixed increased, or decreased attenuation.[23]

The Preabscess State (Pseudoabscess, Focal Lobar Nephronia)

In the continuum of renal infection, we use the term *preabscess state*[7] to refer to that reversable state between focal pyelonephritis and a frank abscess. The term *pseudoabscess* is an excellent alternative term.[6] Similarly, Thornbury[14] has used the term *focal lobar nephronia* to describe this specific entity rather than focal acute pyelonephritis, described above.

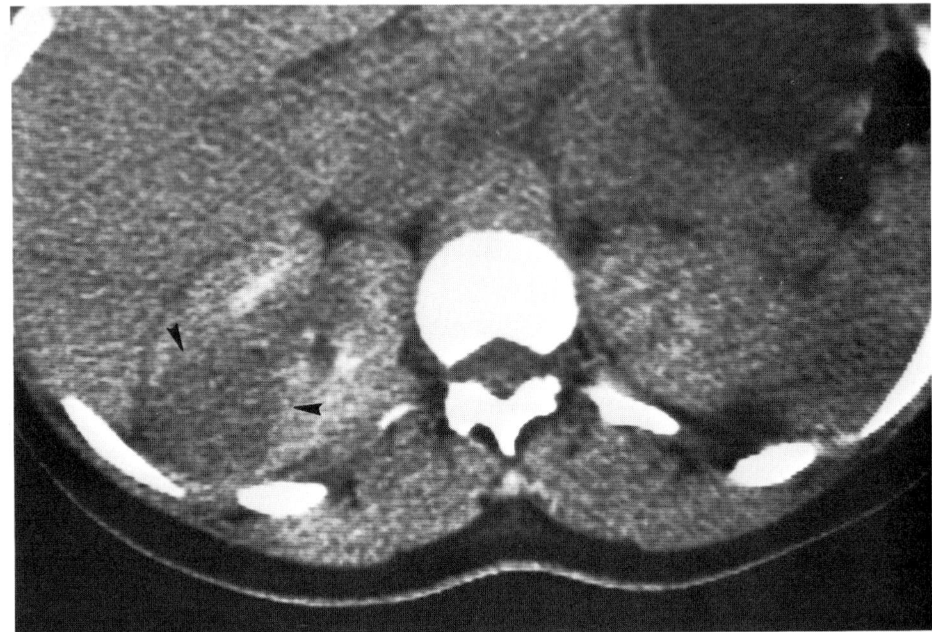

FIG. 4-6.   Focal acute pyelonephritis in a 31-year-old woman with an acute urinary tract infection. Black arrows point to a wedge-shaped area of low attenuation. The rest of the kidney is normal.

On CT, a few small areas with CT numbers close to those of water will be identified within the wedge-shaped or rounded sites of focal pyelonephritis (Fig. 4-7). These wedge-shaped areas may show function on delayed scanning, thus permitting differentiation from an abscess. On occasion, percutaneous aspiration of these areas using ultrasonic or CT guidance can be used to obtain a few drops of fluid for culture and sensitivity. However, by definition, those portions of the kidney involved with the preabscess state are not amenable to therapeutic drainage but may respond to aggressive antibiotic therapy.

With time, these wedge-shaped defects will either become an abscess or, if caught early enough, revert to normal.

Intrarenal Abscess

A renal abscess pathologically represents the most extreme aspect of the spectrum of infection, with liquefaction and destruction of the renal parenchyma. Thus, an abscess is a fluid- or pus-filled cavity without the capability to function except for the surrounding granulation tissue or fibroid capsule. Microscopically, white cells, fluid, and occasionally debris or even a few bacteria are found within its core.

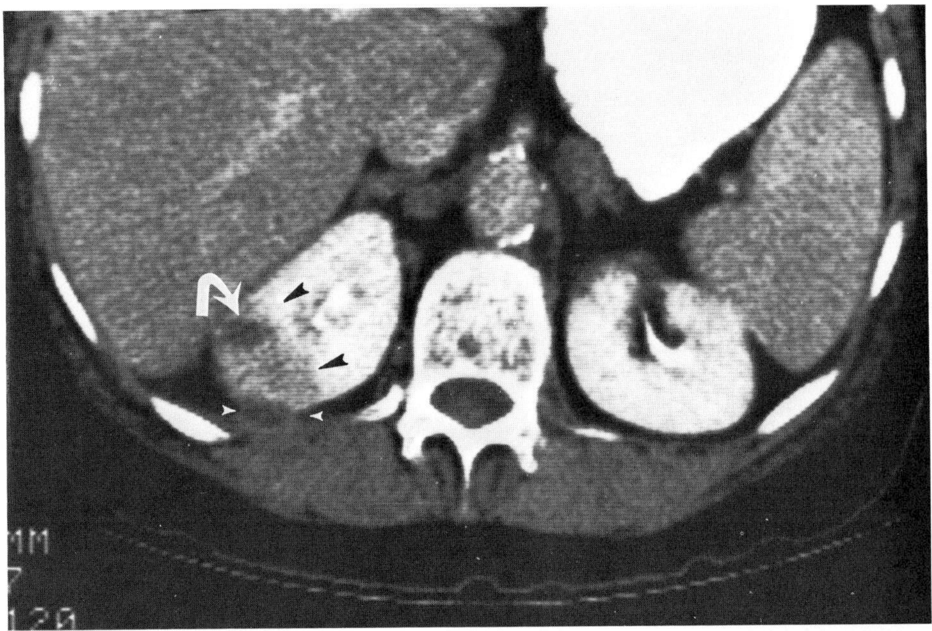

FIG. 4-7.   The preabscess (pseudoabscess or focal lobar nephronia) state. Note the wedge-shaped areas of low attenuation (black arrowheads) without evidence of function. The curved white arrow points to a small area of even lower attentuation, probably representing early liquefaction. With time, this entire area could become a true abscess. At present, the infection is in the in-between state, between a focal pyelonephritis and a frank drainable abscess. Small white arrows point to thickened bridging septae. (From Goldman,[86] with permission.)

Clinically, most intrarenal abscesses are secondary to inoculation with gram-negative organisms, often with renal obstruction. Occasionally, untreated paronychia or tooth abscess, is the etiology, in which case a gram-positive organism such as a staphylococcus will be identified. In drug users, septic emboli can be another etiology. Although classically acutely ill, the patient may present with nonspecific weight loss, low-grade fever, or nausea and vomiting.

There is disagreement in the literature about the best imaging modality for evaluating severe infections in which an abscess is thought to be present.[24,25] Both CT and ultrasound have strong advocates.[26,27] There are no good controlled, prospective studies comparing the two modalities. Ultrasound is chosen by some because of its availability, safety, perceived ease of examination, and supposed lower cost. In fact, CT is less subject to operator dependence in performing and interpreting the examination than ultrasound. The quality of CT examinations is rarely limited by the physical features of the patient, whereas obesity or an unusually cephalad location of the kidneys can result in a technically unsatisfactory ultrasound study. Depending on local reimbursement regulations, the price of a renal ultrasound examination may be

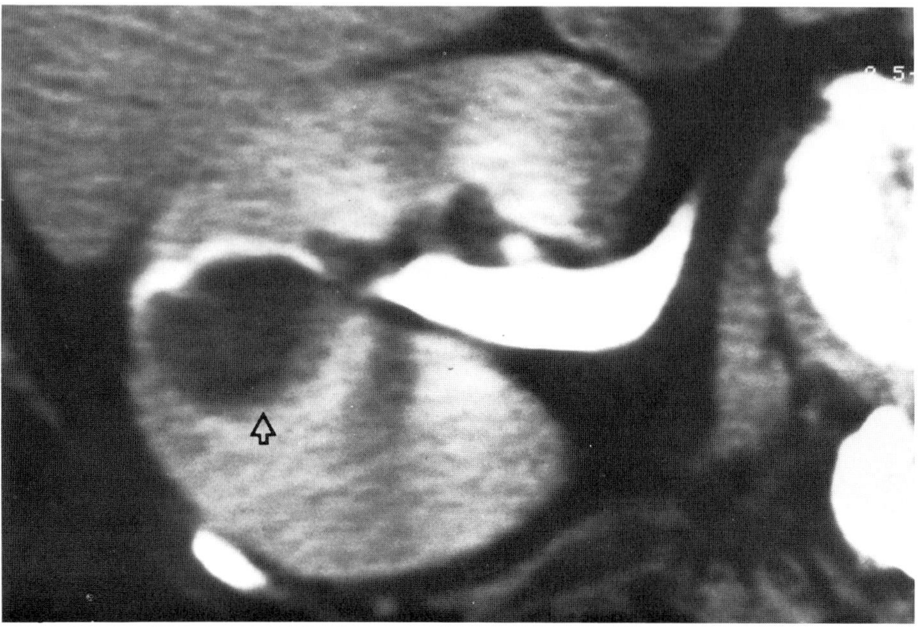

FIG. 4-8.   Frank abscess (arrow) in a 71-year-old woman with septicemia. Note the calyx draped over the abscess and scattered areas of increased attenuation within the abscess cavity, indicative of debris, etc.

equal to or higher than that of a renal CT examination.[27] CT is generally considered to be the more sensitive test.[6,28] In a recent retrospective review, ultrasound failed to depict 7 of 15 intrarenal and extrarenal abscesses and three of five cases of acute bacterial nephritis diagnosed with CT.[9] No lesions detected by other methods were missed by CT, although one was falsely diagnosed as a neoplasm by both modalities. It is possible that in other cases the time interval between the studies played a role, since histologically pyelonephritis can progress and regress rapidly over days. Ultrasound imaging equipment has improved greatly in recent years, but so has CT. Furthermore, CT is more sensitive in demonstrating perinephric and paranephric extension. Thus, current evidence strongly supports using CT as the primary screening test for patients suspected to have a severe renal infection. The lack of specificity of intravenous urography and the high false-negative rate of ultrasound make them less than satisfactory diagnostic tests for renal and perirenal abscesses. The discrepancy in sensitivity between ultrasound and CT may not be important in the clinical management of pyelonephritis, since both are treated with antibiotics and the duration of therapy is based on clinical response. Although conservative treatment of renal abscesses has become more common, some intrarenal and all extrarenal abscesses are managed by percutaneous or surgical drainage. Accurate detection, localization, and delineation of the extent of disease is essential for planning proper therapy. We clearly prefer CT for making the diagnosis of abscess.

The CT definition of an abscess is that of a fairly well-defined area of low attenuation that usually does not meet the criteria for a simple cyst and does not itself enhance (Fig. 4-8). Rarely, an abscess will resemble a simple cyst but with fluid having CT numbers above those of water. More commonly (in 70 to 80 percent of cases), focal or diffuse swelling of the kidney, abnormal enhancement of the surrounding inflamed parenchyma, and inflammatory changes in the perirenal fat are noted (Fig. 4-9).[9,29] Furthermore, careful attention to detail will show the wall to be thickened and/or irregular. In addition, debris is often present within the cavity. Approximately 40 percent have thickening of the Gerota's and/or lateroconal fascia, and 27 percent have extension of the inflammatory process into one of the pararenal spaces. Renal abscesses may rupture into the perirenal and pararenal spaces in up to 23 percent of cases, and occasionally extend through the transversalis fascia into the flank. Perinephric extension probably occurs through the recently described bridging septae.[30] In those cases in which periabscess inflammation is not evident on CT, the clinical history is usually sufficient to make the correct diagnosis,

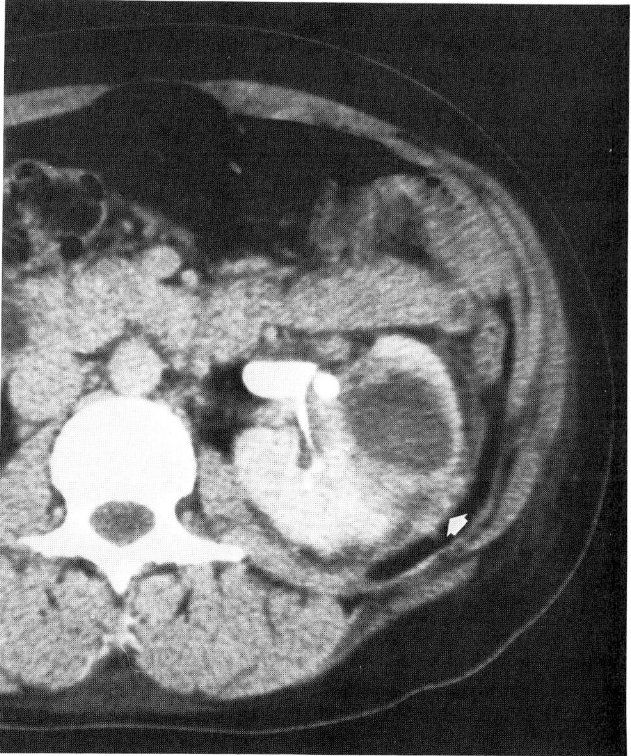

FIG. 4-9.   *E. coli* abscess with perinephric extension (white arrow).

although percutaneous aspiration often is necessary to confirm the presence of infection and to identify the specific pathogen.

On MRI, a hypointense inhomogenous pattern is seen on T_1-weighted images with a similarly inhomogenous but increased intensity pattern on T_2-weighted images.[31,32] If there is an increased protein, even the T_1-weighted images may become more hyperintense.

Emphysematous Pyelonephritis

Emphysematous pyelonephritis is a severe bacterial infection associated with intrarenal gas formation. It is usually caused by mixed floral infection, with *E. coli, Klebsiella, Proteus,* and *Pseudomonas* being the most common organisms.[33] Diabetic patients are especially prone to developing emphysematous infection, with the high glucose in the urine acting as an excellent medium for bacterial growth. Urinary obstruction[34] and impaired immunity are also contributing factors.

Clinically, these patients present with a nonspecific refractory pyelonephritis. Although many of these patients are quite ill, unfortunately, it is not uncommon for these patients to be hospitalized for several days before the severity of the infection is recognized. Careful physical examination may reveal

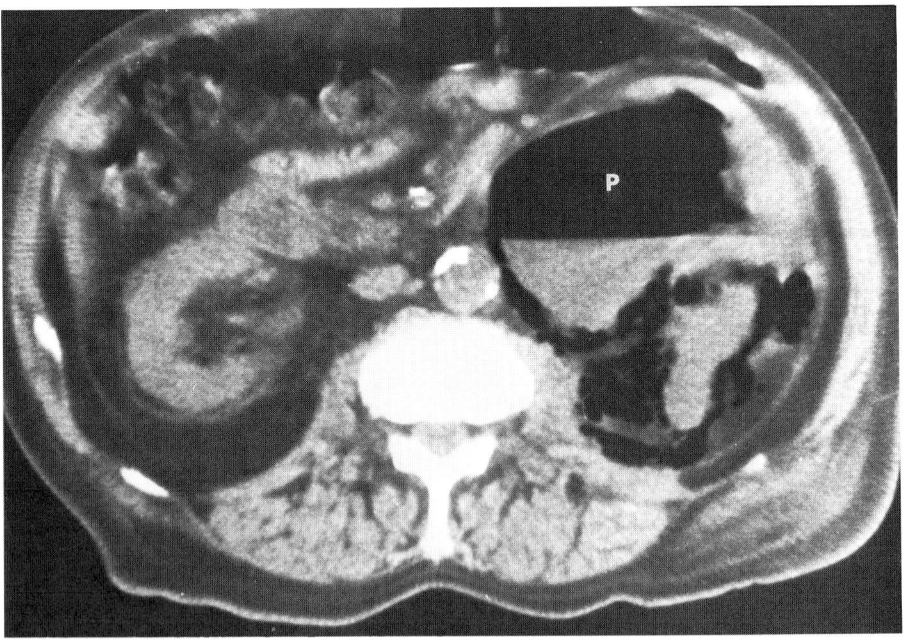

FIG. 4-10.   Emphysematous pyelonephritis with an air-fluid level in the renal pelvis (P) and extensive perinephric emphysema represented as bubbles in the perinephric space. At surgery, the entire renal parenchyma was found to be destroyed.

a crepitant mass,[34] whereas laboratory studies may demonstrate hyperglycemia, leukocytosis, bacteriuria, bacteremia, and/or azotemia.

The pathologic correlate of this life-threatening situation demonstrates a necrotizing pyelonephritis with multiple abscesses and vascular thrombosis.

Because of the high morbidity and mortality associated with emphysematous pyelonephritis, nephrectomy with aggressive intravenous antibiotics is the classic treatment. Recently, a few selected, nontoxic patients have been treated with antibiotics alone or with a combination of percutaneous drainage and antibiotics.[35]

Although plain films will show the air, it may be difficult to determine its exact location. Furthermore, overlying ileus may obscure small amounts of air. CT is ideal for demonstrating whether the air is confined to the calyces, pelvis, perinephric space, subcapsular space, and/or parenchyma (Fig. 4-10). This is far from theoretical, since air confined to the calyces and pelvis is really termed *emphysematous pyelitis*. Similarly, perinephric air should be called *perinephric emphysema*. *Emphysematous pyelonephritis* should be rightfully reserved for the presence of air within the parenchyma, which obviously requires aggressive therapy. At present, CT is the most sensitive modality for identifying even the smallest traces of intrarenal gas and, thus, may yield the first clue for the need of early intervention.[36-43] If used early, CT may be instrumental in salvaging some of these kidneys.

Pyonephrosis

Kidneys obstructed by calculi, strictures, tumors, or extrinsic masses develop hydronephrosis and urinary stasis. The static urine becomes a breeding ground for bacteria, especially in calculi-bearing collecting systems. This can progress to a pyonephrosis, which presents clinically with flank pain and urosepsis.[44] Prompt diagnosis is critical, as effective therapy requires drainage of the obstructed system by percutaneous nephrostomy or retrograde catheterization.

The pyonephrotic kidney is usually nonfunctional or poorly functioning, so the intravenous urogram is not a particularly useful diagnostic tool. Both CT and ultrasound are accurate methods for depicting pyonephrosis.[44-47] Findings on non-contrast-enhanced CT include a dilated collecting system filled with fluid having CT numbers slightly above those of water, debris, and, sometimes, a fluid-debris level. We prefer CT, since it more readily demonstrates the site of obstruction than ultrasound (Fig. 4-11).

MRI can be used to identify the presence of pyonephrosis. Low-intensity dilated calyces and ureter can be seen on T_1-weighted images, with a corresponding high-intensity signal on the T_2-weighted images (Fig. 4-12). Unfortunately, this pattern may be indistinguishable from hydronephrosis unless debris can be identified on the images as a mixed signal. Except for its ability to produce nonreconstructed coronal and sagittal images, it offers little that cannot be obtained by the less expensive CT.

Once the diagnosis has been established, percutaneous drainage can be performed under ultrasonic or fluoroscopic guidance.

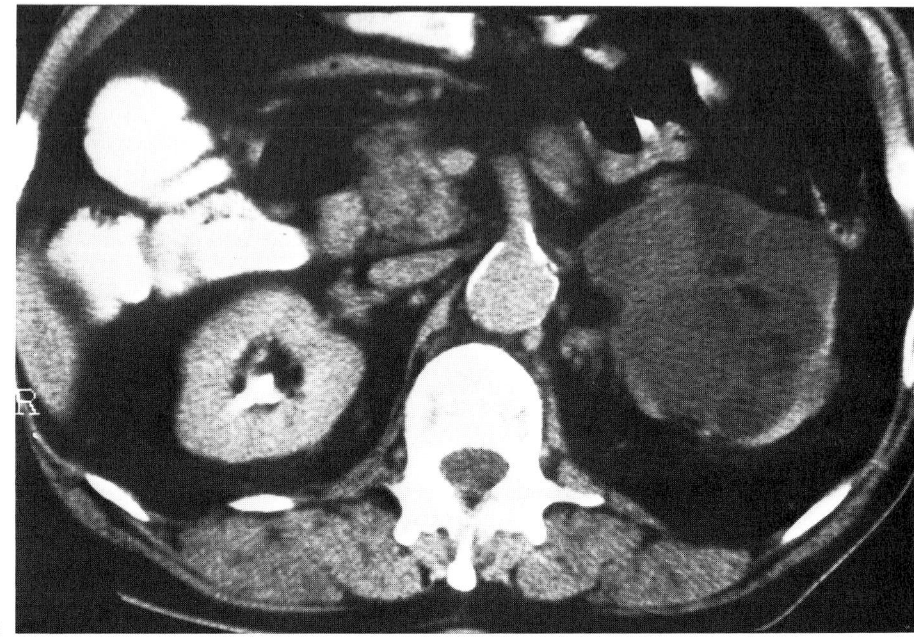

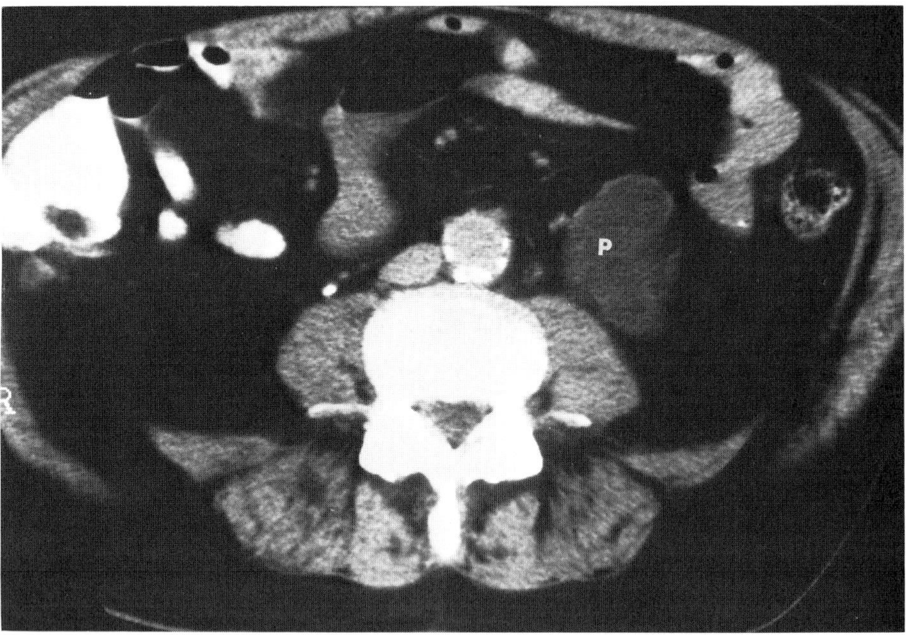

FIG. 4-11.   Right pyonephrosis in a 76-year-old man with chronic renal failure. By carefully tracing the ureter from kidney to bladder the site of obstruction can be identified. (A) At the level of the kidneys, the left kidney is enlarged with thinning of the cortex, medulla, and columns of Bertin. (B) At the level of the pelvis, the left renal pelvis (P) is enlarged and dilated. The normal right ureter is opacified and seen directly in front of the renal psoas muscle. (*Figure continues.*)

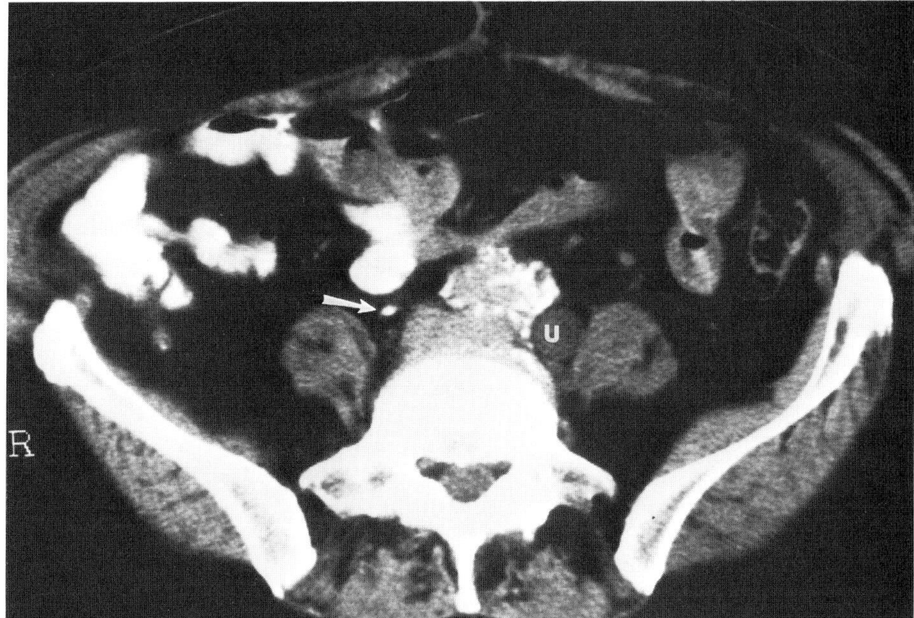

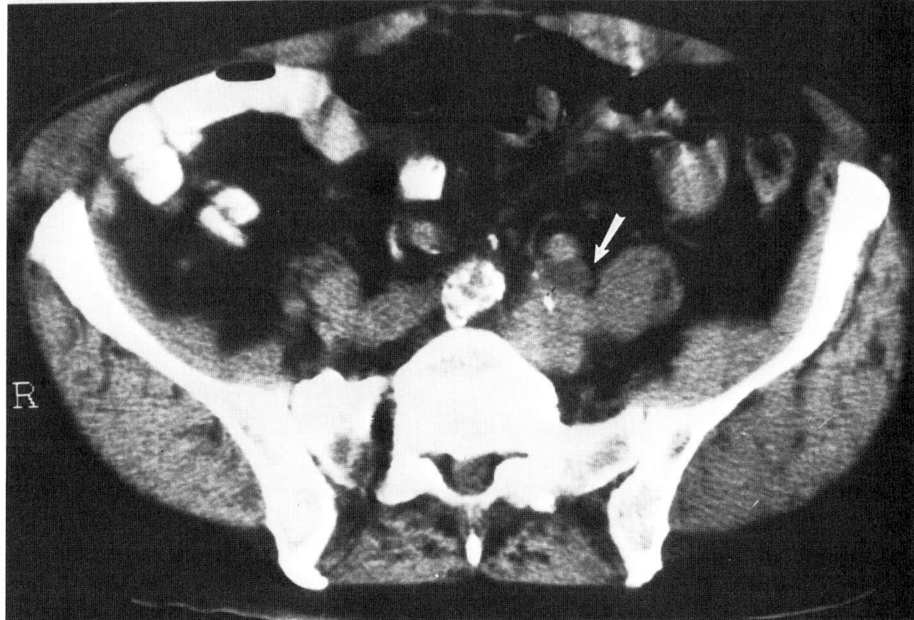

FIG. 4-11 (*Continued*).   (C) At the level of the iliac crest, the left ureter (U) is still dilated. Therefore, the sight of obstruction is below this level. The opacified right ureter (arrow) is normal. (D) At a level a little lower in the pelvis, the left ureter (arrow) is noted to be slightly less dilated, indicating that the site of obstruction is close by. A cut 0.5 cm below this showed the left ureter to be normal.

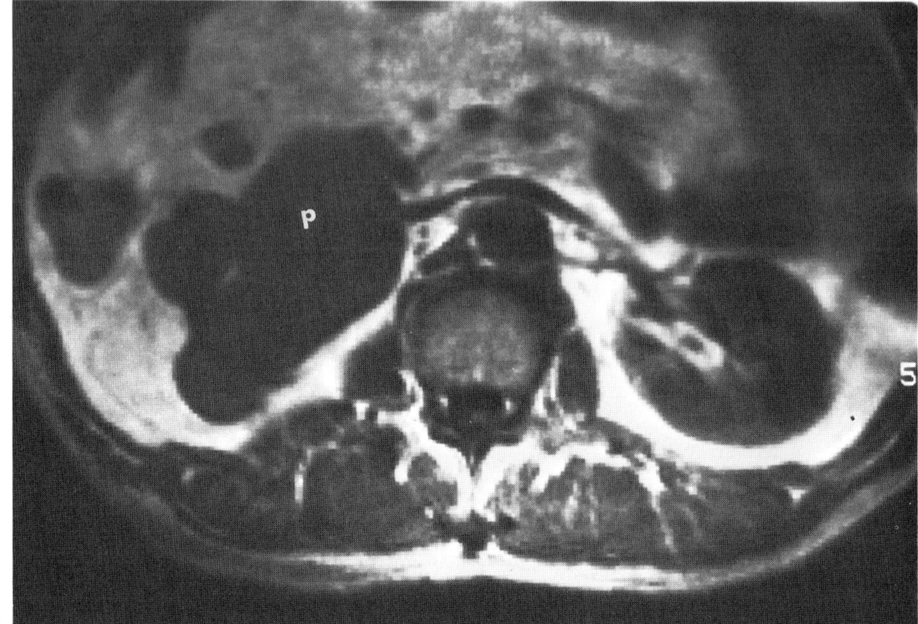

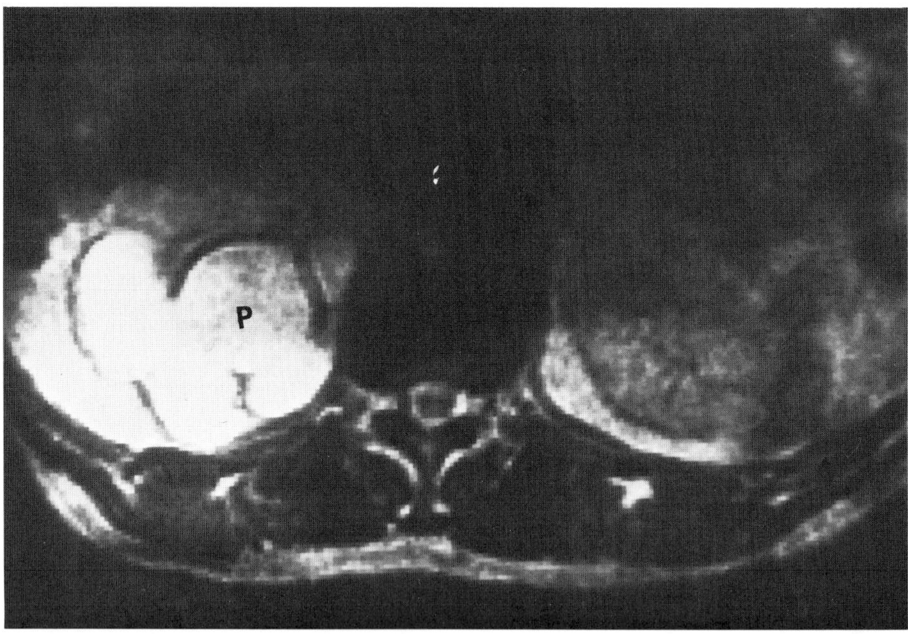

FIG. 4-12. Pyonephrosis in an elderly man with hemoptysis and a lung lesion. (A) The T_1-weighted image shows right pelvis (P) and calyces to be dilated (TE 15 ms; TR .38 s) as does the T_2-weighted image (B) (TE 30 ms; TR 2 s). On these images, no debris is present to differentiate hydronephrosis from pyonephrosis. *E. coli* was present in the urine.

Sequelae of Renal Infections

The increasing use of conservative medical therapy for the treatment of severe renal infections has led to more frequent referrals of these patients for follow-up imaging studies. Swelling and abnormal enhancement of the kidney on intravenous contrast-enhanced CT scans persist for 1 month in most patients despite clinical improvement on appropriate antibiotic therapy, and lasts for several months in a minority.[48] The radiographic severity of the lesion does not predict resolution time; that is, inflammatory changes due to acute bacterial nephritis can persist as long as or longer than those due to an abscess. Our most recent studies have shown that extrarenal inflammation may actually increase in the 2 weeks after diagnosis before subsiding over the next 2 months in most patients (Fig. 4-13).[48] The mechanism for the increasing thickening of the bridging septae of the perirenal space is not known, although it may relate to obstruction or increased flow in the perirenal lymphatic channels that run within the septae.[30] Persistent thickening and stranding of the perirenal fat up to a year following an acute infection has been reported, suggesting that renal infection can cause chronic fibrosis in the surrounding adipose tissue and fascia.

Cortical scars and caliectasis resulting from childhood vesicoureteral reflux are characteristic findings in chronic pyelonephritis, and have been reported in association with nephrolithiasis in adults.[49] Classical teaching and several large clinical series assert that cortical scarring visible on intravenous urography rarely occurs following acute pyelonephritis in the adult with previously normal kidneys. However, global wasting of the kidney without focal scarring has been reported in 6 to 60 percent of intravenous urograms following acute pyelonephritis, especially with pre-existing disease.[50] CT demonstrates that new cortical scars appear in 50 percent or more of patients after acute infections (Fig. 4-14).[48] This high number reflects the greater sensitivity of CT compared to intravenous urography, and also the likelihood that patients referred for CT have more severe infections than the populations on which previously published series of urograms are based.

Another surprising finding in our patients with *S. aureus* abscesses was the ultimate drainage of these abscesses into the calyceal system on follow-up CT examinations (Fig. 4-15).[48] To us, this suggests that some calyceal diverticulae may, in fact, be acquired and not congenital.

Chronic Pyelonephritis (Chronic Atrophic Pyelonephritis, Reflux Nephropathy, Chronic Infection, Abacterial Nephritis)

The classic pathologic finding in chronic pyelonephritis is that of cortical scar overlying a blunt renal calyx. There may be a more generalized loss of parenchyma secondary to fibrosis, most commonly in the upper or lower poles of the kidney. With progression the kidneys become atrophic, although in uninvolved areas compensatory hypertrophy may occur.

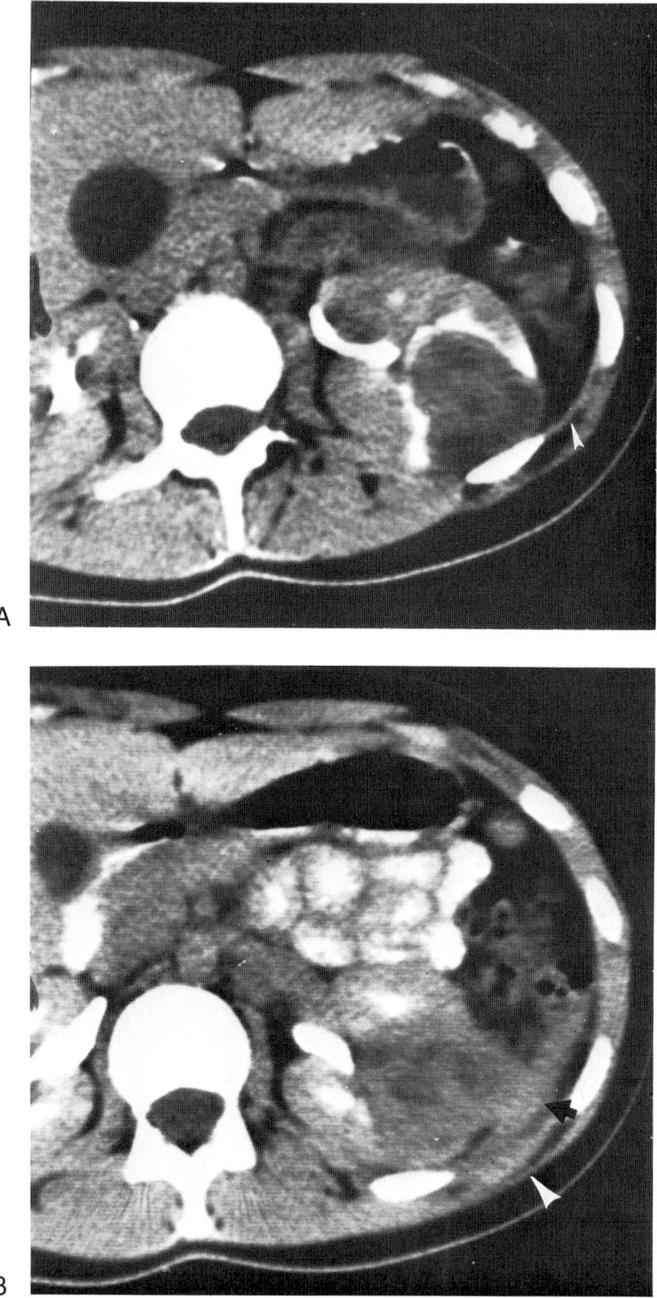

FIG. 4-13.   Sequelae of infection in a 16-year-old girl with a preabscess (pseudoabscess or focal lobar nephronia). Thickening of the transversalis fascia is demonstrated in (A). One week later (B) no change is seen in the abscess but there is an increase in the thickening of Gerota's fascia (black arrow) and the transversalis fascia (white arrow). (*Figure continues.*)

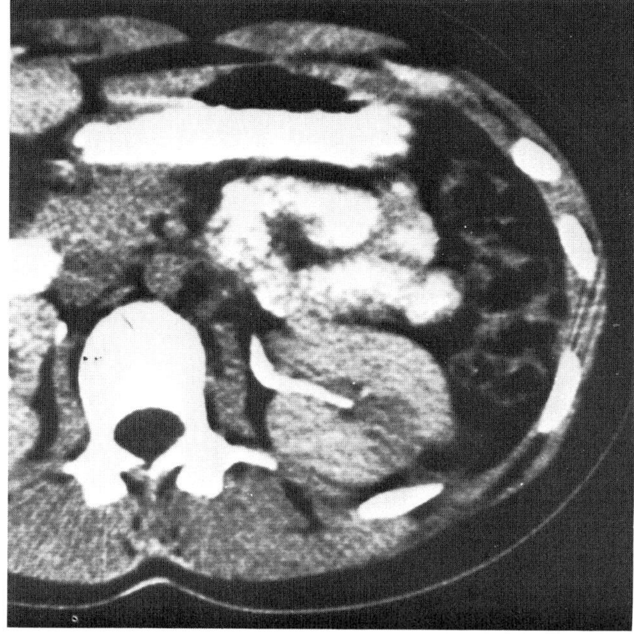

FIG. 4-13 (*Continued*).   (C) Seven and one-half months later, there clearly is loss of renal parenchyma with scar formation. The previous fascial thickening has returned to normal. (From Soulen et al.,[48] with permission.)

It is claimed that nuclear medicine is more sensitive in demonstrating the scars of pyelonephritis.[16,17] However, no large series on this topic has been reported. In fact, we believe CT may well be as sensitive. However, CT is rarely, if ever, used primarily to diagnose chronic pyelonephritis. More often, the diagnosis of chronic pyelonephritis is made on CT studies performed for other reasons. Both unenhanced and enhanced studies will demonstrate the cortical scars, the blunt calyces, the amount of cortical loss, the compensatory hypertrophy, and/or the presence of pelvic or replacement sinus lipomatosis (Figs. 4-16 and 4-17).

Tuberculosis

Tuberculosis is the example par excellence of a granulomatous disease in which the secondary or "fail-safe" system is used in an attempt to isolate the infecting organism, *Mycobacterium tuberculosis*. Invariably, hematogenously spread renal involvement may not become manifest until many years after the initial pulmonary infestation.

The tubercle bacillus first localizes in the glomeruli and cortical arteries. Multiple bilateral asymptomatic small granulomas develop,[51] at which point the progression may stabilize. On the other hand, unchecked, the tubercle

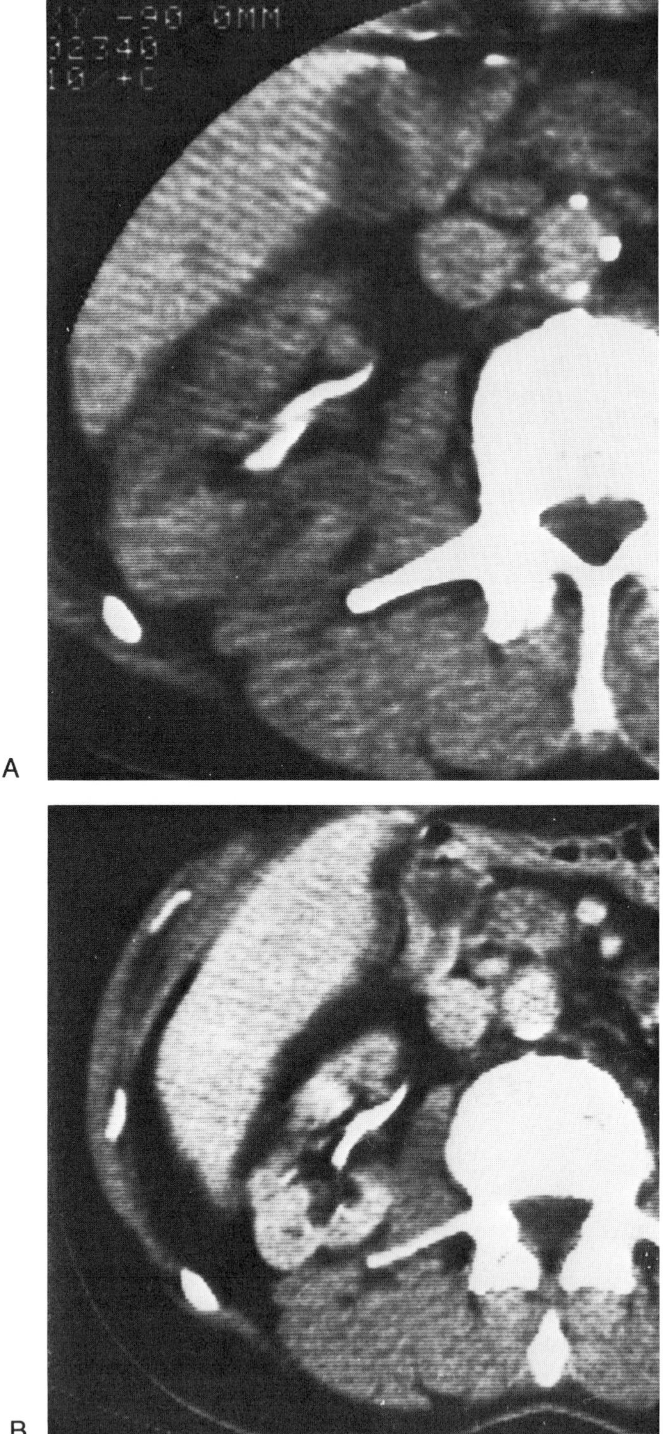

A

B

FIG. 4-14.   Development of renal scars in a 64-year-old woman with flank tenderness and fever. (A) Initial scan in the acute stage shows areas of low attenuation. (B) Scan 4 weeks later shows marked parenchymal shrinkage with scar formation. (From Soulen et al.,[48] with permission.)

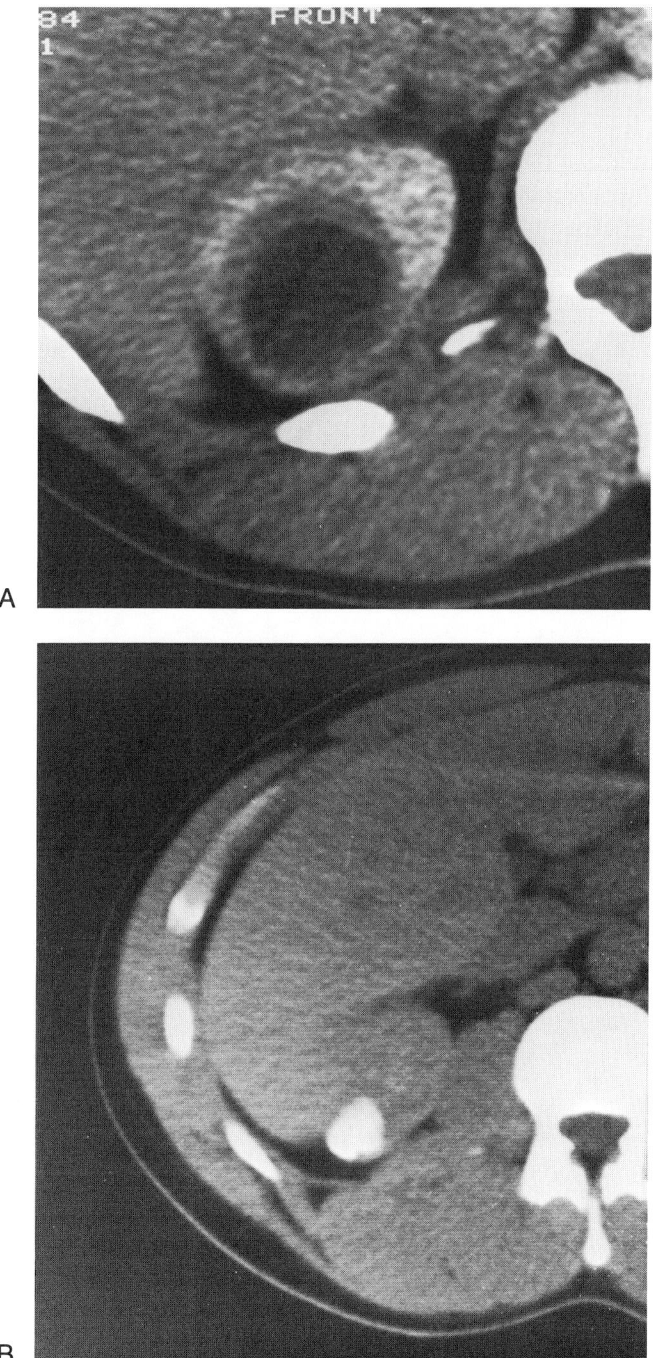

FIG. 4-15. Development of a calyceal "diverticulum" in a 32-year-old man with a staphylococcal abscess. (A) Initial study shows the abscess. Four days later, the patient passed cloudy urine. (B) Delayed films from a follow-up CT scan show filling of the residual small cavity consistent with an "acquired" calyceal diverticulum that drains into the collecting system. (From Soulen et al.,[48] with permission.)

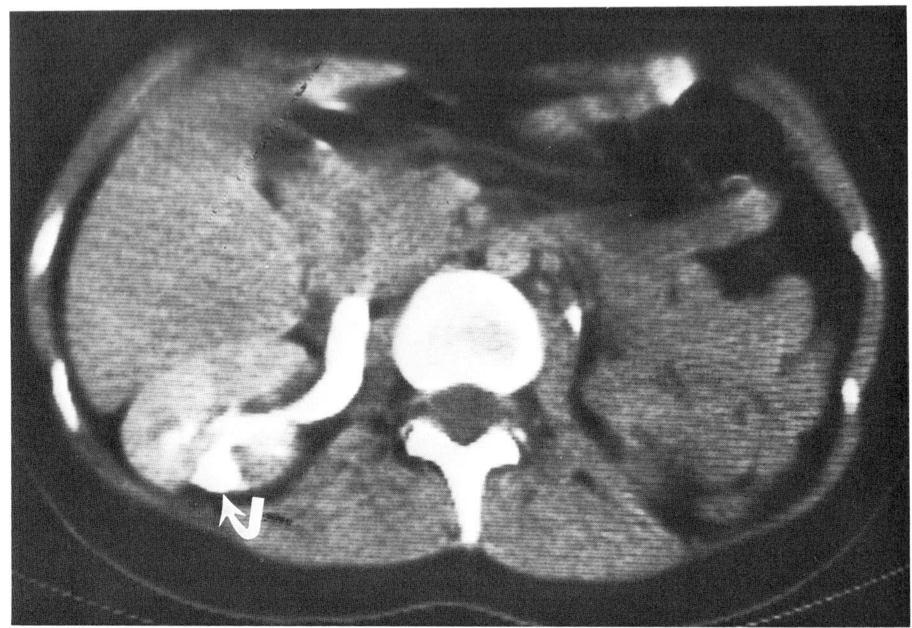

FIG. 4-16.   CT of chronic pyelonephritis as evidenced by a blunt calyx and overlying cortical thinning. (From Goldman,[7] with permission.)

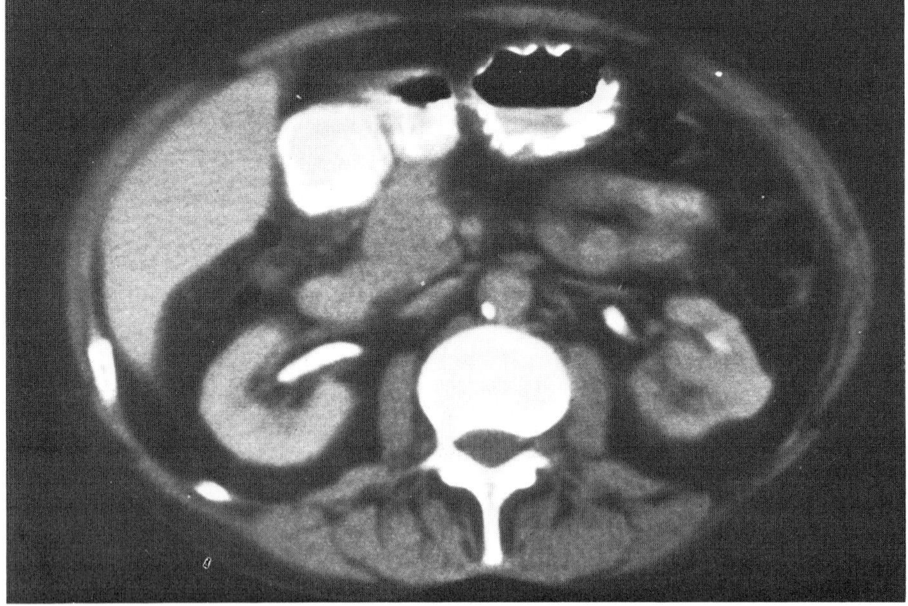

FIG. 4-17.   Long-standing chronic pyelonephritis of the right kidney as evidenced by a marked loss of cortex with multiple scars.

bacillus will cause destruction of the parenchyma first in the tissue surrounding the loop of Henle, resulting in renal papillary necrosis. Teleologically speaking, there is a further attempt to isolate the bacillus by a reactive fibrosis, which leads to infundibular and ureteropelvic-ureterovesical fibrosis. A contracted bladder and pipe-stem ureter are other consequences of this reactive fibrosis. Unfortunately, if still uncontrolled, cortical abscesses, fistulization, and/or caseation may develop, with a small nonfunctioning autonephrectomized kidney the ultimate result.

Clinically, the patient may only have minimal complaints, including frequency, dysuria, nocturia, and pain.[52] Night sweats, fever, and weight loss are reportedly more characteristic, but are often absent. Tuberculosis is one of the more common causes of sterile pyuria.[53]

CT is rarely used primarily to diagnose tuberculosis, but can demonstrate the entire spectrum of tuberculous disease. It can demonstrate the early findings of the infundibular and ureteropelvic stenosis with secondary calyceal obstruction (Fig. 4-18).[51,54] Cortical thinning with occasional fluid-filled levels secondary to collecting system debris can also be readily identified. Renal cortical or medullary cavities (i.e., abscesses) are seen, usually as both regular and irregular low-density areas, but have higher CT numbers secondary to hemorrhage or infection. Often it is difficult to differentiate a hydrocalyx from an abscess (Fig. 4-19). Renal calculi are not uncommon, whereas focal parenchymal calcifications are recognized quite frequently (in 40 percent of cases) and are often recognized on CT without being identifiable on plain film. The renal pelvis may be dilated, but is often narrowed with extensive peripelvic fibrosis. Occasionally, the CT pattern may mimic that of xanthogranulomatous pyelonephritis (Figs. 4-19 and 4-20), but the kidney in the latter is more likely to be enlarged and an obstructing pelvic stone is more common. Not infrequently, perinephric and/or paranephric extension is recognized. Extension medially along and down the psoas[55] and/or iliopsoas muscle (i.e., "the cold abscess") should be looked for. Care should also be exercised in evaluating the nephrographic phase of the CT to determine the extent of renal involvement, and one should be aware that a tuberculoma could mimic an intrarenal tumor. Tuberculosis is a great "mimicker" and can be misdiagnosed as xanthogranulomatous pyelonephritis, pyelonephritis (acute or chronic), a tumor or tumorlike condition, leukoplakia, cholesteatoma, calculous disease, pyonephrosis, and renal papillary necrosis, among other conditions.[52]

Xanthogranulomatous Pyelonephritis

Xanthogranulomatous pyelonephritis is another renal granulomatous disease in which the xanthoma cell, a lipid-laden macrophage, is present in significant numbers. Pathologically, the secondary defense mechanism (i.e., "the failsafe system"), consisting of plasma cells, histiocytes, and macrophages, will be identified. Ideally, these will be surrounded by a fibroblastic encapsulation. In general, xanthogranulomatous pyelonephritis is the result of obstruction

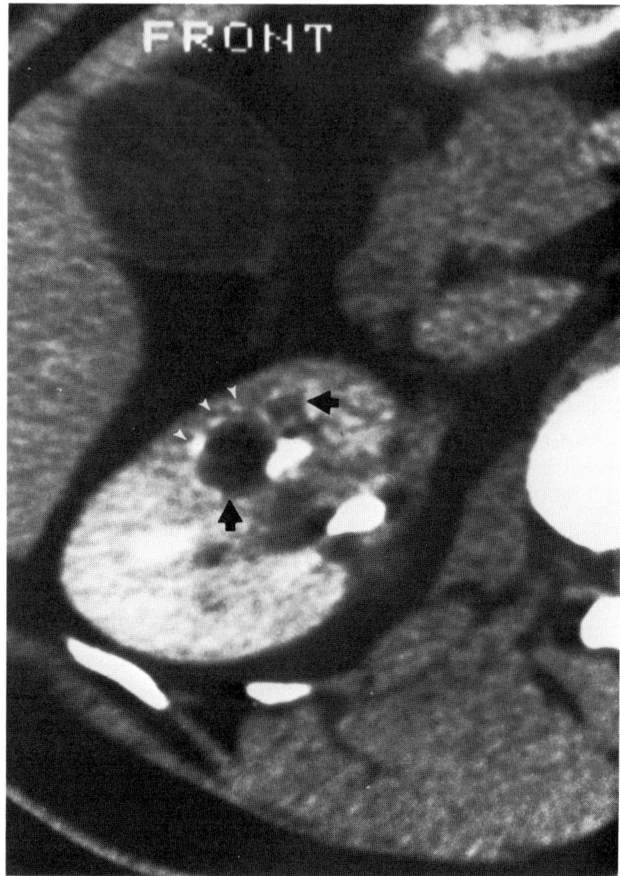

FIG. 4-18.   Early tuberculosis in a 40-year-old man from India involving only a small portion of the kidney. Small white arrowheads point to focal cortical calcifications. Two black arrows point to dilated calyces probably obstructed owing to infundibular narrowing.

of either a calyx or, more commonly, the renal pelvis by a calculus, often a staghorn, with extension of the xanthogranulomatous pyelonephritis from the site of obstruction into the medulla, cortex, perinephric space, and beyond.[56] In general, the kidney's shape remains unchanged but the total renal volume increases markedly. The renal pelvis is usually narrowed and the kidney's parapelvic space and parenchyma are replaced by yellow-orange xanthoma-laden material. Hydro- or pyocaliectasis and renal abscesses are usually present. In the diffuse form, the entire kidney is involved, whereas, in the focal or tumefactive type, only one or two obstructed calyces are involved.[56,57]

Clinically, xanthogranulomatous pyelonephritis can be seen at any age and in either sex, but is more commonly noted in middle-aged women.[58,59] Two general clinical patterns of presentation are seen. In one, there is weight loss,

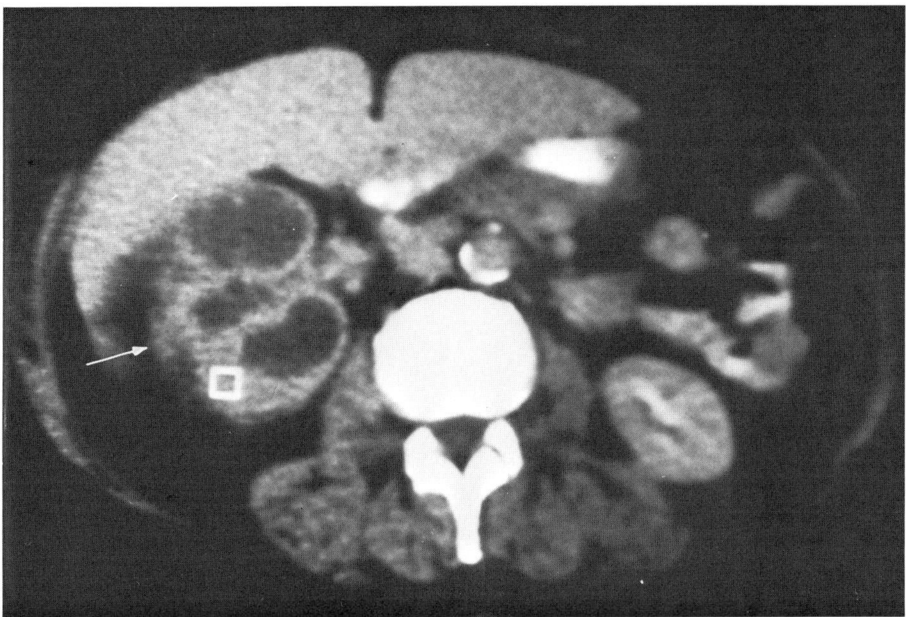

FIG. 4-19.   More advanced case of tuberculosis in an elderly woman who nursed her mother with tuberculosis on the eastern shore of Maryland in the early 1900s. Kidney is slightly enlarged with preservation of its reniform shape. The calyces are enlarged and the renal pelvis obliterated. Arrow points to perinephric involvement.

low-grade fever, and a nonspecific pattern of malaise mimicking a neoplasm. In the other, there may be a superimposed subacute pattern of chills, high-grade fever, etc. Often in diabetics, urinalysis will varyingly show pyuria, proteinuria, and/or microhematuria. Urine cultures often show a spectrum of organisms somewhat different from that obtained from the specimen but usually consisting of *E. coli*, *Proteus*, *Pseudomonus*, and/or *Enterobacter*.[60] Reversible liver enzyme abnormalities, which disappear with nephrectomy, have been reported.

Although characteristic intravenous pyelographic,[61] retrograde pyelographic,[52] arteriographic,[52,56] and ultrasonic patterns have been described, we strongly advocate the use of CT in all suspected cases, especially if surgery is contemplated, because of the high probability of perinephric and paranephric extension. CT demonstrates an enlarged kidney with numerous, rounded, parenchymal areas of low intensity (but without CT numbers in the range of fat) representing dilated calyces and/or abscesses.[56,62] Parenchymal calcifications, renal calculi (obstructing and otherwise), and a small, contracted renal pelvis with peripelvic fibrosis are identified. With contrast, there is usually, but not always, cortical and inflammatory tissue enhancement (Fig. 4-21).[56,63] As with tuberculosis; perinephric, pararenal, psoas and supradiaphragmatic, and gastrointestinal tract extension can usually be identified and categorized, if present (Figs. 4-22 and 4-23).[64–66]

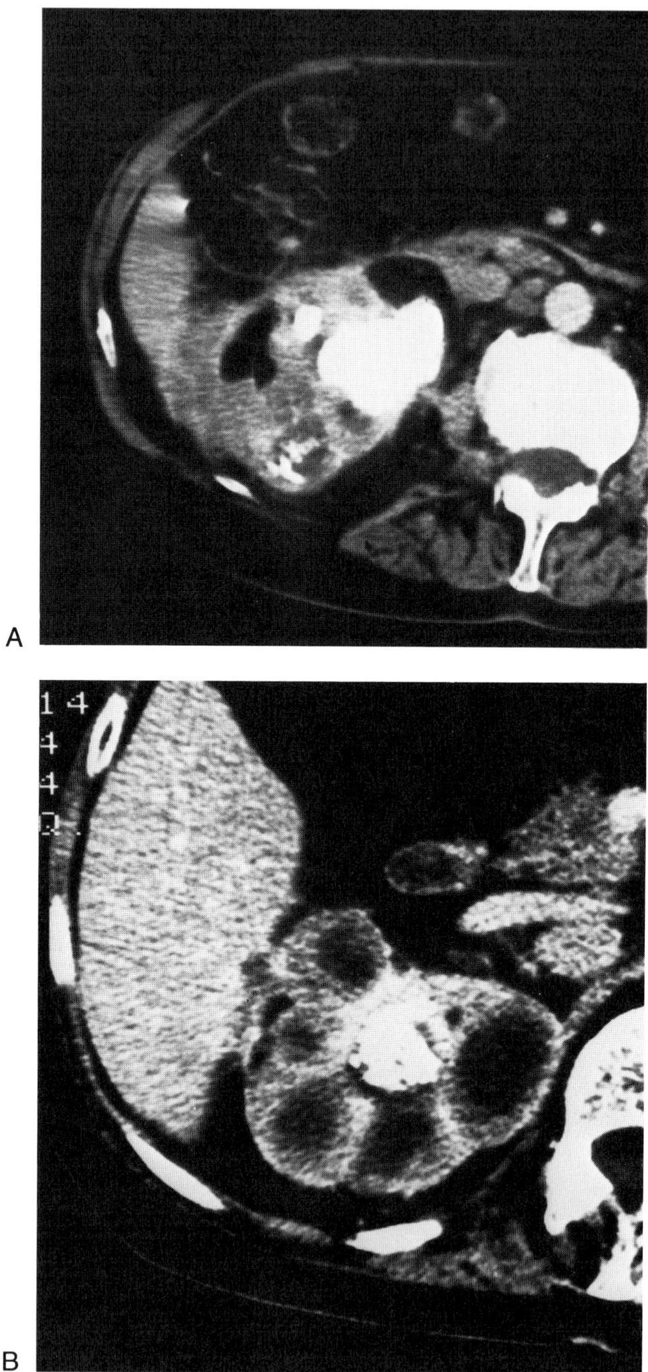

FIG. 4-20.   Xanthogranulomatous pyelonephritis. (A) Level of the pelvis showing the obstructing stone as well as other scattered calcifications in the calyces and parenchyma. (B) Level slightly higher showing the enlarged kidney with preservation of its reniform outline and dilated calyces. The staghorn calculus is again seen.

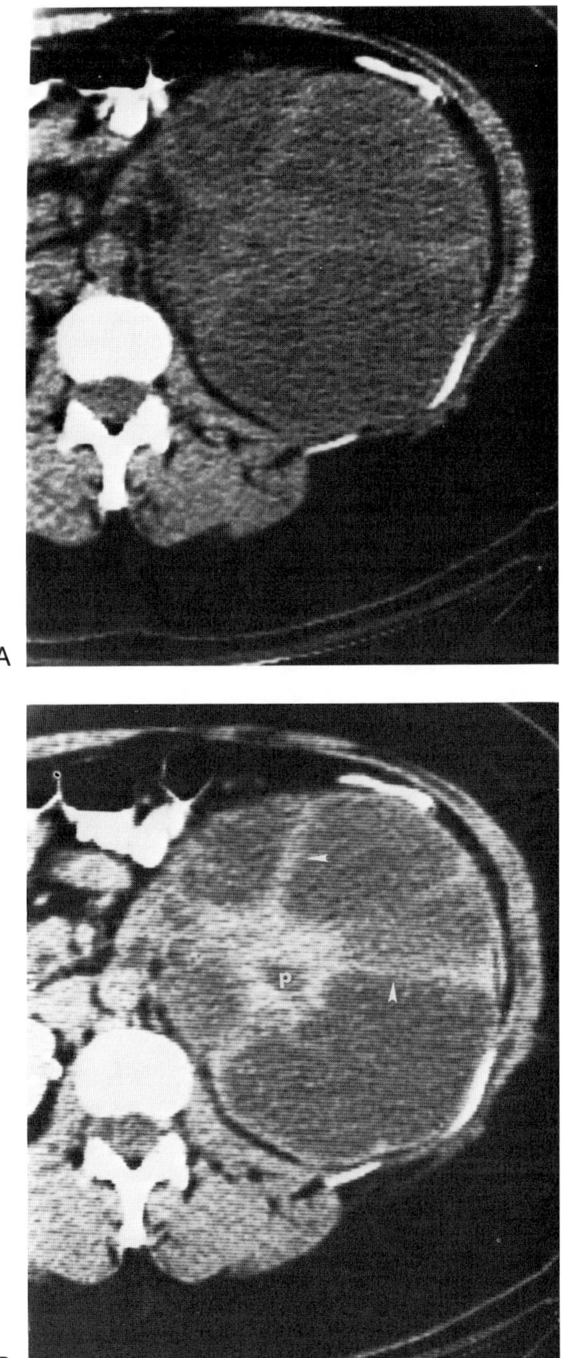

FIG. 4-21.   Xanthogranulomatous pyelonephritis showing evidence of enhancement after contrast injection. (A) CT scan without enhancement. (B) CT after enhancement. Note preservation of the reniform outline with clear definition of the remaining thinned parenchyma and inflammatory tissue (arrows surrounding the dilated calyces) with a small renal pelvis. (From Goldman et al.,[56] with permission.)

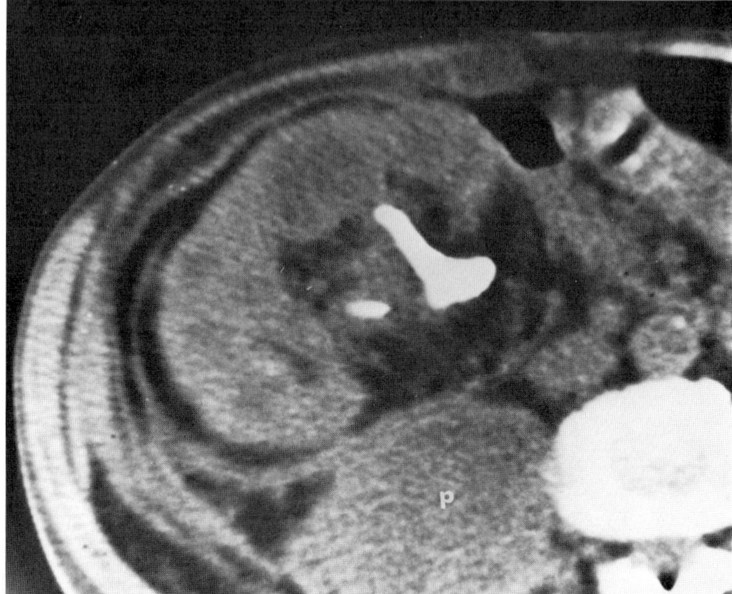

FIG. 4-22.   Xanthogranulomatous pyelonephritis secondary to an obstructing staghorn calculus. Note the psoas abscess (P). (From Goldman et al.,[56] with permission.)

As with CT, on MRI[31,67] the enlarged kidney with its preserved reniform outline is recognized. The parenchymal abscesses and calyces will be of intermediate to low intensity on T_1-weighted sequences (depending on the amount of debris) or of high intensity on T_2-weighted studies. One disadvantage of MRI is its inability to demonstrate either the obstructive renal calculi or other calcifications as readily. On the other hand, MRI is claimed to better identify perinephric or paranephric extension by its high intensity on T_2-weighted images[68] and by its relatively low intensity on T_1-weighted images amid the unaffected normal high-intensity perinephric and paranephric fat.

Echinococcus

Renal involvement of the kidneys can occur by hematogenous or direct spread. Renal symptomatology may occur only after years, commonly presenting with an abdominal mass, flank pain, and burning on urination.[69] There may be no eosinophilia. Only rarely, hydatiduria may be present and the Weinberg and Cassoni tests may be negative as well.

The CT examination will clearly identify the thick-walled, cystic masses and any calcification that is present. Similarly, air or layered debris will also be discernable by CT. Septae, if present, may mimic a multilocular cyst. Both the smaller, lower-density (2 to 15 HU) daughter cysts and the larger high-

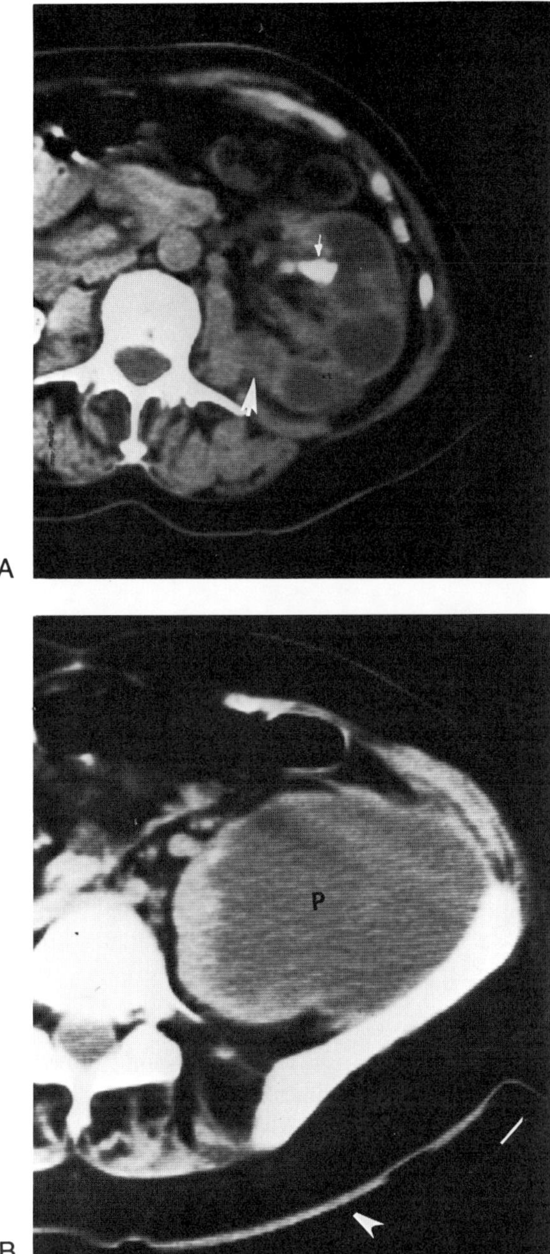

FIG. 4-23.   Xanthogranulomatous pyelonephritis with extension to the ileopsoas muscle. (A) Level of the kidney shows the obstructing stone (small arrow) and the probable site of spread of infection to the psoas (large arrow). (B) Level of the iliac crest showing abscess involving ileopsoas. The infection from the kidney could be clearly followed from the kidney down the psoas into the bony pelvis. (From Goldman et al.,[56] with permission.)

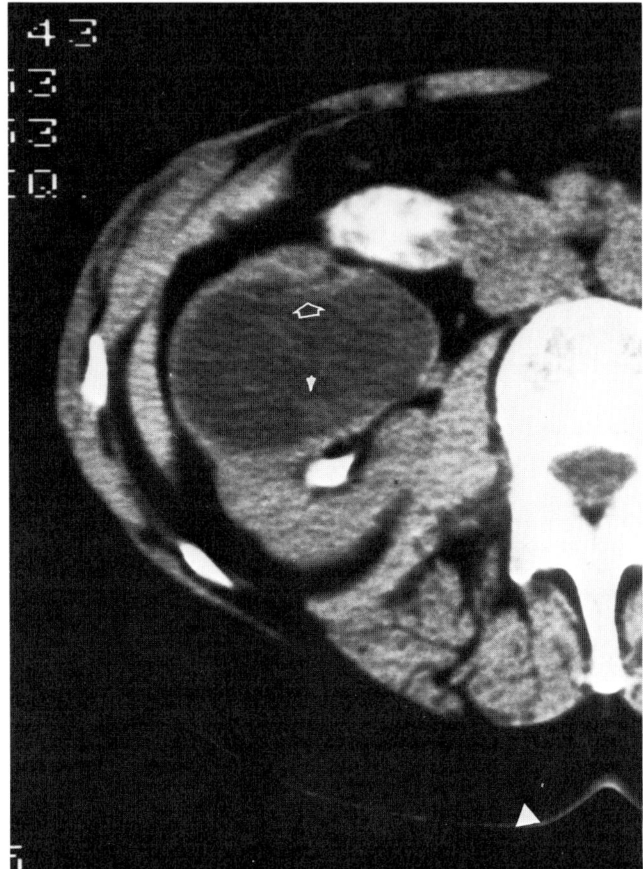

FIG. 4-24.   Infected cyst in 50-year-old black woman. Open arrow points to an area of cyst wall thickening that mimics a tumor. Solid arrowhead points to debris within cyst.

density (15 to 40 HU) mother cysts are believed to be distinguishable by some.[70,71] CT also is ideal to demonstrate other areas of echinococcosis, such as the liver, abdomen, or chest.

Actinomycosis

Actinomyces israelii, a gram-positive filamentous anaerobe, rarely affects the kidney; however, when involved, the spread to the kidney is by the hematogenous or direct contiguous route. It can present as a diffuse pyelonephritis, a pyonephrosis, or chronic suppuration with cortical abscess.[72–75] Fistulous tracts are common. CT is ideal for demonstrating the extent of disease and for determining whether the disease is confined to above or below the diaphragm.[75,76]

Aspergillosis

Aspergillus is a human saprophyte that usually affects the kidney when disseminated in those patients who are immunosuppressed, have diabetes or cancer, or are receiving steroids. In rare instances, involvement of the kidney can occur via the ascending route from the bladder.[77] Zirinsky[78] reported a case of a patient with a multilocular mass found on ultrasound who had enlarged para-aortic lymph nodes and focal calcifications on CT.

Pancreatitis

Involvement of the perinephric space by pancreatitis is readily identifiable by CT. When pancreatitis extends into the kidney itself[79] the left kidney is more often affected than the right.[80] The involvement may mimic a mass or an abscess with perinephric involvement.

Renal Fistula

Inflammatory kidney disease can develop fistulae almost anywhere, including the gastrointestinal tract, skin, and lung. The causes are multiple, and include inflammation, neoplasm, surgical complications, foreign body, and trauma. In these often quite ill patients, multiple imaging modalities including CT, are necessary to evaluate the extent of the problem.[81]

Renal Papillary Necrosis

CT does not have a primary role in the diagnosis of renal papillary necrosis. Occasionally, the sloughed papilla is noted within the contrast-filled calyx, as is the calcification, if present. An obstructing ureteric sloughed papilla with punctate calcifications has been reported.[82]

Cholesteatoma

Cholesteatoma is believed to be an inflammatory process involving desquamation of keratinized, squamous metaplastic tissue from the collecting system mucosa. Infection, obstruction, calculi, and vitamin A deficiency have been variously implicated. Its CT pattern is incompletely described, although a case with high CT numbers in the cholesteatoma has been reported.[83]

Infected Cysts

Demonstrating the presence of infection in a renal cyst can be difficult, and no one radiographic technique is fool-proof. These patients may or may not be symptomatic.[84,85] On CT, signs include cyst-wall thickening or calcification (Fig. 4-24). The presence of debris is also a clue, although it can be indistinguishable from hemorrhage. The use of a gallium or indium white blood cell count can be helpful.

CONCLUSION

Although there are a multiplicity of infectious processes that affect the kidney, there are really only two major defense mechanisms (primary and secondary) available with which the body may respond. As such, many of the acute processes look similar. Even more striking are the granulomatous infections, which have a myriad of features in common. There are, however, slight differences that can serve as clues in differentiating most of these entities from each other. One great difficulty in our basic understanding of these infectious processes is the lack of a uniformly accepted terminology. Although there is a multiplicity of imaging modalities, CT plays a significant and often vital role in the diagnosis and management of patients with renal infection. MRI, at present, plays only a limited role and is relegated to a few highly select situations.

REFERENCES

1. Balfé DM, Stanley RJ, McClennan BL: The CT spectrum of renal inflammatory disease. p. 167. In Siegelman SS, Gatewood OMB, Goldman SM (eds): Computed Tomograhy of the Kidneys and Adrenals. Churchill Livingstone, New York, 1984

2. Hill GS, Clark RL: A comparative angiographic, microangiographic, and histologic study of experimental pyelonephritis. Invest Radiol 7:33, 1972

3. Morehouse HT, Weiner SN, Hoffman-Tretin JC: Inflammatory disease of the kidney. Semin Ultrasound CT MR 7:246, 1986

4. Lee JKT, McClennan BL, Melson GL, Stanley RJ: Acute focal bacterial nephritis: Emphasis on gray scale sonography and computed tomography. AJR 135:87, 1980

5. Wegenke JD, Malek GH, Alder AJ, Olson JG. Acute lobar nephronia. J Urol 135:343, 1986

6. Oyen R, Baert AL, Marchal G: CT and US in acute inflammatory kidney disease. Proceedings, 17th International Congress of Radiology, Paris, 1989

7. Goldman SM: Acute and chronic urinary infection: Present concepts and controversies. Urol Radiol 10:17, 1988

8. Hodson CJ, Maling TM, McManamon JJ, Lewis MG: The pathogenesis of reflux nephropathy (chronic atrophic pyelonephritis). Br J Radiol (suppl) 48:1, 1975

9. Soulen MC, Fishman EG, Goldman SM, Gatewood OMB: Bacterial renal infection: Role of CT. Radiology 171:703, 1989

10. Gold RP, McClennan BL, Rottenberg RR: CT appearance of acute inflammatory disease of the renal interstitium. AJR 141:343, 1983

11. Roberts JA: Pyelonephritis, cortical abscess, and perinephric abscess. Urol Clin North Am 13:637, 1986

12. Fair WR, McClennan BL, Jost RG: Are excretory urograms necessary in evaluating women with urinary tract infection? J Urol 121:313, 1979

13. Wicks JD, Thornbury JR: Acute renal infections in adults. Radiol Clin North Am 17:245, 1979

14. Thornbury JR: Perirenal anatomy: Normal and abnormal. Radiol Clin North Am 17:321, 1979

15. Silver TM, Kass EJ, Thornbury JR: The radiological spectrum of acute pyelonephritis in adults and adolescents. Radiology 118:67, 1976

16. Sty JR, Wells RG, Starshak RJ, Schroeder BA: Imaging in acute renal infection in children. AJR 148:471, 1987

17. Conway JJ: The role of nuclear medicine: Possibilities and practicalities. p. 183. In Uroradiology Syllabus. Uroradiological Society Meeting, Naples, FL, September, 1989

18. Morehouse HT, Weiner SN, Hoffman JC: Imaging of inflammatory disease of the kidney. AJR 143:135, 1985

19. Ishikawa I, Saito Y, Onouchi Z, et al: Delayed contrast enhancement in acute focal bacterial nephritis: CT features. J Comput Assist Tomogr 9:894, 1985

20. Davidson AJ, Talner LB: Urographic and angiographic abnormalities in adult-onset acute bacterial nephritis. Radiology 106:249, 1973

21. Davidson AJ: Radiology of the Kidney. WB Saunders, Philadelphia, 1985, p. 282

22. Hoffman EP, Mindelzun RE, Anderson RU: Computed tomography in acute pyelonephritis associated with diabetes. Radiology 135:691, 1980

23. Rigsby CM, Rosenfield AJ, Glickman MG, Hodson J: Hemorrhagic focal bacterial nephritis: Findings on gray-scale sonography and CT. AJR 146:1173, 1986

24. Browning RD, Smith LP, Wenzel DJ, et al: Sonography and computed tomography of urinary tract infection. Arch Intern Med 145:841, 1985

25. Jeffrey RB, Federle MP: CT and ultrasonography of acute renal abnormalities. Radiol Clin North Am 21:515, 1983

26. Jeffrey RB: Bacterial renal infection: Role of CT. (letter) Radiology 173:574, 1989

27. Soulen MC, Fishman EK, Goldman SM: Bacterial renal infection: Role of CT. (reply) Radiology 173:575, 1989

28. Hoddick W, Jeffrey RB, Goldberg HI, et al: CT and sonography of severe renal and perirenal infections. AJR 140:517, 1983

29. Gerzof SG, Gale ME: Computed tomography and ultrasonography for diagnosis and treatment of renal and retroperitoneal abscesses. Urol Clin North Am 9:185, 1982

30. Kunin M. Bridging septa of the perinephric space: Anatomic, pathologic, and diagnostic considerations. Radiology 158:555, 1986

31. LiPuma JP: Magnetic resonance imaging of the kidney. Radiol Clin North Am 22:925, 1984

32. Hamlin DJ, Ackerman N, Kaude JV, et al: Magnetic resonance imaging of renal abscess in an experimental animal model. Acta Radiol Diagn 26:315, 1985

33. Langston CS, Pfister RC: Renal emphysema. A case report and review of the literature. AJR 110:778, 1970

34. Michaeli J, Mogle P, Perlberg S, et al: Emphysematous pyelonephritis, review article. J Urol 131:203, 1984

35. Hall JRW, Choa RG, Wells IP: Percutaneous drainage in emphysematous pyelonephritis— an alternative to major surgery. Clin Radiol 39:622, 1988

36. Kim DS, Woesner ME, Howard TF, Olson LK. Emphysematous pyelonephritis demonstrated by computed tomography. AJR 132:287, 1979

37. Vas W, Carlin B, Salimi Z, et al: CT diagnosis of emphysematous pyelonephritis. Comput Radiol 9:37, 1985

38. Olzabal A, Velasco M, Martinez A, et al: Emphysematous pyelonephritis. Urology 29:950, 1987

39. Allen HA III, Walsh JW, Brewer WH, et al: Sonography of emphysematous pyelonephritis. J Ultrasound Med 3:533, 1984

40. Graham JN, Berlin BB, Graydon RG: Case profile: Computed tomography in emphysematous pyelonephritis. Urology 27:277, 1986

41. Leekam RN, Shankar L, Bayley TA: Emphysematous pyelonephritis as seen on technetium 99m DTPA renal imaging. Clin Nucl Med 12:140, 1987

42. Lachance S, Wicklund R, Carey T, Totonchi M: Emphysematous pyelonephritis complicated by hemorrhage diagnosed by computerized tomography scan. J Urol 134:940, 1985

43. Lautin EM, Gordon PM, Friedman AC, et al: Emphysematous pyelonephritis: Optimal diagnosis and treatment. Urol Radiol 1:93, 1979

44. Piccirillo M, Rigsby CM, Rosenfield AT: Sonography of renal inflammatory disease. Urol Radiol 9:66, 1987

45. Yoder IC, Lindfors KK, Pfister RC: Diagnosis and treatment of pyonephrosis. Radiol Clin North Am 22:407, 1984

46. Subramanyam BR, Raghavendra BN, Bosniak MA, et al: Sonography of pyonephrosis: A prospective study. AJR 140:991, 1983

47. Coleman BG, Arger PH, Mulhern CB Jr, et al: Pyonephrosis: Sonography in the diagnosis and management. AJR 137:939, 1981

48. Soulen MC, Fishman EK, Goldman SM: Sequelae of acute renal infections: CT evaluation. Radiology 173:423, 1989

49. Newhouse JH, Amis ES Jr: The relationship between renal scarring and stone disease. AJR 151:1153, 1988

50. Mihindukulasuriya JCL, Maskell R, Polak A: A study of fifty-eight patients with renal scarring associated with urinary tract infection. Q J Med 194:165, 1980

51. Goldman SM, Fishman EK, Hartman DS, et al: Computed tomography of renal tuberculosis and its pathological correlates. J Comput Assist Tomogr 9:771, 1985

52. Goldman SM, Gatewood OMB: Inflammatory renal disease. p. 607. In Lang EK (ed): Selection of Imaging Studies in Urology. Problems in Urology. Vol. 3. JB Lippincott, Philadelphia

53. Gow JB: Genitourinary tuberculosis. p. 1037. In Walsh PC, Gittes RF, Perlmutter AD (eds): Campbell's Urology. 5th Ed. WB Saunders, Philadelphia, 1986

54. Premkumar A, Lattimer J, Newhouse JH: CT and sonography of advanced urinary tract tuberculosis. AJR 148:65, 1987

55. Bergner DM, Roth JK Jr, Lang EK: The role of computerized tomography in the management of bilateral tuberculous psoas abscess. J Urol 124:1020, 1982

56. Goldman SM, Hartman DS, Fishman EK, et al: CT of xanthogranulomatous pyelonephritis: Radiological-pathological correlation. AJR 141:963, 1984

57. Elder JS, Marshall FF: Focal xanthogranulomatous pyelonephritis in adulthood. Johns Hopkins Med Bull 146:141, 1980

58. Rosi P, Selli C, Carin M, et al: Xanthogranulomatous pyelonephritis: Clinical experience with 62 cases. Eur Urol 12:96, 1986

59. Grainger RG, Longstaff AJ, Parsons MA: Xanthogranulomatous pyelonephritis: A reappraisal. Lancet 1:1398,

60. Malek RS, Elder JS: Xanthogranulomatous pyelonephritis: A critical analysis of 26 cases and the literature. J Urol 119:589, 1978

61. Beackley MC, Ranniger K, Roth FJ: Xanthogranulomatous pyelonephritis. AJR 121:500, 1974

62. Subramanyam BR, Megibow AJ, Raghavendra BN, Bosniak MA. Diffuse xanthogranulomatous pyelonephritis: Analysis of computed tomography and sonography. Urol Radiol 4:5, 1982

63. Claes H, Vereeken R, Oyen R, Van Damme B: Xanthogranulomatous pyelonephritis with emphasis on computerized tomographic scan. Urology 29:389, 1987

64. Parsons MA, Harris SC, Grainger RG, et al: Fistula and sinus formation in xanthogranulomatous pyelonephritis. A clinico-pathological review and report of four cases. Br J Urol 58:488, 1986

65. Cheatle TR, Waldron RP, Arkell DG: Xanthogranulomatous pyelonephritis associated with pyeloduodenal fistula. Br J Surg 72:764, 1985

66. Sussman SK, Gallmann WH, Cohan RH, et al: CT findings in xanthogranulomatous pyelonephritis with coexistent renocolic fistula. J Comput Assist Tomogr 11:1088, 1987

67. Mulopulos GP, Patel SK, Pessis D: MR imaging of xanthogranulomatous pyelonephritis. J Comput Assist Tomogr 10:154, 1986

68. Feldberg MAM, Driessen KP, Witkamp TD, et al: Xanthogranulomatous pyelonephritis: Comparison of extent using computed tomography and magnetic resonance imaging in one case. Urol Radiol 10:92, 1988

69. Hertz M, Zissin R, Dresnik Z, et al: Echinococcus of the urinary tract: Radiologic findings. Urol Radiol 6:175, 1984

70. Petrillo G, Tomaselli S, Greco S: Renal echinococcosis: Case report. J Comput Assist Tomogr 5:912, 1981

71. Kalovidouris A, Pissiotis C, Pontifex A, Gouliamos A: CT characterization of multivesicular hydated cysts. J Comput Assist Tomogr 10:428, 1986

72. Patel BJ, Moskowitz H, Hashma TA: Unilateral renal actinomycosis. Urology 21:172, 1983

73. Ellis LR, Kenny GM, Nellans RE: Urogenital aspets of actinomycosis. J Urol 122:132, 1979

74. Anhalt M, Scott R Jr: Primary unilateral renal actinomycosis: Case report. J Urol 103:126, 1970

75. Denton AE III: Computed tomographic findings in thoracic and renal actinomycosis: Case report and review of the literature. J Am Osteopath Assoc 85:57, 1985

76. Allen HA III, Scatarige JC, Kim MH: Actinomycosis: CT findings in six patients. AJR 149:1255, 1987

77. Flechner SM, McAninch JW: Aspergillosis of the urinary tract: Ascending route of infection and evolving patterns of disease. J Urol 125:598, 1981

78. Zirinsky K, Auh Y, Hartman BJ, et al: Computed tomography of renal aspergillosis. J Comput Assist Tomogr 11:177, 1987

79. Rauch RF, Korobkin M, Silverman PM, Dunnick NR: Subcapsular pancreatic pseudocyst of the kidney. J Comput Assist Tomogr 7:536, 1983

80. Nicholson RC: Abnormalities of the perinephric fascia and fat in pancreatitis. Radiology 139:125, 1981

81. Cohen EL, Greenstein AJ, Katz SE: Nephrocolocutaneous fistula: Use of CT to aid diagnosis. Comput Radiol 7:291, 1983

82. Andriole GL, Bahnson RR: Computed tomographic diagnosis of ureteral obstruction caused by a sloughed papilla. Urol Radiol 9:45, 1987

83. Wills JS, Pollack HM, Curtis JA: Cholesteatoma of the upper urinary tract. AJR 136:941, 1981

84. Goldman SM: Simple renal cyst. p. 6. In Hartman DS, Davidson AJ (eds): Renal Cystic Disease. Fascicle I, Chapter 1. AFIP Atlas of Radiologic Pathologic Correlations. WB Saunders, Philadelphia, 1989

85. Goldman SM, Hartman DS: The simple renal cyst. p. 1092. In Pollack H (ed): Clinical Urography. 5th Ed. WB Saunders, Philadelphia, 1990

86. Goldman SM: Radiological diagnosis and assessment of inflammatory diseases. p. 325. In Lang EK (ed): Percutaneous and Interventional Urology and Radiology. Springer-Verlag, New York, 1986

5 CT and MRI of Metastatic Disease to the Urinary Tract

JOHN P. VOLPE
PETER L. CHOYKE

A new, unsuspected renal mass in a cancer patient, discovered during routine radiographic examinations, is usually met with consternation by radiologists and clinicians. Does this lesion represent a primary renal tumor, or is it a metastasis from the patient's known primary malignancy? This question arises with increasing frequency as oncologic patients are screened more often with modern sectional imaging techniques. The purpose of this chapter is to increase the reader's familiarity with renal metastases by reviewing the mechanisms of metastases to the urinary tract, describing the range of appearances of urinary tract metastases on CT and MRI examinations, and presenting guidelines for radiologic management of such lesions.

The urinary tract, of which the kidney is the major component, is the fifth leading site of metastases in the body.[1] Metastases are found in 2 to 20 percent of autopsies performed on patients dying of cancer.[1-4] Renal metastases, unlike these in bone, brain, liver, and lung, tend to be asymptomatic and are rarely a cause of life-threatening bleeding or azotemia.[2,5] Ureteral metastases, however, with accompanying narrowing and obstruction, are a significant cause of morbidity and mortality.[6] Bladder metastases are rare but their occurrence is usually accompanied by dysuria or bleeding.

Despite its importance in homeostasis and its large blood supply, the urinary tract is an uncommon site of metastases. It would appear that the urinary tract is somewhat "privileged" in this respect. The theoretical reasons for this are discussed in the following section.

MECHANISM OF METASTASIS

How does a tumor spread to the urinary tract? The answer to this question is complex and is not yet fully understood. A metastasis derives from a complicated series of tumor-host interactions, and its formation involves both a systematic process of dissemination and chance mechanisms. The process of metastasis can be described in a series of sequential steps known as the metastatic cascade, consisting of tumor formation, dissemination, arrest, and growth.[7]

The first event in the cascade is the formation of a primary neoplasm somewhere within the body. Through neovascularization, the tumor establishes an independent source of nutrition and proceeds to invade local tissue and, in particular, blood and lymphatic vessels, thereby allowing the second step of the cascade, dissemination, to occur.[8] Only a minority of cells that enter the circulation result in metastases. Such cells are vulnerable to host-defense mechanisms, as well as mechanical shearing forces. Cancer cells are less flexible and therefore more vulnerable to mechanical compression within microvascular beds. In experimental models, less than 0.1 percent of disseminated tumor cells survive to produce metastases.[9] Those cells that survive this passage will lodge in the microvascular bed of the target organ. The cells adhere to the vascular endothelium and basement membranes, allowing migration and growth into the target parenchyma.[10] The arrest phase and subsequent growth phase of the metastatic cascade are characterized by population of cells that are antigenically and biochemically distinct from their primary neoplasm.[11,12] For instance, a metastatic phenotype that produces a proteolytic enzyme, such as type IV collagenase (important in injuring vascular basement membranes), will be favored in the metastatic cascade over another cell type that does not. Tumor angiogenesis factor (TAF) is another humoral substance necessary for successful growth of the metastasis.[11] Contrary to common intuition, metastases can grow (and respond to chemotherapy) quite differently from the primary tumor and have different biochemical profiles.

The host tissue is not defenseless against implantation. Tumor cell lysis may be mediated by local immune response, tissue oxygenation, and acid-base conditions.[7] Since the degree of neovascularity controls the delivery of nutrients, clearance of metabolites, and oxygen supply, inhibitors of TAF secreted by the host tissue may significantly attenuate tumor growth.[12]

One of the oldest theories of metastasis was postulated by Paget in 1896 and is known as the "seed and soil" principle. This theory stated that a site-specific metastasis was the consequence of a fertile environment (the soil) in which compatible tumor cells (the seed) could proliferate.[13] Metastases to the urinary tract are unusual and generally occur late, after the appearance of multiple metastases elsewhere in the body.[5] From this, it can be surmised that the microenvironment of the urinary tract is unfavorable to the development of metastases. In the particular case of the kidney, this is likely due to a combination of immune surveillance, shearing forces at the glomerulus, and inhibition of tumorigenic growth promoters. These natural defenses can be overwhelmed, however, by particularly aggressive metastatic phenotypes or by an excessive number of cells presented to the kidney.

Metastatic lesions arising from disseminated tumor cells are commonly small, multiple, and slow growing until a volume of 0.5 to 2 cm^3 is attained.[13] At this size, they may easily be confused with cysts or simply overlooked. With this in mind, we will consider the appearances of metastases on CT and MRI following a brief review of techniques to optimize detection.

IMAGING OF METASTASES TO THE URINARY TRACT

Metastases to the urinary tract can be encountered with practically any imaging modality directed at the kidney. Urography and pyelography are important as diagnostic tools but are not routinely employed to monitor oncology patients. Sonography is quite useful in the identification and characterization of renal masses but is ineffective in evaluation of the ureters and retroperitoneum. CT and, to a lesser extent, MRI, have emerged as primary means of evaluation of depicting and aiding in the evaluation of metastases to the urinary tract and will be the focus of the remainder of the technical discussion of this chapter.

Techniques

CT should be performed before and after intravenous (IV) contrast administration when possible. This permits evaluation of the abdominal viscera, as well as the retroperitoneum, in seeking metastatic deposits. Moreover, if administered as a bolus with rapid sequence scanning during the injection phase, the presence of enhancement can greatly aid in the distinction between a solid mass and cystic disease of the kidney.[14,15] Thin sections (5 mm or less) should be employed for selected lesions. The entire ureter should be traced with contiguous 10-mm-thick sections. Evaluation of the bladder should be performed last when sufficient contrast material has entered the bladder. Occasionally, it is useful to place the patient in the prone or oblique position in order to highlight certain areas of the bladder with the more dependent contrast material. Some have advocated the use of air insufflation or mineral oil instillation for better demarcation of the bladder wall; we have found these techniques generally unnecessary. Tumors on the neck or the dome of the bladder may be difficult to image with CT.[16] Cystoscopy is usually required to confirm the nature of a lesion identified radiographically.[17]

MRI provides an alternative in specific circumstances, especially when multiplanar scanning is needed. MRI should be performed with T_1- and T_2-weighted images in the axial plane through the kidneys. Multiplanar imaging is useful, particularly in the coronal plane. The ureters are difficult to evaluate on MRI because they do not lie in one plane and can therefore be confused with vessels and bowel in nonaxial sections. The complex anatomy and spherical shape of the bladder make it amenable to imaging in multiple planes. The axial, coronal, and sagittal views are considered complementary in evaluation of the bladder. T_1-weighted or "proton density" (i.e., TR 250 to 1,000 ms and TE 15 to 30 ms) are useful when imaging the bladder. Thin sections (3 to 5 mm) are helpful in reducing partial volume effects. Intravenous paramagnetic contrast agents such as gadolinium DTPA (Gd-DTPA) may be useful in detecting lesions, but their value has not been demonstrated in a prospective study. Gd-DTPA, however, appears quite useful in the assessment of renal lymphoma, especially in the presence of pre-existing renal failure when iodinated contrast material should be avoided. At this time, the administration of Gd-DTPA in the presence of compromised renal function has not been fully approved by the Food and Drug Administration (FDA) and should be employed with caution. The role of gradient echo techniques, although promising, has not yet been elucidated.

CT has many advantages over MRI in the evaluation of metastases to the urinary tract. These include better spatial resolution, a bowel opacifying agent, and general availability. Advantages of MRI include its multiplanar capabilities, which are most useful in evaluating the bladder, and the absence of ionizing radiation. Given the comparative costs and marginal benefit in this patient population, MRI must be considered "gilding the lily" in most cases.[18–20] Nevertheless, in patients who are allergic to contrast medium or in patients in whom multiplanar views are deemed desirable, MRI has a limited but important role.

KIDNEY METASTASES

Renal metastases have been reported with practically every malignancy. The most common primary lesions are lung cancer, colon cancer, stomach cancer, and breast cancer, reflecting the frequent occurrence of these primaries.[1,2,5] Disproportionate representation is seen with melanoma, which accounted for 35 to 40 percent of renal metastases in two series, and with uterine, ovarian, and testicular neoplasms.[3,21] The latter can be explained by the relative frequency of renal hilar adenopathy that accompanies these primaries and results in contiguous invasion of the renal pelvis and renal parenchyma.

Clinically, symptomatic metastases to the kidney are rare; the most common complaints are hematuria and flank pain.[2] Although albuminuria and evaluation of BUN and creatinine may be seen, most patients with renal metastases retain good renal function.[5] Some reports have focused on massive hematuria and renal dysfunction as a result of renal metastases, for example, from choriocarcinoma and osteogenic sarcoma.[22,23] Cytologic examination of the urine is simple, inexpensive, and, although rarely positive, may obviate the need for biopsy.[21] Squamous cell carcinoma and melanoma seem to yield better cytologic samples than do other primary tumors, in our experience.

Like many diseases that affect the kidney, metastases often spread hematogenously. Thus, the appearance of metastases corresponds to a segmental vascular distribution and is round or wedge shaped, similar to the pattern in renal infection or infarction. Most renal metatases are found in the periphery of the kidney, corresponding to entrapment in the cortical glomeruli.[24] Not infrequently, an inflammatory or neoplastic wedge-shaped lesion encompassing the cortex and medulla is seen simulating the appearance of acute focal bacterial nephritis[14] (Figs. 5-1 and 5-2). More often, however, one or more discrete peripheral masses are seen (Fig. 5-3). Bilaterality is common and is seen in up to 60 percent of cases.[23] Lesions are generally multiple, although single metastases can be seen in up to one-third of cases[25–27] (Fig. 5-4).

Metastatic lesions are most often homogeneous in enhancement, although necrotic areas can be noted. Administration of IV contrast will produce enhancement (5 to 15 HU), although rarely to the same degree as renal parenchyma.[27,28] Colon cancer growing within the kidney can produce a large

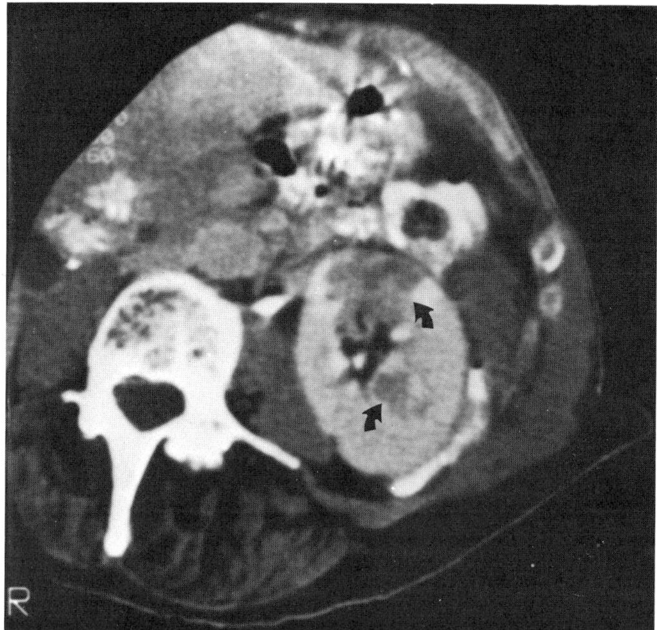

FIG. 5-1.   Renal metastases from uterine sarcoma. The larger of the two lesions (arrows) is wedge shaped and inhomogeneously enhancing. (From Choyke et al.,[27] with permission.)

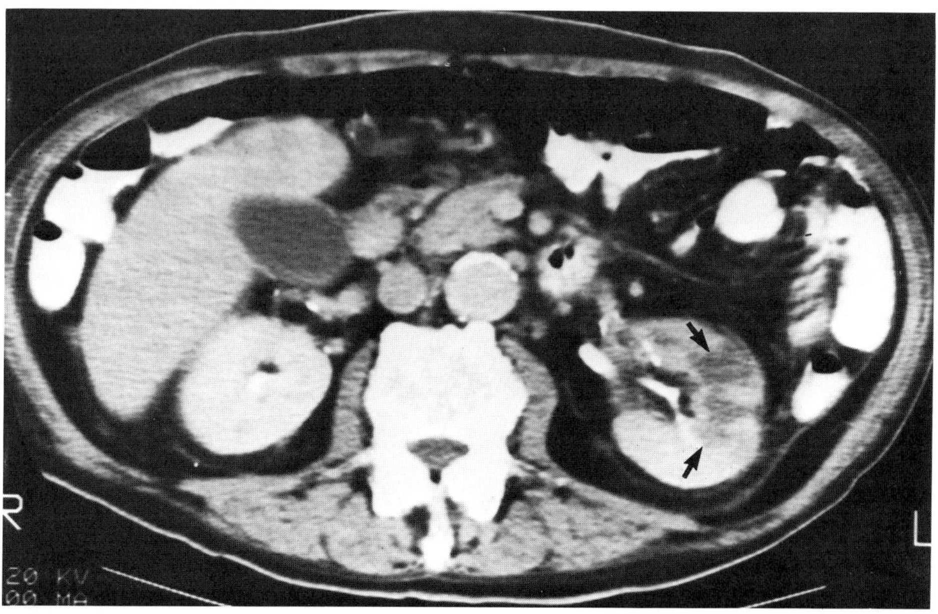

FIG. 5-2.   Renal metastases from squamous cell lung carcinoma. Note the linear infiltrative appearance (arrows) of the lesions.

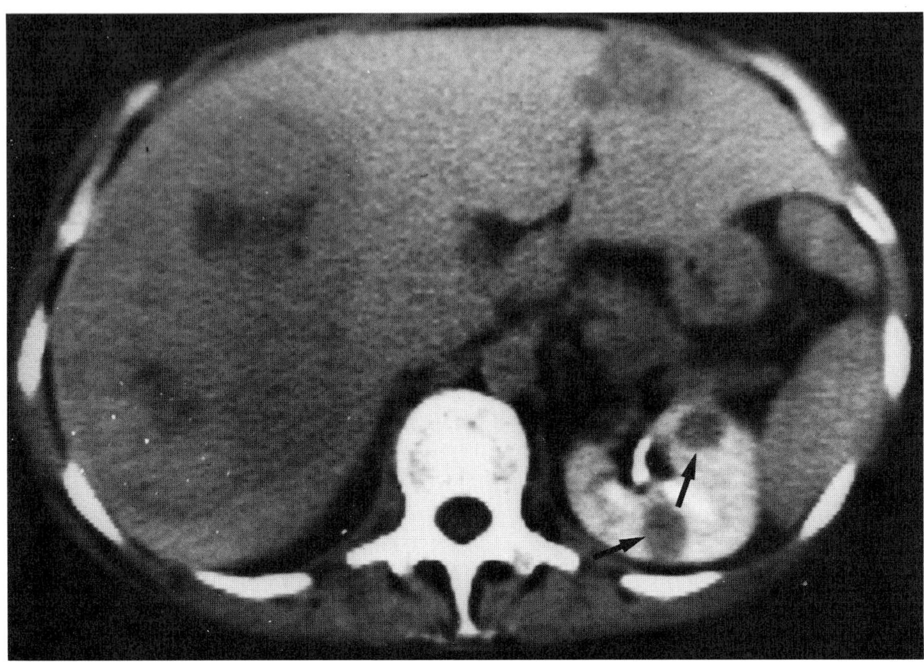

FIG. 5-3.   Renal and hepatic metastases from breast cancer. Note that the round peripheral lesions in the left kidney (arrows) could be mistaken for renal cysts. (From Choyke et al.,[27] with permission.)

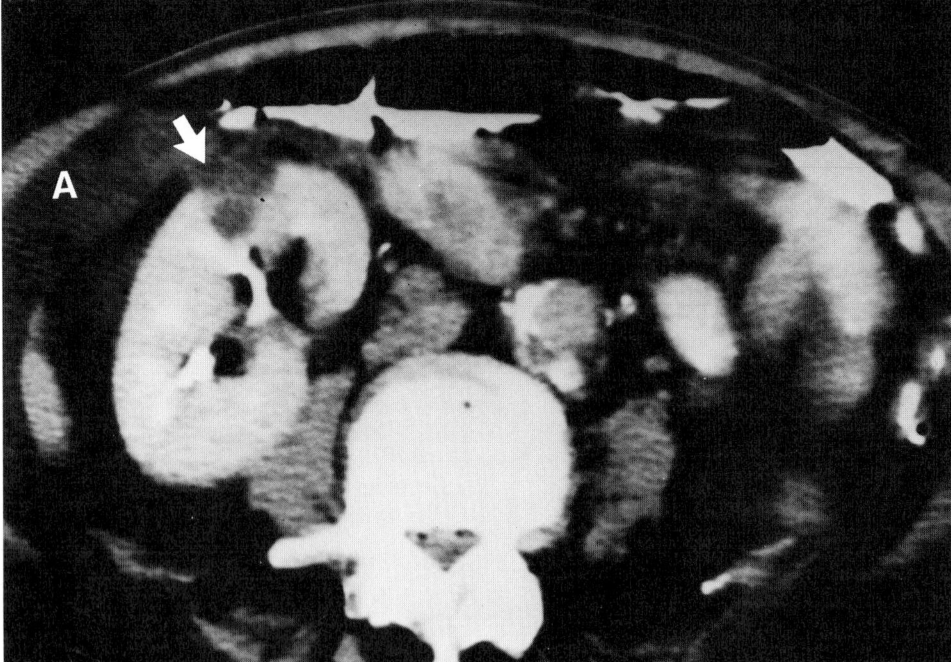

FIG. 5-4.   Single renal metastasis arising from an esophageal carcinoma. Note wedge-shaped appearance with a bulging external contour (arrow). Ascites (A) is present.

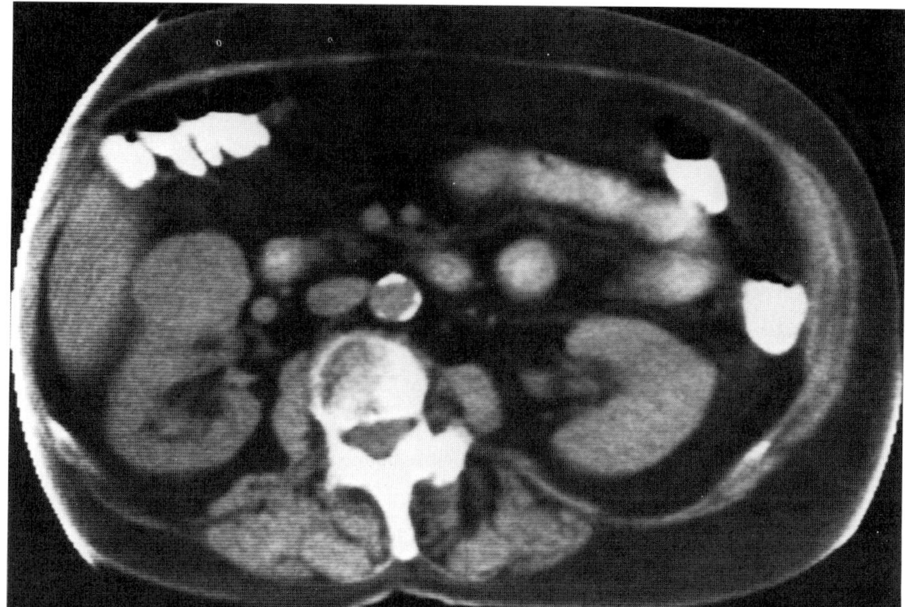

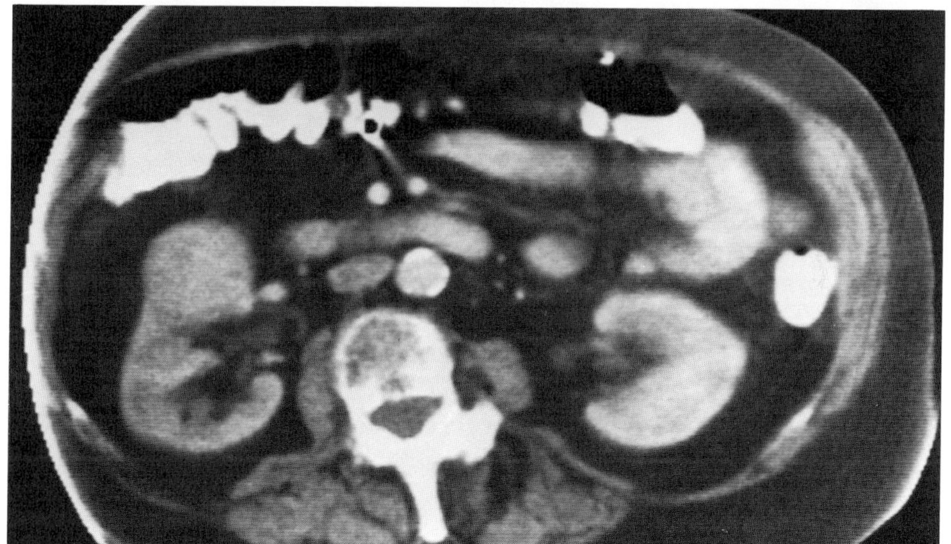

FIG. 5-5.   Large exophytic mass arising from colon adenocarcinoma. Note this tumor before (A) and after contrast (B) mimics the appearance of renal cell carcinoma. (From Choyke et al.,[27] with permission.)

exophytic mass, possibly mistaken for a renal cell carcinoma (Fig. 5-5). Calcifications can be seen in deposits of osteogenic sarcoma and in lesions treated with chemotherapy[29] (Fig. 5-6). Direct spread into the perinephric space has been noted with melanoma and lung cancers, particularly squamous cell carcinoma, but there is no reason to believe that this phenomenon is unique to

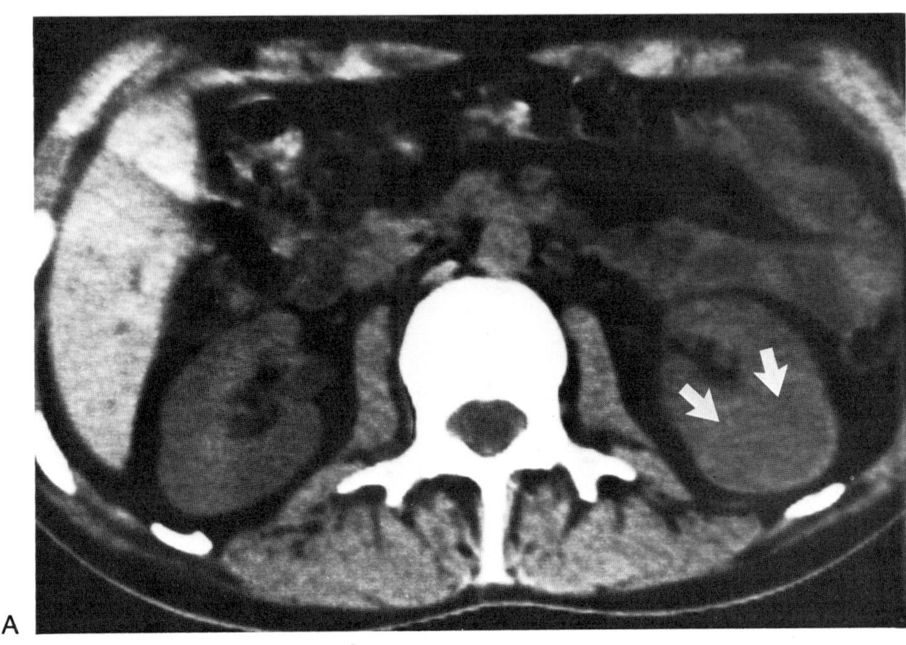

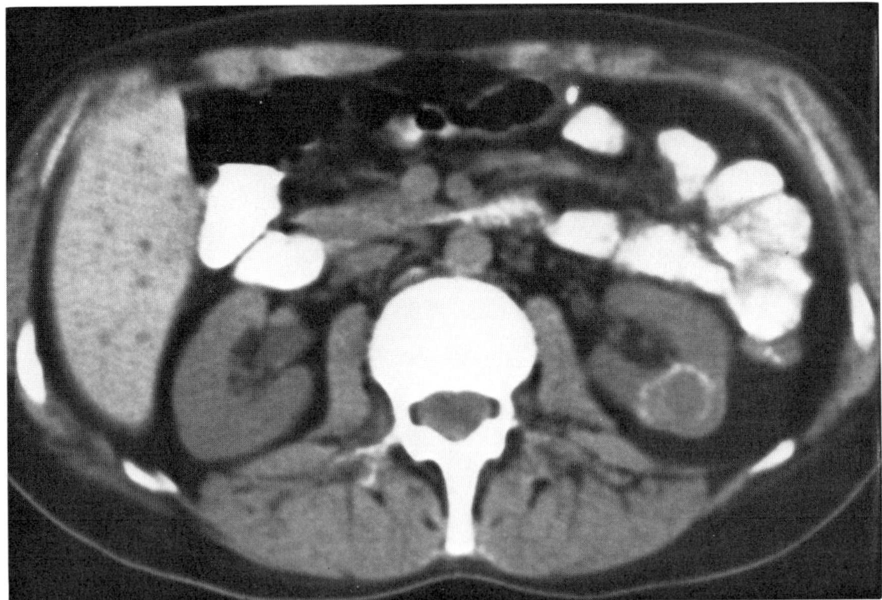

FIG. 5-6.   Renal metastases from seminoma of the testis. (A) Noncontrast scan demonstrates an enlargement of both kidneys with a globular contour in the left kidney consistent with a renal metastasis (arrows). (B) One year later, following several cycles of chemotherapy, a ringlike calcification can be seen. (*Figure continues.*)

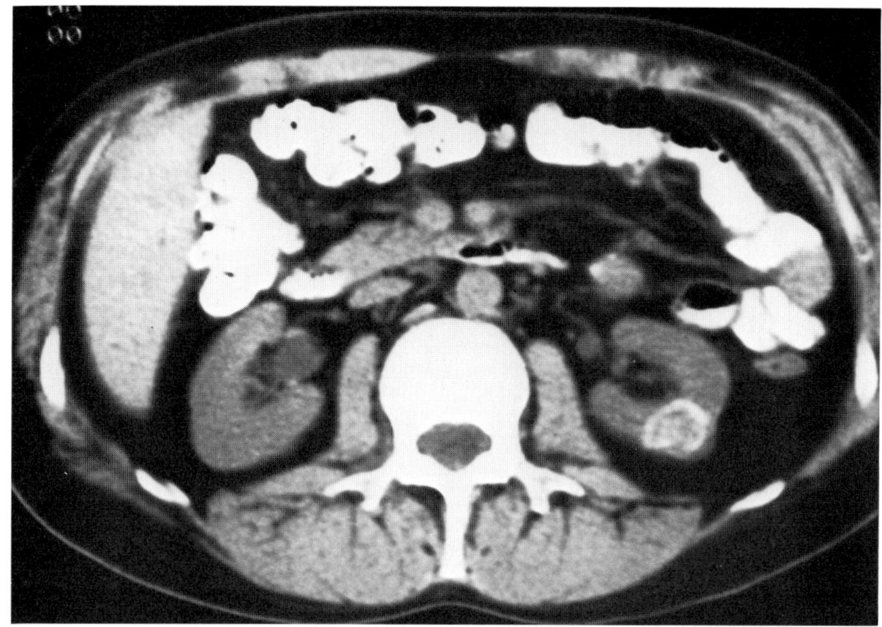

FIG. 5-6 (*Continued*). (C) Four years later, CT shows dense calcification of lesion.

these primaries.[27,30] The perinephric space has a rich network of lymphatics that permit the propagation of the tumor (Figs. 5-7 and 5-8). Interestingly, Gerota's fascia seems to interfere with the spread of tumor.

A distinction must be made between distant hematogenous metastases and local extension of tumor.[31] The latter is more frequent with tumors that involve the para-aortic and paracaval lymph nodes and the kidney contiguously. Examples of this include ovarian and testicular neoplasms, as well as melanoma and lymphoma. Direct organ invasion can be seen with colonic, hepatic, adrenal, and gastric primaries that violate Gerota's fascia and secondarily invade the kidney. The opposite pathway is probably more common; renal cell carcinomas can invade adjacent structures such as liver, bowel, and pancreas.

One of the most important problems presented by a renal mass in a cancer patient is whether this represents metastases or a new primary tumor. At autopsy, renal metastases are found more than twice as frequently as primary renal cell cancers.[32,25] In a patient with a known history of cancer in another organ, a focal renal lesion is statistically four times as likely to represent a metastasis.[27,33] A patient with widespread metastasis from another primary tumor is even more likely to have a renal metastasis than a second (renal) primary tumor. The converse may be true in a patient with a remote history of cancer and no other evidence of disease.

During treatment, renal metastases may not respond to therapy in the same manner as metastases to other organs such as liver or lung, based on the

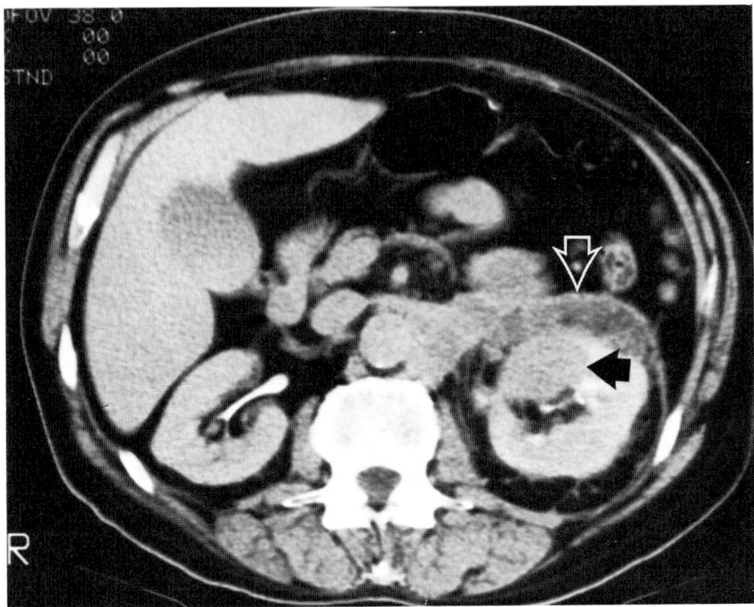

FIG. 5-7.   Perinephric extension of renal metastases in a patient with lung cancer. Note renal lesion (solid arrow) and contiguous spread to the perinephric space (open arrow). (From Choyke et al.,[27] with permission.)

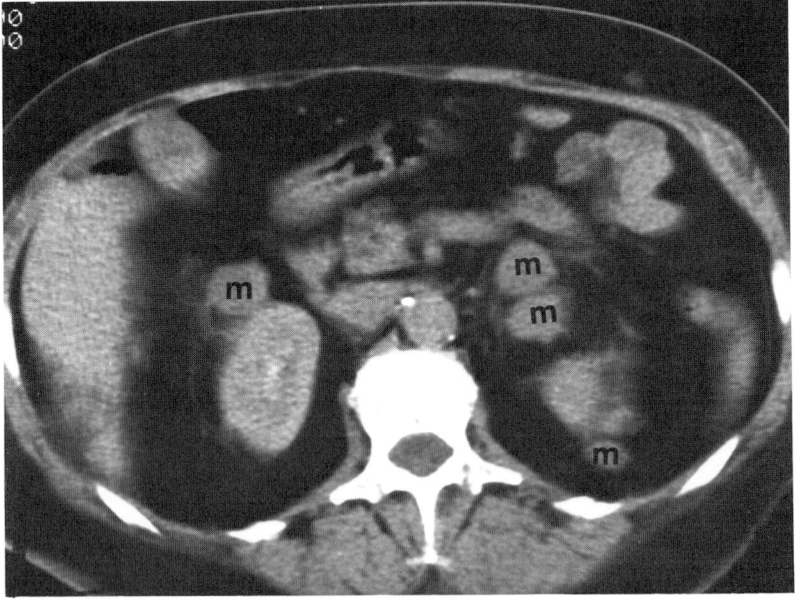

FIG. 5-8.   Perinephric extension from melanoma. Note multiple melanotic nodules in the perinephric space (m).

heterogeneous nature of site-specific cell lines.[7] Moreover, the primary lesion may share neither the growth nor response rates of the metastases.[11] In cases in which the signal characteristics on MRI of a suspected metastatic lesion and the primary tumor are the same, the lesion has been assumed to be a metastasis. This formulation is not reliable. First, MRI findings are often non-specific and variations in signal can be seen in both primary and secondary neoplasms. Conversely, since heterogeneity in cell type and growth patterns is expected, the lack of similar signal characteristics between the primary lesion and its metastases should not dissuade one from the diagnosis of metastasis.

URETERAL METASTASES

Metastases to the ureter, which receives its blood supply from branches of the renal, gonadal, common iliac, and vesicular arteries, may spread hematogenously or in the lymphatics.[34] The most common primary carcinomas to disseminate to the ureter are breast, stomach, colon, skin (malignant melanoma), and lung in decreasing order of frequency.[6,35]

Isolated intraluminal ureteral metastases are rare and usually appear as single, focal lesions that involve a portion of the ureteral wall. Circumferential metastases are more common.[36] At autopsy 25 to 60 percent of cases demonstrate bilateral involvement.[35]

Ureteral or periureteral metastasis may provoke an intense fibroblastic reaction in surrounding tissues known as malignant retroperitoneal fibrosis, which may lead to ureteral obstruction. This may also occur through tumor encasement of the ureteral wall.[37] Lesions are rarely symptomatic, with pain in the back or flank the commonest complaint. Up to 50 percent of patients will demonstrate renal dysfunction with elevated BUN and creatinine.[38] Hematuria rarely occurs, as metastases tend to spare the mucosa; however, advanced melanoma may cause melanuria and positive urine cytology. With a greater than 30 percent false-negative rate, though, cytology is inadequate as a screen for metastatic disease.[39]

CT has been cited as helpful in 90 percent of cases of ureteral obstruction.[40] Bosniak et al.[34] reported on 36 patients with ureteral obstruction and hydronephrosis, of whom 22 patients were found by CT to have metastatic ureteral involvement; in 18 cases this was the first known metastasis, and in 4, the first manifestation of cancer. CT manifestations vary from a large mass with retroperitoneal invasion to focal lesions that merely stenose and thicken the wall of the ureter.[37,41] To date, MRI has had little role in the evaluation of the ureter.

Nearly 90 percent of cases with metastasis to the ureter are associated with generalized secondary lesions when diagnosed and have a poor prognosis. Surgery is seldom justified in these patients, although palliative measures are suggested.[6] Retrograde urography and internal stent placement during cystoscopy have become the standard method of treatment; if a catheter cannot be placed cystoscopically, a percutaneous nephrostomy may be needed.

Residual tumor in a ureteral stump following radical nephrectomy for renal cancer may be a source of renal cell metastases.[21] Most of these lesions probably represent residual tumor left behind from a tumor already invading the urothelium but not removed at surgery.

BLADDER METASTASES

Metastases to the bladder at autopsy are found in fewer than 4 percent of cases.[1,2,42] The most common primary neoplasms associated with bladder metastases are, in decreasing frequency, melanoma, stomach, breast, and lung.[42–44] Dissemination to the bladder is traditionally thought to occur via implantation of venous or lymphatic emboli.[45] More commonly, one sees contiguous spread of tumor from adjacent organs such as the prostate, uterus, cervix, or sigmoid colon.[2,42,44]

The majority of metastatic bladder lesions are clinically silent. Hematuria, back pain, and symptoms of bladder irritation (frequency, nocturia, and dysuria) have been reported.[45,46] As with melanoma anywhere in the urinary tract, melanuria may be seen when it involves the bladder.[47] The diagnosis of bladder involvement is almost always made late in the course of the disease, a manifestation of more widespread metastases. Urine cytologic examination is occasionally useful in the diagnosis but more often gives false-negative results.

CT or MRI appearance of bladder metastases includes one or more nodules projecting into the lumen of the bladder or diffuse thickening of an area of bladder wall (Fig. 5-9). Enhancement can be seen but is not necessary for the diagnosis. Cystoscopy with biopsy is usually required to confirm the diagnosis.[17]

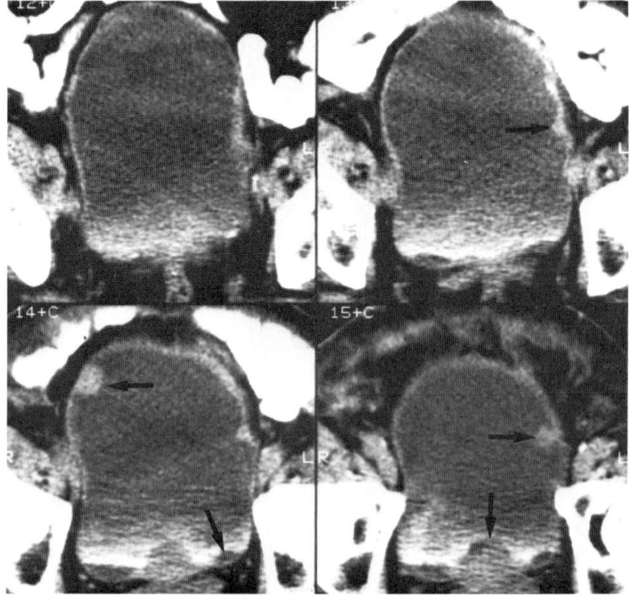

FIG. 5-9.   Multiple bladder metastases in a patient with melanoma. Note multiple polyplike masses arising from the bladder wall (arrows).

LYMPHOPROLIFERATIVE DISEASE

Kidney lymphoma is historically considered separately from other metastatic diseases of the urinary tract because its behavior is considered unique. With increasing knowledge about nonlymphomatous metastases, it is recognized that the patterns of spread associated with lymphoma are not unique. Nevertheless, for purposes of clarity, we will discuss lymphomas in this section.

Renal lymphoma at autopsy is common, with reports of up to 34 percent involvement in older studies.[48] Non-Hodgkin's lymphoma is more common than Hodgkin's disease. The genituourinary tract is rarely the first manifestation of lymphoma in the body.[49] Lymphoma spreads to the kidney, ureter, and bladder, most commonly via hematogenous dissemination or from lymphatics that massively invade the perinephric space and secondarily invade the periureteric space[50] (Fig. 5-10). Despite huge masses of neoplasm, collecting system dilatation is often not as great as expected, owing to the phenomenon of nondilated obstructive uropathy in which the renal failure is due to absence of normal ureteral peristalsis.

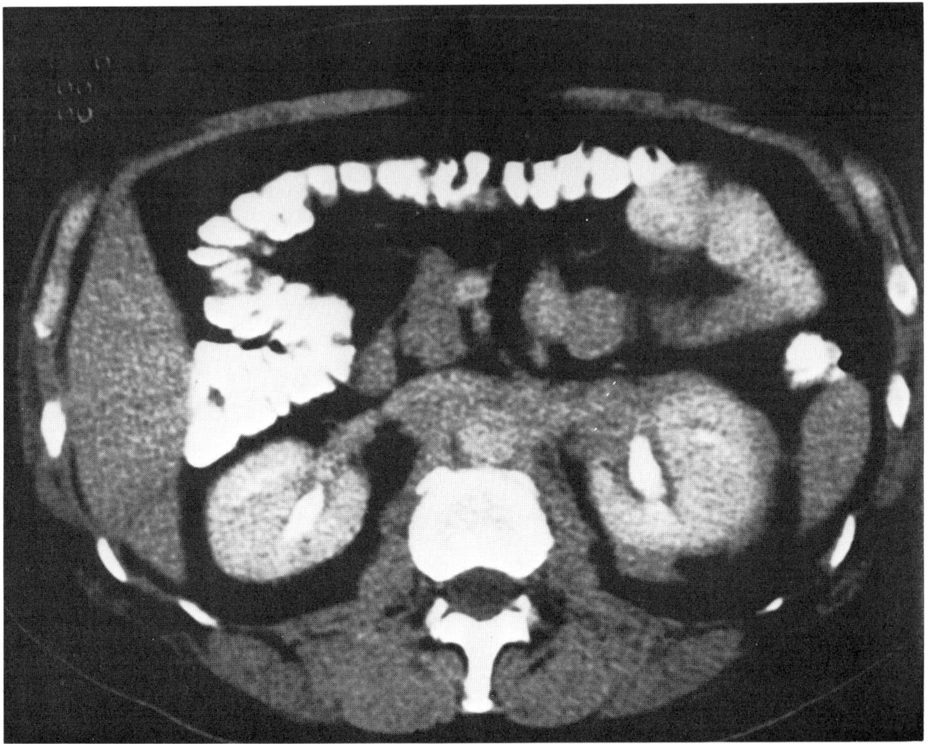

FIG. 5-10.   Non-Hodgkin's lymphoma directly invading kidney via adjacent lymphadenopathy. Note extensive adenopathy with secondary invasion of the left renal sinus.

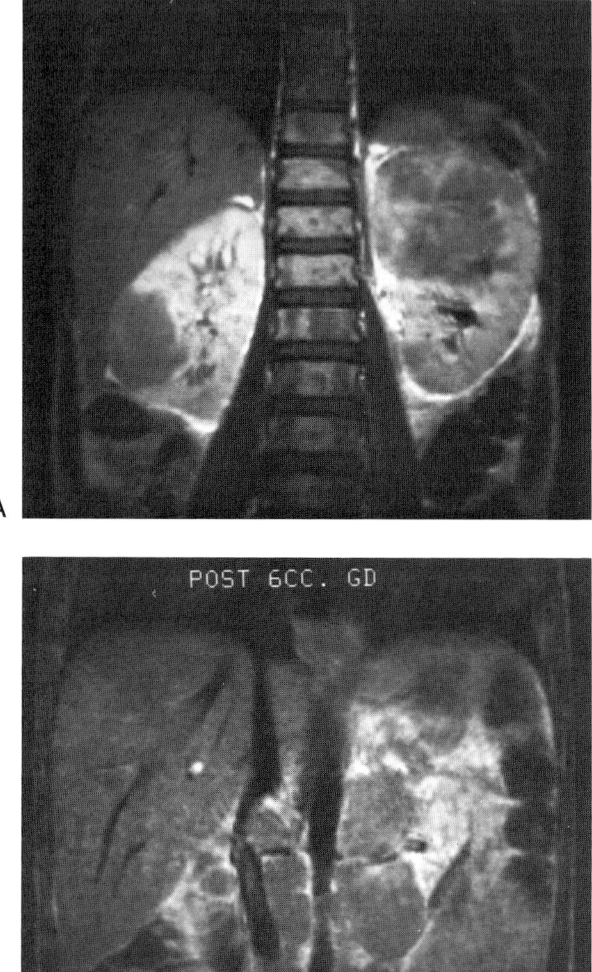

FIG. 5-11.   (A & B) Gadolinium-DTPA enhanced T_1-weighted scan demonstrating multiple lymphomatous masses in a patient with Wiscott-Aldrich syndrome. Mottled bone marrow enhancement is likely due to lymphoma infiltration. (Bone marrow aspirate of iliac crest was positive.)

Hematogenous spread of lymphoma most commonly produces multiple solid masses in the periphery of the kidney. On CT, these lesions are rounded and poorly enhancing and can be mistaken for cortical cysts.[51,52] This assumption can be inadvertantly supported by sonography, since lymphomatous nodules can be quite sonolucent.[53] On MRI, lymphomatous masses generally appear more solid, and Gd-DTPA enhancement can produce quite striking

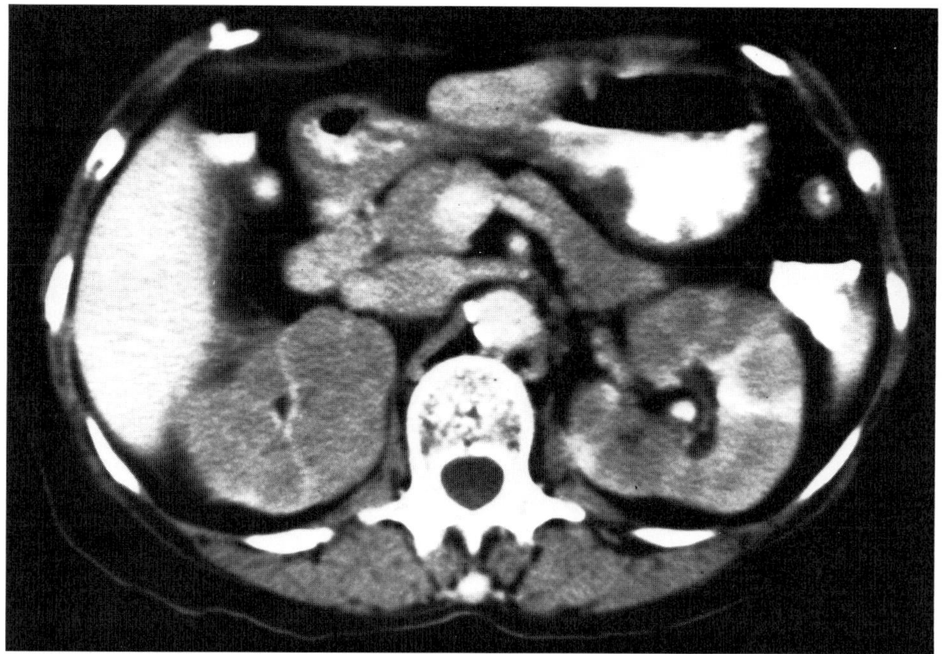

FIG. 5-12.   Multiple lymphomatous metastases of the kidney on CT. Note poorly enhancing masses bilaterally.

depiction of the extent of renal involvement[54] (Fig. 5-11). Multinodular lymphoma can produce renal insufficiency; however, this is often rapidly responsive to chemotherapy.[55] Multinodular renal lymphoma need not be associated with renal hilar lymphadenopathy, as the mechanism of spread can often be purely hematogenous in origin, but it is rarely the only site of disease in these instances (Fig. 5-12).

An important but less common pattern of urinary tract metatasis in lymphomas, myelomas, and leukemias is diffuse infiltration of renal parenchyma.[56] Leukemic infiltration is more common with lymphocytic cell types than by those of myelogenous origin. Renal function may only be compromised late in the disease. The hallmark of renal infiltration is diffuse enlargement of the kidneys with retention of the normal reniform shape.[57] The intensity of the nephrogram is decreased urographically, and on CT the calyces are often compressed by the cellular infiltrate and edema (Fig. 5-13). Function is delayed and the kidneys concentrate poorly. It is important, however, to distinguish lymphoproliferative infiltration from other causes of renal enlargement in patients with lymphoproliferative disorders, including interstitial nephritis (due to amphotericin or other drugs), pyelonephritis, and renal vein thrombosis, all of which can mimic secondary infiltration.[58] Gallium citrate scans are commonly nonspecific. Dramatic improvements in renal function can be seen with therapy.

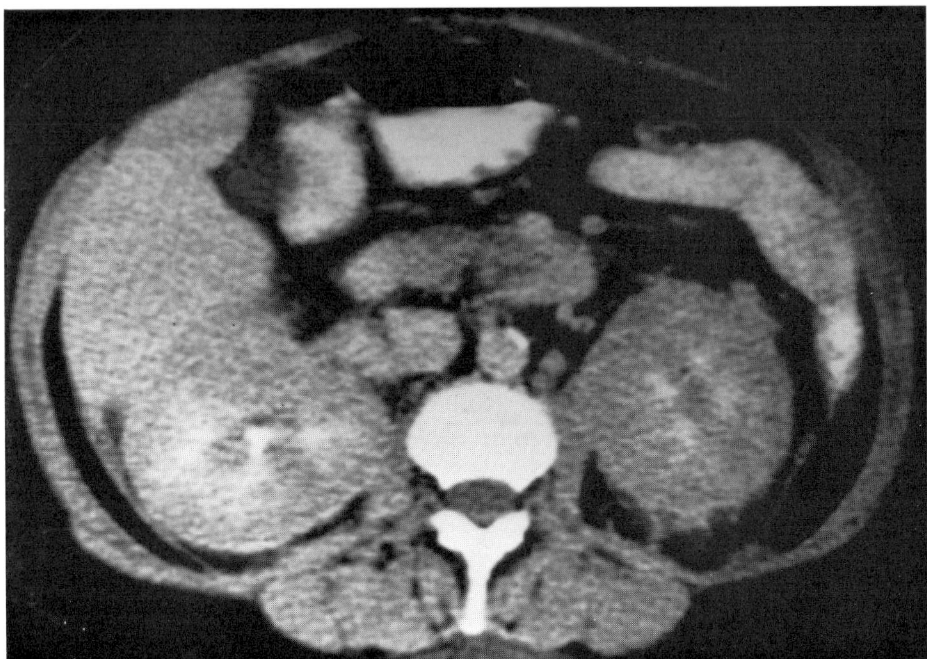

FIG. 5-13. Diffuse lymphomatous infiltration. Note bilateral renal enlargement with poor nephrogram. This pattern could either represent a confluence of multiple separate nodules as seen in Figure 5-12 or diffuse interstitial infiltration.

Ureter and Bladder

Malignant lymphoma is the third leading cause of metastases to the ureter.[38] It is invariably associated with retroperitoneal adenopathy but can appear as an isolated lesion (Fig. 5-14). Treatment can result in retroperitoneal fibrosis.

Patients with bladder lymphoma typically present with hematuria. Lymphomatous nodules are commonly multiple; however, the most frequent involvement by lymphoma or leukemia is microscopic.[59] Non-Hodgkin's lymphoma is more frequent than Hodgkin's disease[55] Extramedullary plasmacytomas have been described but are rarely associated with multiple myeloma.

ROLE OF BIOPSY

The decision to perform a biopsy must always be predicated on the individual clinical situation. Since renal metastases generally occur late in the disease, when widespread disease is often present, the differentiation of a new primary tumor from yet another metastasis involving the kidney will usually not contribute to patient management. In the special case of lymphoma, the additional presence of solid organ involvement (as opposed to lymphadenopathy alone)

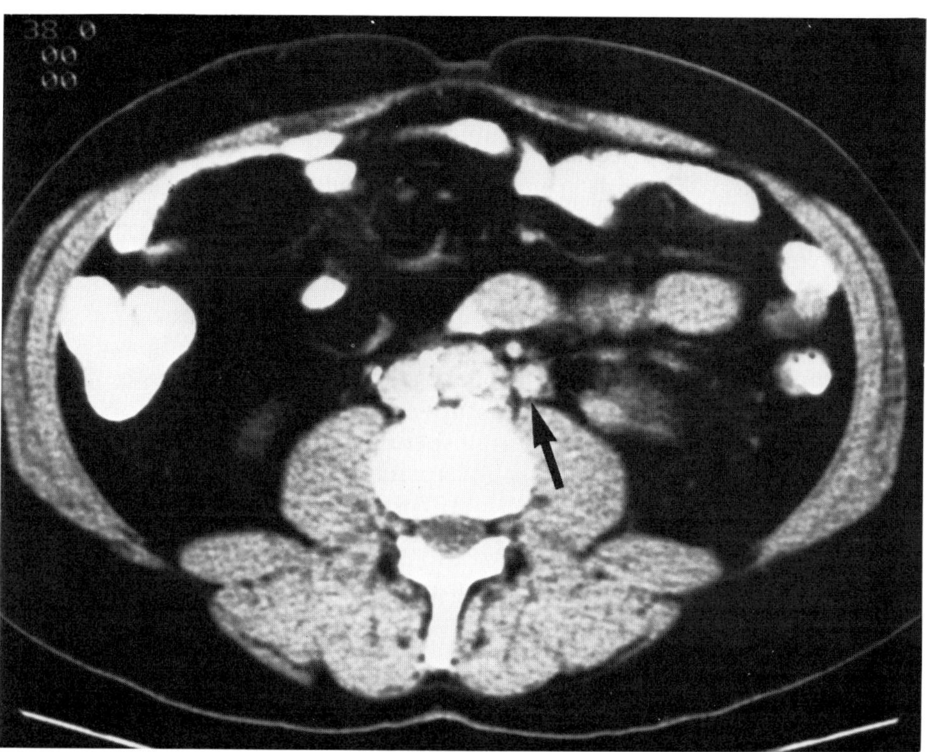

FIG. 5-14.   Ureteral metastasis arising from lymphoma. Note periureteric thickening on left side (arrow). Lymphangiographic contrast medium is seen in the retroperitoneal lymph nodes.

may have therapeutic ramifications. In cases in which the appearance of metastases is typical (i.e., multiple round or wedge-shaped lesions and bilateral involvement), the need for a biopsy may be obviated.

Patients with a *distant history* of tumor in whom a new renal mass is the sole manifestation of disease in the body will require an accurate diagnosis, since the early stages of renal cancer are theoretically curable, whereas a renal metastasis carries a relatively poor prognosis. A percutaneous biopsy could forestall an unnecessary nephrectomy in such cases. There are several important parts to a successful renal biopsy in this setting: patient selection as discussed, an adequate sample, and an informed and competent cytologist. Biopsies should be performed under the direct guidance of ultrasound or CT with 20- to 22-gauge thin-wall needles. Attempts should be made to avoid the more necrotic centers of the target lesion and direct the needle to the more vital lesion periphery. Several passes should be obtained to avoid sampling error. Complications are rare and tract seeding is exceedingly unusual.[60,61] It is crucial to inform the cytologist or pathologist of the history and to have available previous tissue samples for comparison, since metastatic lesions, particularly adenocarcinomas, can be mistaken for renal cell carcinomas.

SUMMARY

Metastases to the urinary tract are an increasingly frequent clinical problem and result from increased longevity, heightened surveillance, and improved recognition in cancer patients.[62] Most urinary tract metastases are clinically silent but occasionally result in massive life-threatening hematuria or severe pain. The radiographic appearances of metastases in the kidney range from solitary and exophytic, mimicking primary renal cancers, to multifocal bilateral or infiltrative. Perinephric involvement is seen in melanoma, lung cancers, and lymphomas. Ureteral and bladder involvement can be detected by CT or MRI. Although intraluminal involvement is rare, extrinsic or contiguous spread is more common and can result in obstruction of the urinary tract. Urinary tract metastases are an unusual but important clinical problem for which a combination of conventional urographic techniques as well as ultrasound, CT, or MRI are necessary for diagnosis and management.

REFERENCES

1. Abrams HL, Spiro R, Goldstein N: Metastases in carcinoma: Analysis of 1,000 autopsied cases. Cancer 3:74, 1950
2. Klinger ME: Secondary tumors of the genitourinary tract. J Urol 65:144, 1951
3. Bracken BR, Chica G, Johnson DE, Luna M: Secondary renal neoplasms: An autopsy study. South Med J 72:806, 1979
4. Galluzzi S, Payne PM: Bronchial carcinoma: A statistical study of 741 necropsies with specific references to the distribution of blood-born metastases. Br J Cancer 9:511, 1955
5. Wagle DG, Moore RH, Murphy GP: Secondary carcinomas of the kidney. J Urol 114:30, 1975
6. Babaian RJ, Johnson DE, Ayala AG, Sie ET: Secondary tumors of ureter. Urology 14:341, 1979
7. Sanchez J, Baker V, Miller DM: Basic mechanisms of metastasis. Am J Med Sci 292:376, 1986
8. Weiss L, Orr WF, Honn KV: Interactions of cancer with the microvasculature during metastasis. FASEB J 2:12, 1988
9. Hagmar B, Ryd W, Erkell LJ: Why do tumors metastasize? An overview of current research. Tumour Biol 5:141, 1984
10. Liotta LA: Mechanisms of cancer invasion and metastasis. Important Adv Oncol 28:41, 1985
11. Terranova VP, Hic S, Diflorio RM, Lyall RM: Tumor cell metastasis. CRC Crit Rev Oncol Hematol 5:87, 1986
12. Fidler IJ: Review: Biologic heterogeneity of cancer metastases. Breast Cancer Res Treatm 9:17, 1987
13. Schirrmacher V: Cancer metastasis: Experimental approaches, theoretical concepts, and impacts for treatment strategies. Adv Cancer Res 43:1, 1985
14. Nishitani H, Onitsuka H, Kawahira K, et al: Computed tomography of renal metastases. J Comput Assist Tomogr 8:727, 1984
15. Zeman RK Cronan JJ, Rosenfield AT, et al: Renal cell carcinoma: Dynamic thin-section CT assessment of vascular invasion and tumor vascularity. Radiology 167:383, 1988
16. Salo J, Alfthan O: Transurethral ultrasound versus CT scan. Prog Clin Biol Res 260:237, 1988

17. Silverstein LI, Plaine L, Favis JE, Kabokow B: Breast carcinoma metastatic to bladder. Urology 29:544, 1987

18. Quint LE, Glazer GM, Chenevert TL, et al: In vivo and in vitro MR imaging of renal tumors: Histopathologic correlation and pulse sequence optimization. Radiology 169:359, 1988

19. Hricak H, Thoen RF, Carroll PR: Detection and staging of renal neoplasms: A reassessment of MR imaging. Radiology 166:643, 1988

20. Fein AB, Lee JK, Balfe DM, et al: Diagnosis and staging of renal cell carcinoma: A comparison of MR imaging and CT. AJR 148:749, 1987

21. Petersen RO: Urologic Pathology. JB Lippincott, Philadelphia, 1986

22. Smith EB, Dunnick NR, Nelson P, Hammond CB: Renal metastases of malignant gestational trophoblastic disease: The use of intravenous urography in staging. Gynecol Oncol 20:317, 1985

23. Nieh PT, Waltman AC, Althauson AF: Therapeutic embolization of symptomatic renal tumors: J Urol 117:378, 1977

24. Thomas JL, Barnes PA, Bernadino ME, Lewis E: Diagnostic approaches to adrenal and renal metastases. Radiol Clin North Am 20:531, 1982

25. Becker WE, Schellhammer PF: Renal metastases from carcinoma of the lung. Br J Urol 58:494, 1986

26. Bosniak MA, Stern W, Lopez F, et al: Metastatic neoplasm to the kidney. Radiology 92:989, 1969

27. Choyke PL, White ME, Zeman RK, et al: Renal metastasis: Clinicopathologic and radiologic correlation. Radiology 162:359, 1987

28. Bhatt GM, Bernadino ME, Graham SD Jr: CT diagnosis of renal metastases. J Comput Assist Tomogr 7:1032, 1983

29. Goldstein C, Ambos JA, Bosniak MA: Multiple ossified metastases to the kidney from osteogenic sarcoma. AJR 128:148, 1977

30. Shirkhoda A: Computed tomography of perirenal metastases. J Comput Assist Tomogr 10:435, 1986

31. Roberts DI: Secondary neoplasms of the genito-urinary tract. Br J Urol 50:68, 1978

32. Newsam JE, Tulloch SW: Metastatic tumors in the kidney. Br J Urol 38:1, 1966

33. Honda H, Coffman CE, Flickinger FW, et al: CT analysis of metastatic neoplasms to the kidney: Comparison with primary renal cell carcinoma. RSNA Scientific Program. Radiology 169:193, 1988

34. Bosniak MA, Megibow AJ, Ambos JS, et al: Computed tomography of ureteral obstruction. AJR 138:1107, 1982

35. Ambos JS, Bosniak MA, Megibow A, Raghavendra B: Ureteral involvement by metastatic disease. Urol Radiol 1:105, 1979

36. Fitch WP, Robinson JR, Radwin HM: Metastatic carcinoma of the ureter. Arch Surg 111:874, 1976

37. Puech JL, Song MY, Joffre F: Ureteral metastases: CT findings. Eur J Radiol 7:103, 1987

38. Cohen WM, Freed SZ, Hasson J: Metastatic cancer to the ureter: A review of the literature and case presentation. J Urol 112:188, 1974

39. Kenny PJ: CT of ureteral tumors. J Comput Assist Tomogr 11:102, 1987

40. Fein AB, McClennan BL: Solitary filling defects of the ureter. Semin Roentgenol 21:201, 1986

41. Megibow AJ, Mitnick JS, Bosniak MA: The contribution of computed tomography to the evaluation of the obstructed ureter. Urol Radiol 4:95, 1982

42. Melicow MM: Tumors of the urinary bladder: A clinicopathological analysis of over 2,500 specimens and biopsies. J Urol 74:498, 1955

43. Bartone FF: Metastatic melanoma of the bladder. J Urol 91:151, 1964

44. Ganem EJ, Batal JT: Secondary malignant tumors of the urinary bladder metastatic from primary foci in distant organs. J Urol 75:965, 1956

45. Pontes JES, Oldford JR: Metastatic breast carcinoma to the bladder. J Urol 104:839, 1970

46. Haid M, Ignatoff J, Khandekar JD, et al: Urinary bladder metastases from breast carcinoma. Cancer 46:229, 1980

47. Stein BS: Malignant melanoma of the genitourinary tract. J Urol 132:859, 1984

48. Richmond J, Sherman RS, Diamond HD, Craver CF: Renal lesions associated with malignant lymphomas. Am J Med 32:184, 1962

49. Martinez-Maldonado M, De Arellano GAR: Renal involvement in malignant lymphomas: A survey of 49 cases. J Urol 95:485, 1966

50. Hartman DS, Davis CJ, Goldman SM, et al: Renal lymphoma. Radiologic-pathologic correlation of 21 cases. Radiology 144:757, 1982

51. Rubin BE: Computed tomography in the evaluation of renal lymphoma. J Comput Assist Tomogr 3:759, 1979

52. Chilcote WA, Barkowski KGP: Computed tomography in renal lymphoma. J Comput Assist Tomogr 7:439, 1983

53. Hartman DS, Davidson AJ, Davis CJ, Goldman SM: Infiltrative renal lesions: CT-sonographic-pathologic correlation. AJR 150:1061, 1988

54. Richards MA: Magnetic resonance imaging in lymphoma. Cancer Surv 6:315, 1987

55. Miyake O, Namiki M, Sonod T, Kitamura H: Secondary involvement of genitourinary organs in malignant lymphoma. Urol Int 42:360, 1987

56. Ambos JA, Bosniak MA, Madayag MA, Lefleur RS: Infiltrating neoplasms of the kidney. AJR 129:859, 1977

57. Lalli AF: Lymphoma and the urinary tract. Radiology 93:1051, 1969

58. Weimar G, Culp DA, Koening S, Nasayana A: Urogenital involvement by malignant lymphomas. J Urol 125:230, 1981

59. Sufrin G, Keogh B, Moore RH, Murphy GP: Secondary involvement of the bladder in malignant lymphoma. J Urol 118:251, 1987

60. Ferrucci JT, Wittenberg J, Mueller PR, et al: Diagnosis of abdominal malignancy by radiologic fine-needle aspiration biopsy. AJR 134:323, 1980

61. Livraghi T, Damascelli B, Lombardi C, Spagnoli I: Risk in fine-needle abdominal biopsy. J Clin Ultrasound 11:77, 1983

62. Mitnick JS, Bosniak MA, Rothberg M, et al: Metastatic neoplasm to the kidney studied by computed tomography and sonography. J Comput Assist Tomogr 9:43, 1985

6 CT and MRI of Upper Urinary Tract Obstruction

PHILIP J. KENNEY

Obstruction of the urinary tract may occur at any level from the calyx to the urethral meatus. This discussion concentrates on ureteral obstruction. It should be recognized that lower urinary tract obstruction can result in similar changes in the upper tracts. Nevertheless, lower tract obstruction will be distinguishable from upper tract obstruction by such features as bilaterality of upper tract changes, bladder distention and/or bladder wall hypertrophy, and voiding abnormalities.[1]

Today, many diagnostic procedures can detect upper urinary tract obstruction. The value of CT and MRI can only be appreciated with an understanding of the capabilities and limitations of the other diagnostic techniques available. Acute ureteral obstruction causes a typical symptom complex, including renal colic. Intravenous (IV) urography is usually diagnostic in such cases. Occasionally, sonography or retrograde pyelography may be useful, but rarely are CT or MRI needed. Chronic ureteral obstruction commonly has an insidious nonspecific presentation. Obstruction causes loss of renal function. Eventually this causes nonvisualization of the kidney at urography, but nonvisualization can result from many other causes. IV urography remains the most cost-effective radiologic method for initial evaluation of urinary tract abnormalities, including hematuria and suspected obstruction. However, it is often inadequate, especially in cases of long-standing obstruction. Even if hydronephrosis is identified on the IV pyelogram (IVP), the exact site and etiology of the obstruction are often obscure.

Sonography is useful in screening cases of suspected obstruction and in further evaluating kidneys that function poorly at urography.[2] Sonography does not rely on function of the kidney. Sonography examines the kidney in a "resting state," not in a diuretic state as stimulated by contrast. It can accurately detect or exclude ureteral obstruction. Sonography has a reported accuracy of up to 98 percent in detecting hydronephrosis in nonfunctioning kidneys.[3] Its sensitivity and specificity are over 90 percent in patients with an elevated serum creatinine of uncertain cause.[4] Sonography is also useful because it is widely available and relatively inexpensive and has no significant ill effects. Thus, it is especially useful as a screening procedure. Nevertheless, sonography has serious limitations. Obstruction is diagnosed by sonography when there is dilatation of the collecting system, pelvis, or ureter. Obstruction that has not resulted in dilatation will be missed on sonography.[5,6] Blunted calyces caused by papillary necrosis or chronic pyelonephritis, or a capacious extrarenal pelvis may be misconstrued as hydronephrosis, as may a dilated nonobstructed system.[2,7] A much more common limitation of sonography is this: *while ultrasound is very good at detecting hydronephrosis, it is not very effective at identifying the cause, since the obstructed region often is obscured by bowel gas anteriorly and bone posteriorly.*

The retrograde pyelogram and percutaneous nephrostogram are invasive techniques that have important roles in the diagnosis of upper urinary tract obstruction. Both are highly accurate, when technically successful, at detecting not only obstruction but also the site and, often, the etiology. These techniques are especially useful, since relief of the obstruction can be achieved by stent or nephrostomy placement. Nevertheless, these procedures are relatively expensive, require some anesthesia, and may result in infection or hemorrhage. Unsuccessful attempts are not rare. While extremely useful, these techniques are best reserved for patients known to have obstruction, based on prior diagnostic procedures. They are not screening procedures.

CT OF OBSTRUCTION

Role of CT

With all the above points in mind, it is clear that the role of CT is limited. Most cases of obstruction can be diagnosed and treated without need for CT. CT is more expensive and less widely available than urography and sonography. What is its proper role? While CT will never be a screening tool and is useful only in selected cases, it has advantages that make it a very powerful tool for detecting the site and etiology of obstruction, especially when renal function is poor.[8,9]

CT is noninvasive, and the risks of the radiation exposure and contrast are no greater than with urography. It is accessible for most patients in the United States. It is easily performed in reproducible fashion. It does not require function of the kidney in order to visualize the urinary tract, and gas and bone do not obscure abnormalities. It shows not only the urinary tract but all surrounding structures. Although contrast material is not needed to visualize the urinary tract, CT can show abnormal patterns of contrast excretion. CT can be useful, therefore, not only to detect obstruction but to visualize the cause directly. In one study, CT allowed correct diagnosis in all 14 cases of unilaterally nonfunctioning kidneys.[8] CT can distinguish among an absent kidney, a non-functioning hydronephrotic kidney, or an infarcted kidney better than sonography. In another report, correct diagnosis of the cause of ureteral obstruction was made on CT in 92 percent of 36 cases of hydronephrosis of uncertain etiology.[9] It was possible to distinguish intrinsic from extrinsic tumors accurately and to distinguish calculi from soft tissue masses. Because of all these factors, CT can be extremely useful in further evaluating cases of suspected ureteral obstruction when previous screening procedures have been inadequate, before the use of more invasive procedures, or when such procedures (especially retrograde pyelography) have failed.

An important factor that guides clinical management of obstructive uropathy is the presence of salvageable renal tissue. While more quantitative and physiologic tests such as radionuclide scans are more definitive, CT can show parenchymal thickness. If a mere shell is present, it is unlikely that there is recoverable function.

Technique

Attention to a few technical details is necessary to obtain diagnostic images of the kidney and ureter. Adequate images of the kidney and ureter are usually obtained with 10-mm-thick contiguous slices (Figs. 6-1 and 6-2). CT scans of the lower abdomen and pelvis are often performed with an interslice gap. While the presence of hydronephrosis can usually be detected with such technique, the exact site and cause of obstruction may be missed. Thin sections (5 mm usually suffices) help in detecting small calculi or intrinsic tumors; thin sections are also needed to get accurate density readings of small lesions. The entire ureter should be imaged. Sometimes this requires slices to the perineum, as in the case of urinary anomalies.[10]

Contrast enhancement is not necessary to detect hydronephrosis or to visualize the dilated ureter, and contrast medium should not be administered when there is significant renal insufficiency. Nevertheless, contrast is useful when possible. Delayed excretion makes the presence of obstruction more obvious. Enhancement of the ureteral wall can make it more recognizable, and ureteral tumors will be enhanced making them more visible.[11] The use of contrast can help avoid confusing an extrarenal pelvis with hydronephrosis. When there is residual function, contrast may fill the obstructed ureter, permitting a clearer definition of the site of obstruction. This will often require performance of delayed scans (30 to 60 minutes or more after contrast injection) to allow filling of the ureter (Fig. 6-3). If there is a filling defect in the ureter, noncontrast scans should be done in order to determine whether one is dealing with calculus or tumor. Calculi may be obscured by the contrast.

Routine filming technique is usually sufficient. However, wide (bone) windows may help visualize small soft tissue masses surrounded by contrast.[12] Magnified views may also help in viewing small ureteral lesions.

Normal Anatomy

The normal renal pelvis is variable in size, but the calyces are usually not apparent on CT (Fig. 6-1). The kidney parenchyma should have symmetric thickness and contrast enhancement. In the early dynamic phase, cortico-

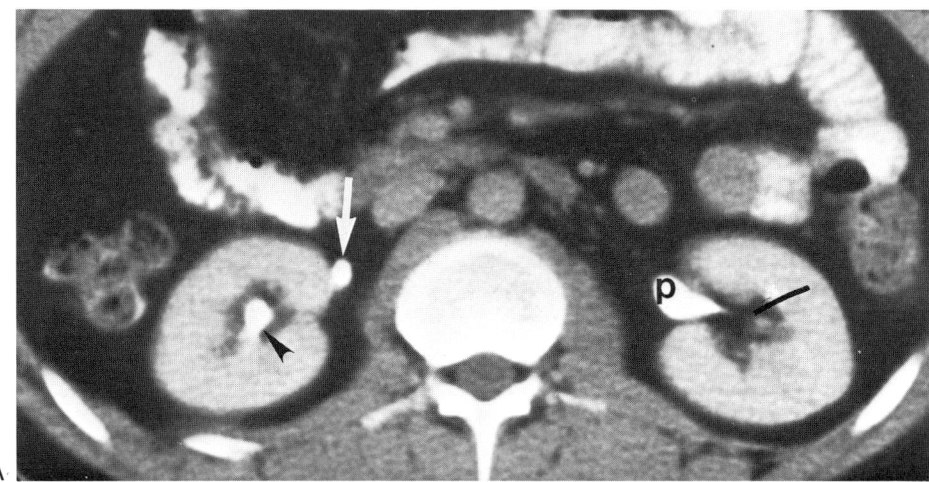

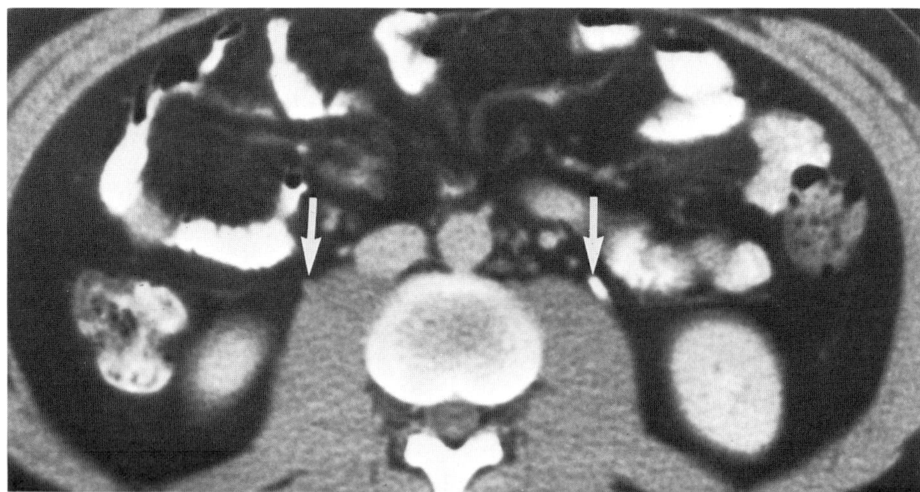

FIG. 6-1. Normal renal and ureteral anatomy. (A) In this normal patient, there is symmetric enhancement of the renal parenchyma, filling of the left renal pelvis (p), and proximal right ureter (arrow). The lower pole major calyx is seen on the right (arrowhead) but the minor calyces on the left are not apparent. (B) More inferiorly, the ureters (arrows) course anterior to the psoas muscle. The right ureter appears unenhanced, due to a normal peristaltic contraction. *(Figure continues.)*

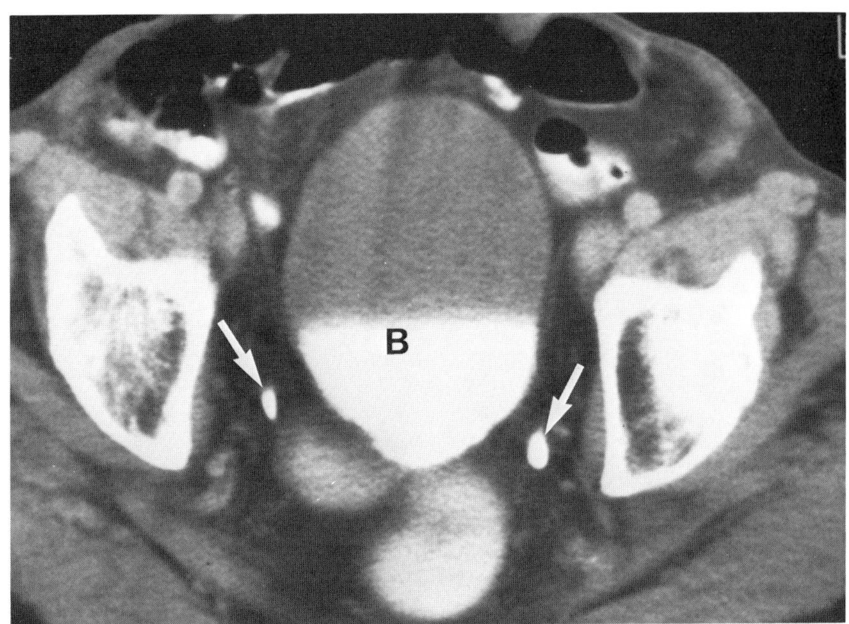

C

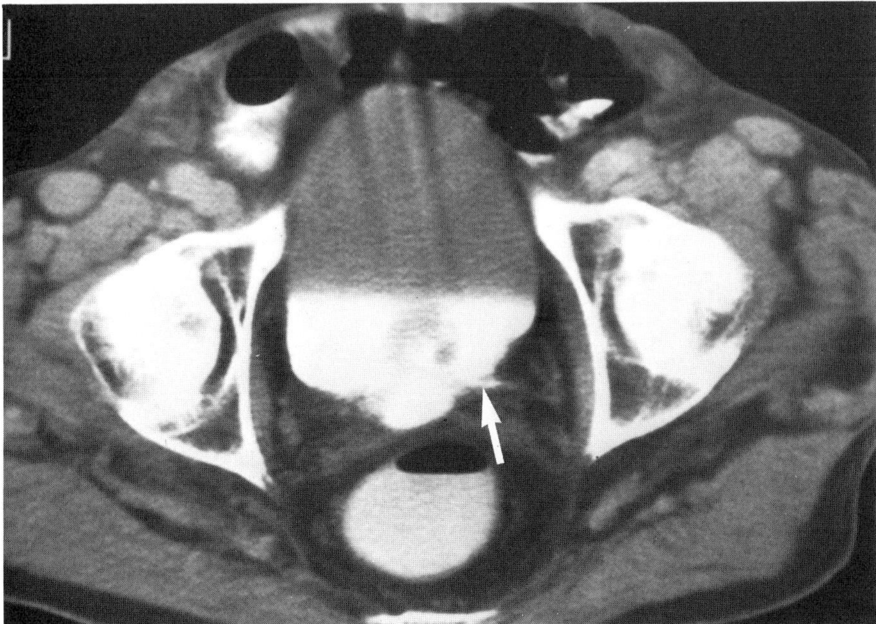

D

FIG. 6-1 *(Continued).*   (C) The ureters (arrows) are seen in the midpelvis, nearing the bladder (B). (D) The right ureterovesical junction (arrow) can be seen in this patient.

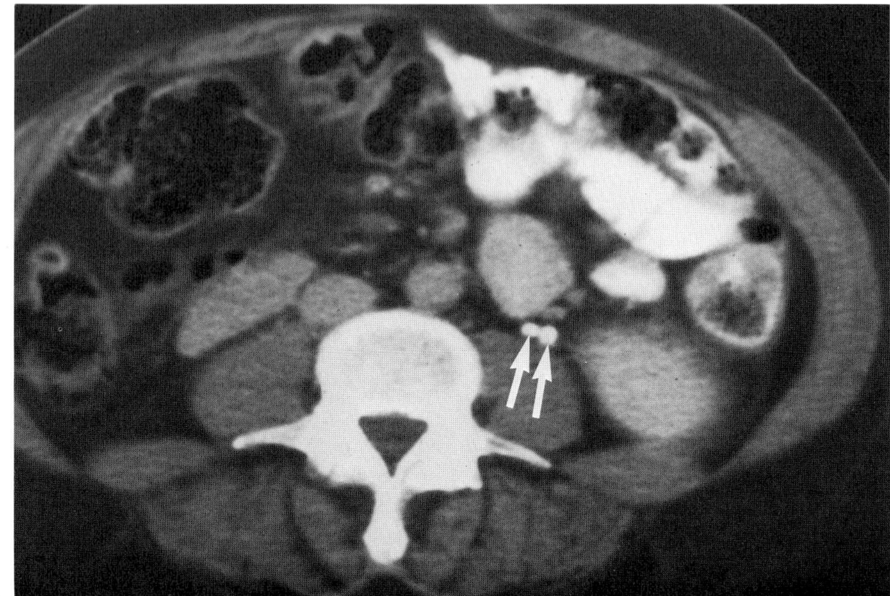

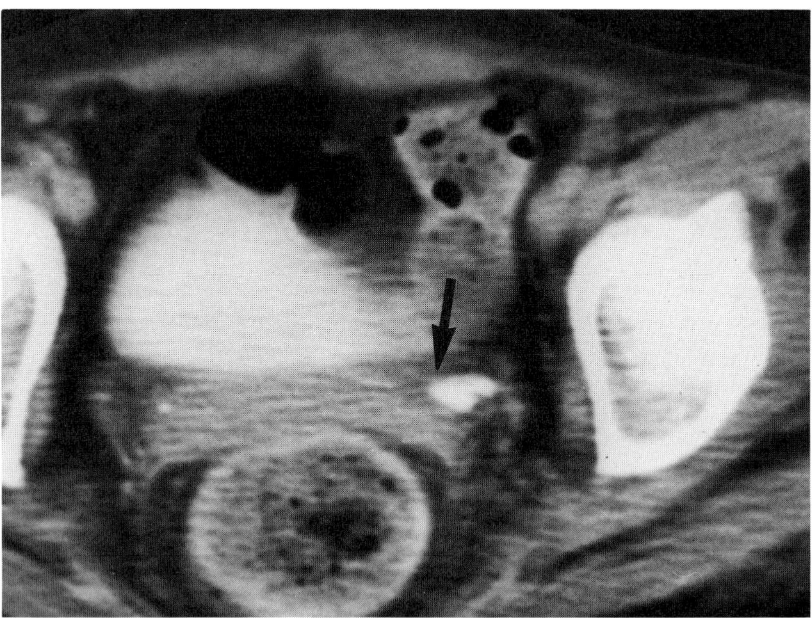

FIG. 6-2. This patient has a duplicated left ureter. Right nephrectomy was performed in the past. (A) Two normal ureters (arrows) are clearly seen coursing together anterior to the psoas. (B) The ureters join at the ureterovesical junction with a single ureteral orifice (arrow).

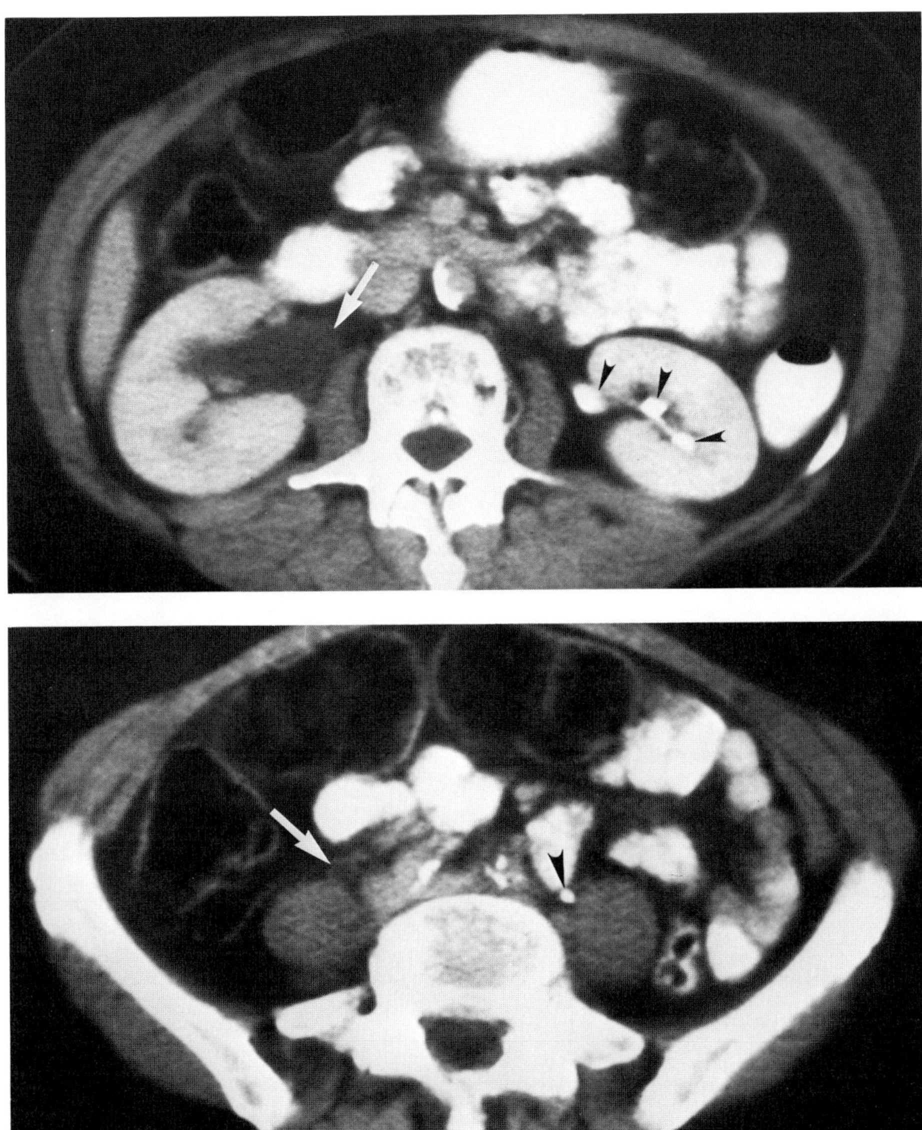

FIG. 6-3. This 62-year-old woman received radiation therapy 2 years previously for cervical carcinoma. (A) An image of the kidneys 2 minutes after a bolus of intravenous contrast shows enhancement of renal parenchyma of normal thickness bilaterally; the calyces and pelvis on the left are normal. On the right, a dilated pelvis (arrow) is present with delayed opacification. (B) At the pelvic brim, the unopacified dilated right ureter (arrow) can be seen as well as the normal left ureter (arrowhead). *(Figure continues.)*

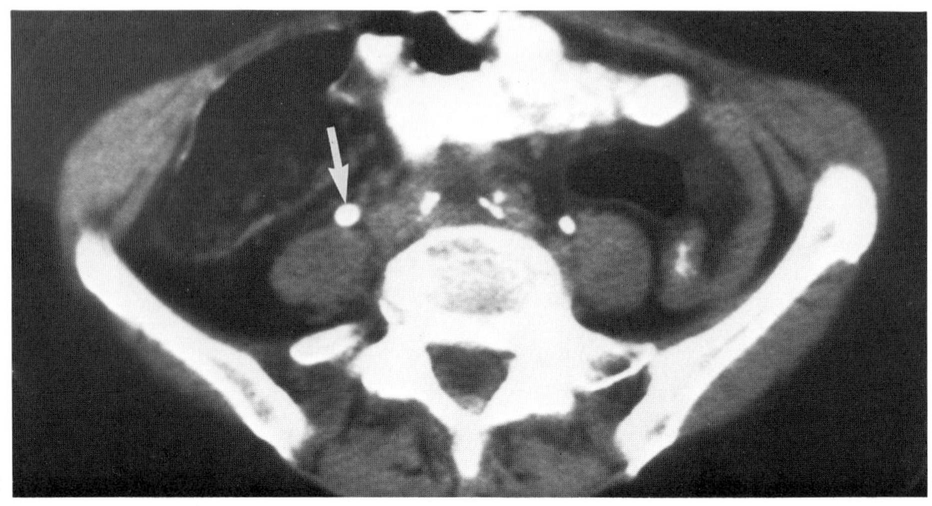

C

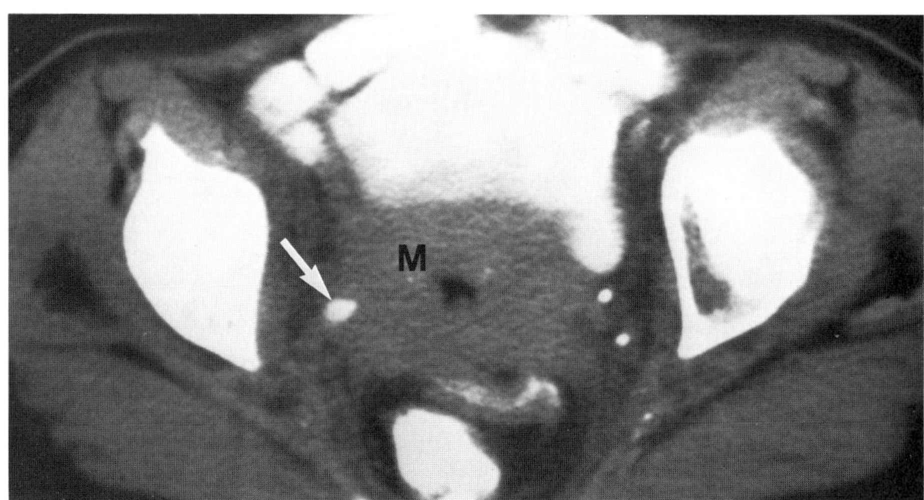

D

FIG. 6-3 *(Continued).*   (C) One hour after contrast injection, the right ureter (arrow) is filled with contrast (B). (D) In the pelvis, delayed view shows the right ureter (arrow) obstructed by a soft tissue mass (M) due to recurrent cervical carcinoma.

medullary differentiation is normal. Appearance of contrast in the collecting system should occur at the same time on both sides.

The normal ureter originates in the most inferior portion of the renal pelvis and passes inferiorly anterior to the psoas muscle. It drapes over the iliac vessels as it enters the pelvis. On contrast-enhanced scans, the ureter is readily seen as a white dot in the expected location (Fig. 6-1). Because of peristalsis, the ureter may be seen on some slices but not on others (Fig. 6-1B). The unenhanced normal ureter is unrecognizable, but a dilated ureter can be followed from the pelvis down along this course (Figs. 6-3 and 6-4). With ureteral duplication, two ureters will exit the renal sinus and follow closely together until they join or enter the bladder (Fig. 6-2). If there is ureteral ectopy, the ureter may be seen entering the bladder neck, urethra, seminal vesicle, vagina, and so forth[10] (Fig. 6-5).

CT Findings of Obstruction

The earliest CT findings of ureteral obstruction are dilatation of calyces, pelvis, and ureter and delayed opacification of these structures. If the obstruction is mild or not of long duration, the dilated ureter may fill with contrast on delayed views (Fig. 6-3). Eventually there is loss of renal function, and no enhancement of the hydronephrotic system occurs. Although abnormal enhancement patterns in obstructed kidneys have been described, they are not diagnostically accurate by themselves.[13] With long-standing severe obstruction, there will be thinning of renal parenchyma, resulting in a shell of tissue surrounding a hydronephrotic sac. Unlike simple cysts, the rim of cortex surrounding such a sac will be enhanced[8] (Fig. 6-4). Such a kidney may be either large or small. In addition to functional changes and dilatation, CT will clearly show the point of obstruction and the obstructing lesion. The ureter will be dilated to the point of obstruction, but will be normal or inapparent below (Fig. 6-4). At this site, a lesion will be seen, and its characteristics can indicate the diagnosis.

Calculi

Urinary calculi are one of the most common causes of upper urinary tract obstruction. CT is only necessary in a limited number of cases, since most calculi are apparent on plain radiographs, urography, and direct pyelography. CT may be used to prove that a calcification lies in the ureter when the kidney is nonfunctioning (Fig. 6-4). This may be especially worthwhile if retrograde pyelography has failed. CT is useful for evaluating radiolucent calculi.[14] On urography and pyelography, these may simulate ureteral tumors. Cytology is notoriously unreliable in such situations, since false-positive results are common with well-differentiated tumors, and false-positive results can result from chronic inflammation. Carefully done CT (thin sections, pre- and postcontrast) will show that the lesion is a calculus, since all calculi are much more dense than soft tissue. Urate calculi are reported to have Hounsfield numbers of 100 to 300.[11,14–16] Radiopaque stones such as calcium oxalate and struvite have higher densities, 300 to 800 HU. Ureteral tumors are in the 20- to 40-HU range. Some investigators have suggested that CT density readings may be useful to determine stone composition.[15,16] This has not been shown to be clinically useful, however. One of the greatest potential difficulties with

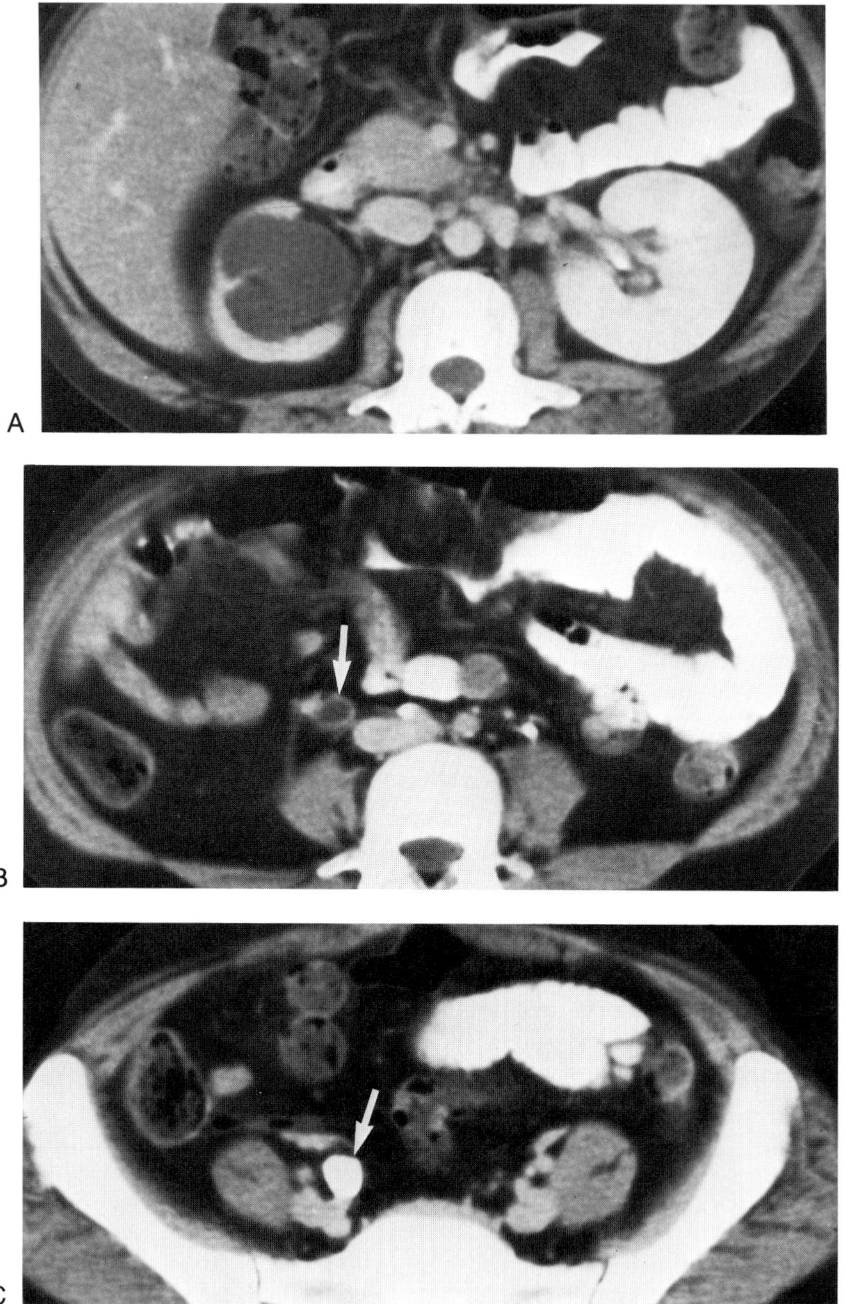

FIG. 6-4. Right hydronephrosis was detected on sonography in this 45-year-old diabetic woman. A 1 × 2-cm calcification was present in the right lower quadrant on plain radiographs. (A) CT scan shows marked cortical atrophy on the right with a dilated, unenhanced collecting system. Note that the rim of residual parenchyma is enhanced. (B) The dilated, right ureter (arrow) can be followed. (C) A calculus (arrow) lies within the right ureter. This was the cause of obstruction, since the ureter was not dilated below this level.

126

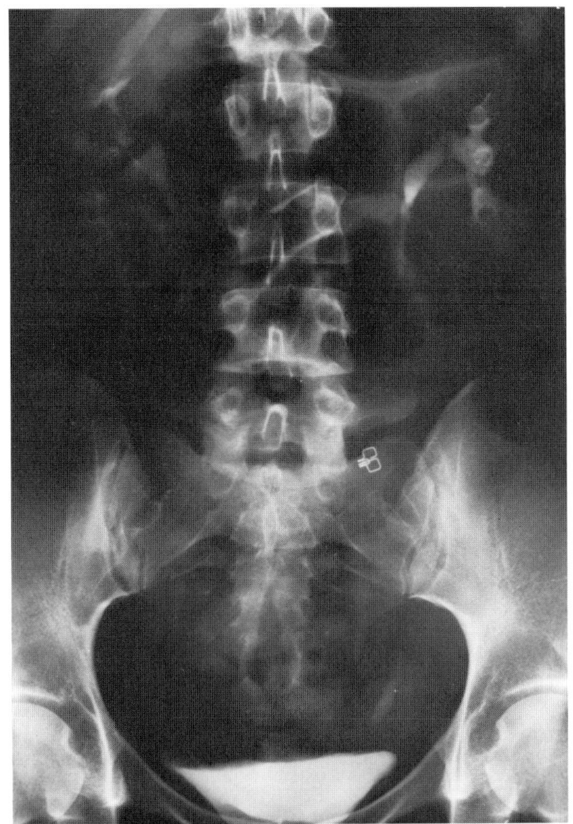

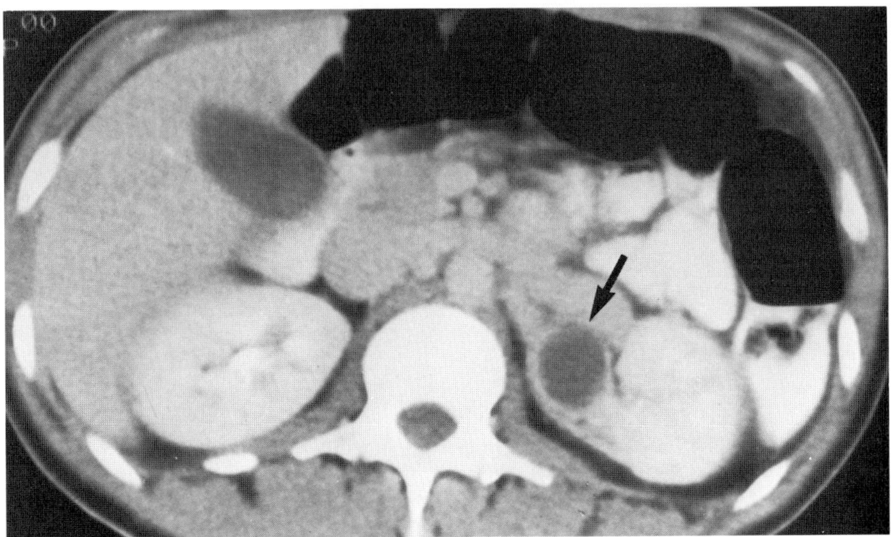

FIG. 6-5. Fever and pelvic pain were the presenting symptoms in this 31-year-old woman. (A) Intravenous urogram shows slightly subtle mass effect suggesting a non-visualized left upper pole. The bladder is normal. (B) CT was requested to rule out abscess. A 2.5-cm cystic area (arrow) is shown in the medial upper left kidney. *(Figure continues.)*

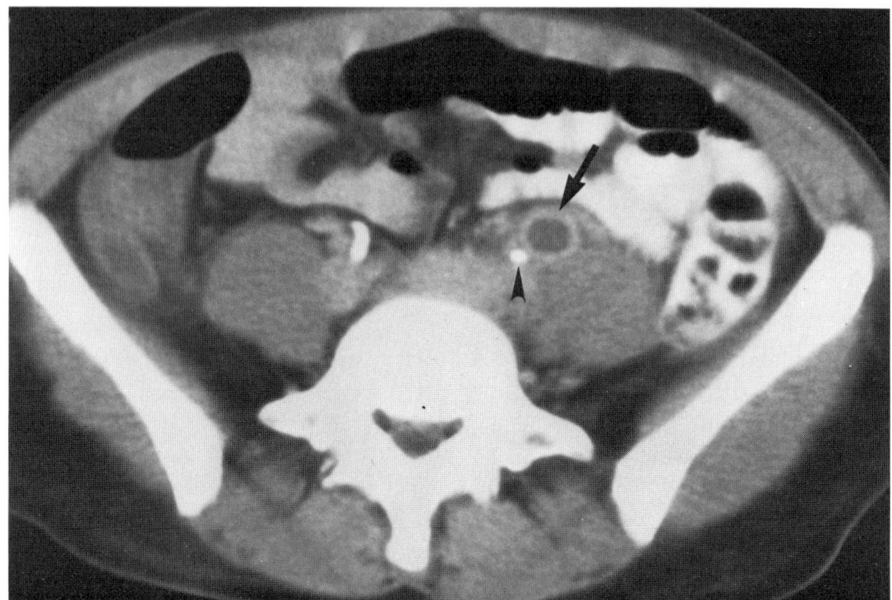

C

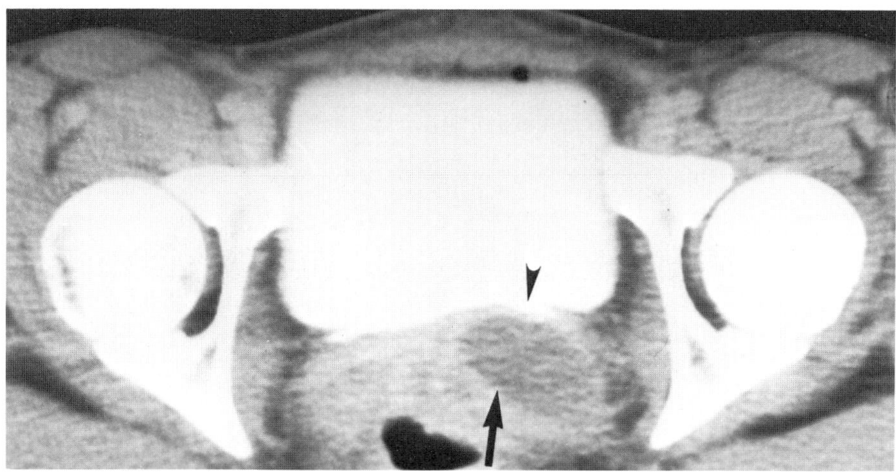

D

FIG. 6-5 *(Continued)*.   (C) A dilated tubular structure (arrow) courses from the cystic structure alongside the left ureter (arrowhead). (D) There is no intravesical ureterocele; the tubular structure (arrow) ends in the vagina. Note the normal left ureteral orifice (arrowhead). Surgery confirmed the diagnosis of complete duplication of the ureter with an obstructed ectopic upper pole ureter ending in the vagina.

this is the high incidence of stones of mixed composition.[11] Nevertheless, CT is useful because all stones, including radiolucent calculi, appear "pure white" on CT scans filmed with standard abdominal windows[11] (Fig. 6-6). Noncontrast scans must be done if a stone is suspected, since contrast medium will obscure the stone (see the section, *Technique*).

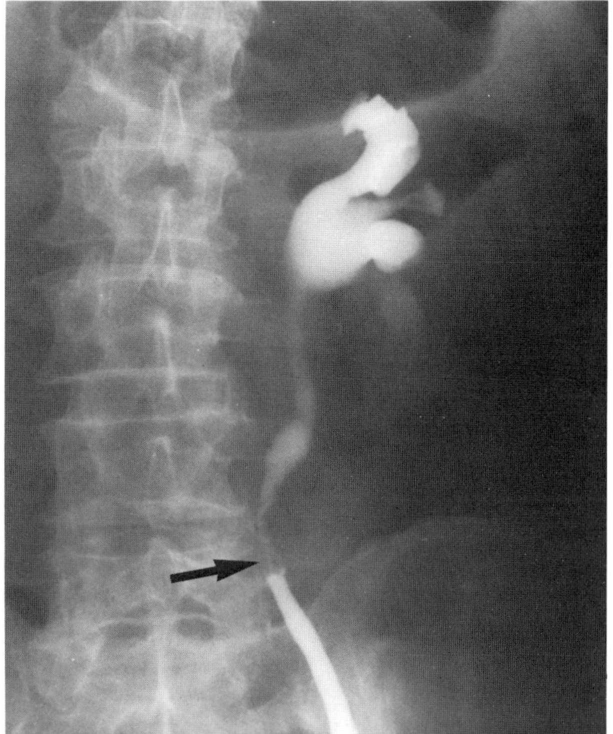

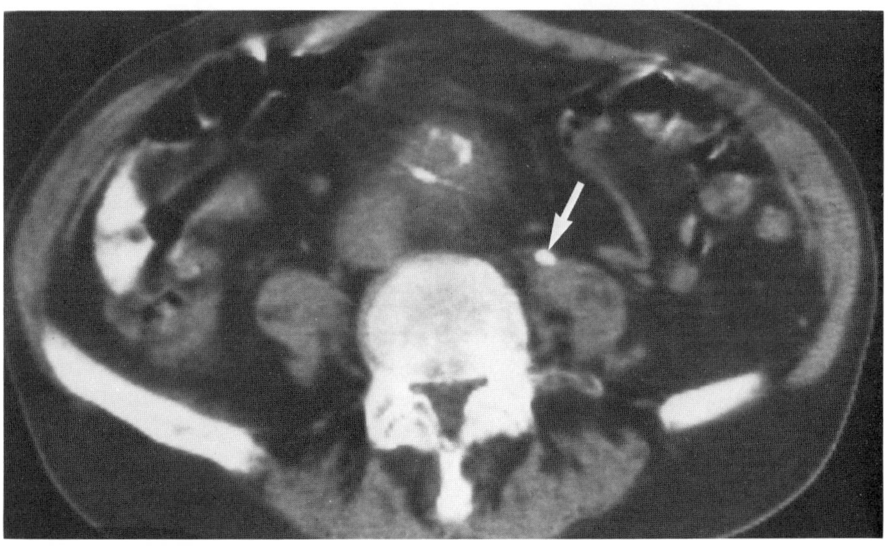

FIG. 6-6. This 70-year-old man had a palpable aortic aneurysm and mild renal insufficiency. Intravenous urogram showed left hydronephrosis but poor visualization of the left ureter. No radiopaque calculi were seen. (A) Retrograde pyelogram shows a filling defect (arrow). Cytology was "atypical," and the serum urate level was high. (B) Noncontrast CT at the level of the filling defect shows a calculus (arrow), subsequently unremoved by ureterolithotomy.

Upper Urinary Tract Uroepithelial Tumors

While intrinsic ureteral tumors are not common, they can present diagnostic difficulties. Signs and symptoms are nonspecific. Upper urinary tract uroepithelial tumors often are missed on urography.[17] Cytology has limited sensitivity, with 30 percent false-negative results.[18] When a filling defect is detected on urography, retrograde pyelography often is diagnostic (72 to 85 percent)[19,20] but sometimes fails. As noted above, CT is capable of distinguishing stone from tumor. Ureteral tumors have soft tissue density (20 to 50 HU) and can enhance slightly after contrast (30 to 90 HU).[11,12] Blood clot has somewhat higher density (50 to 60 HU) than unenhanced renal parenchyma but is not enhanced and a clot will not persist in the same location in the urinary tract.[11,14] Ureteral tumors are usually transitional cell and typically are small, round, filling defects confined within the ureter or renal pelvis[12,21] (Fig. 6-7). Occasionally more infiltrative lesions occur and invade adjacent structures. Concentric thickening of the ureteral wall may also be seen.[21] Multifocal lesions are common. Probably the circumstance in which CT is most valuable is in the patient with severe hydronephrosis, such that urography is nondiagnostic (Fig. 6-7). CT will reliably detect a ureteral tumor in such a patient. In addition, many patients who present in such a fashion will not have a ureteral tumor, but some other obstructive lesion that can be diagnosed by CT. Many such patients will not require retrograde pyelography. CT is especially useful in patients with negative urine cytology, or in whom ureteral tumor was not a strong clinical suspicion, or in whom retrograde pyelography failed. CT may serendipitously detect upper urinary tract tumors in patients being evaluated for bladder cancer. CT is also useful for staging ureteral tumors, since it can distinguish localized from advanced disease with more than 95 percent accuracy.[21]

Extrinsic Masses

Primary uroepithelial tumors are usually small and confined within the pelvis or ureter. They are distinguished by CT from extrinsic masses, which are usually large and not confined within the ureter. Extrinsic masses may cause obstruction by compression or invasion of the ureter (Figs. 6-3, 6-8, and 6-9). CT can show not only evidence of obstruction, but also the mass itself. Any neoplasm that arises in, invades, or metastasizes to the retroperitoneum can cause obstruction. Inflammatory masses (e.g., retroperitoneal abscess, Crohn's disease, retroperitoneal fibrosis) can also cause ureteral obstruction. The CT appearance of such lesions has been well covered in other texts.[22,23] CT has been shown to be highly accurate in detecting obstruction and the obstructing mass in such cases.[1,9] The CT features of the mass may allow correct diagnosis of the lesion, but it is not possible in all cases to distinguish inflammatory from neoplastic masses. CT-directed biopsy may be done, however.

CT has become a standard method of staging and following patients with

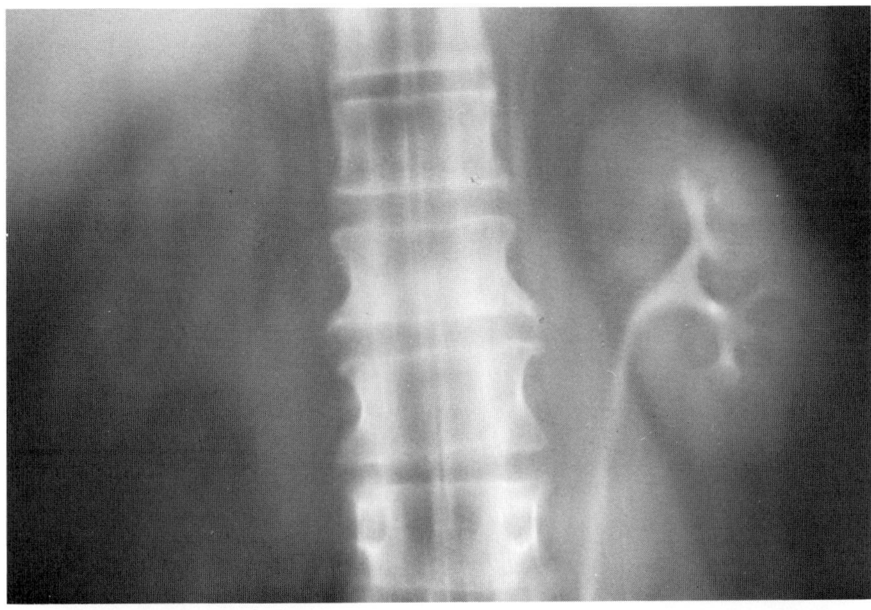

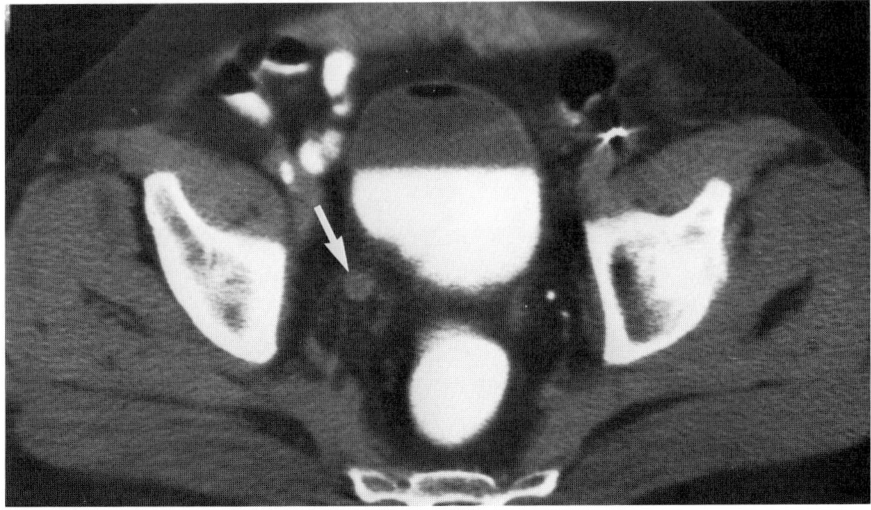

FIG. 6-7.   This 73-year-old man had severe hydronephrosis. (A) Intravenous urogram done to investigate hematuria revealed a nonvisualizing right kidney. No calculi were detected. Sonography confirmed hydronephrosis but was otherwise unrevealing. (B) CT showed a dilated right ureter (arrow). In the pelvis, the ureter is filled with soft tissue density, typical of a primary ureteral tumor. Note the indistinctness of the ureteral wall—tumor and wall have the same density. *(Figure continues.)*

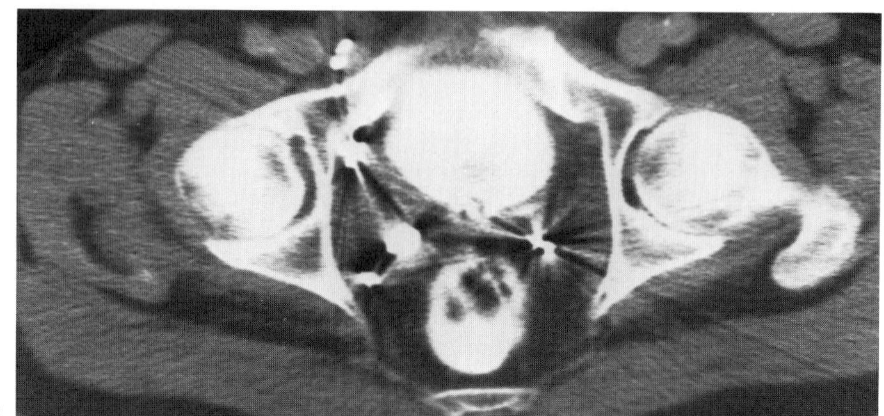

C

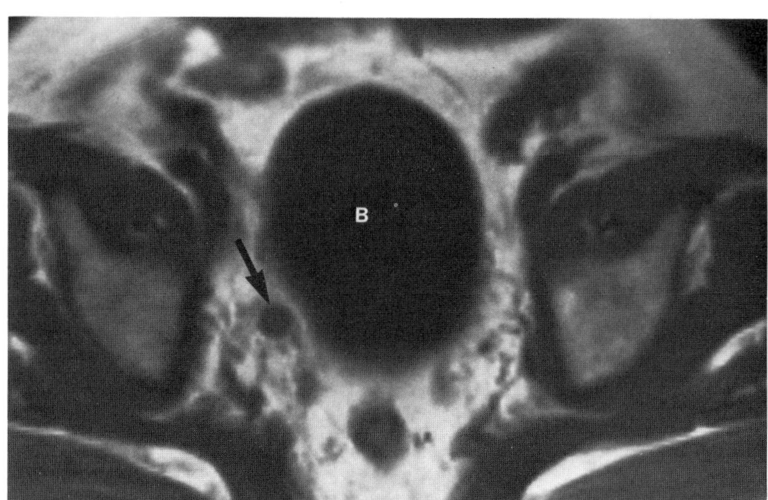

D

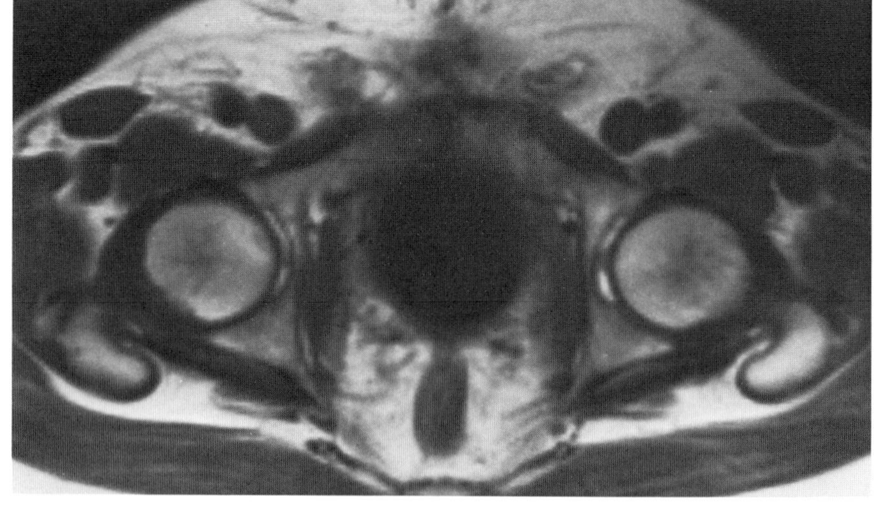

E

FIG. 6-7 *(Continued)*.   (C) Clips from prior prostatectomy cause significant artifact in the low pelvis. (D) T_1-weighted MRI (same level as Fig. B) also shows dilated right ureter (arrow) with medium signal intensity. The lesion was hyperintense on T_2 weighted scan. B, bladder. (E) Lower in the pelvis, note the virtual absence of clip artifact. Ureteral tumor was resected by nephroureterectomy.

abdominal neoplasms. It has also become commonly used for evaluating abdominal inflammatory processes. Thus, it is often the case that unsuspected upper urinary tract obstruction is first discovered on CT, frequently as a sign of recurrent tumor (Figs. 6-3 and 6-9). CT is quite useful in such cases because it can accurately determine the extent of the disease as well as detect the obstruction (Fig. 6-8).

Ureteral Strictures and Congenital Anomalies

When hydronephrosis is discovered on CT, the dilated urine-filled ureter can be followed on sequential slices until there is a change in caliber, indicating the point of obstruction. If, even with careful technique, no stone or tumor is identified, the diagnosis is most often ureteral stricture. This can be either

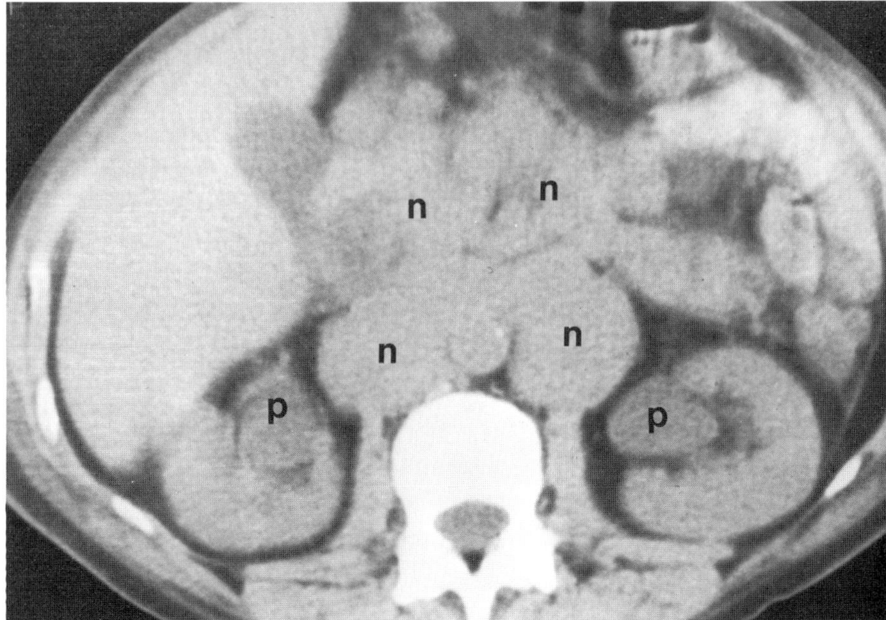

FIG. 6-8.   Several years after treatment of non-Hodgkin's lymphoma, this patient presented in renal failure. Bilateral hydronephrosis is evident on this noncontrast CT, as well as extensive lymphadenopathy (n), the cause of the obstruction. p, pelvis.

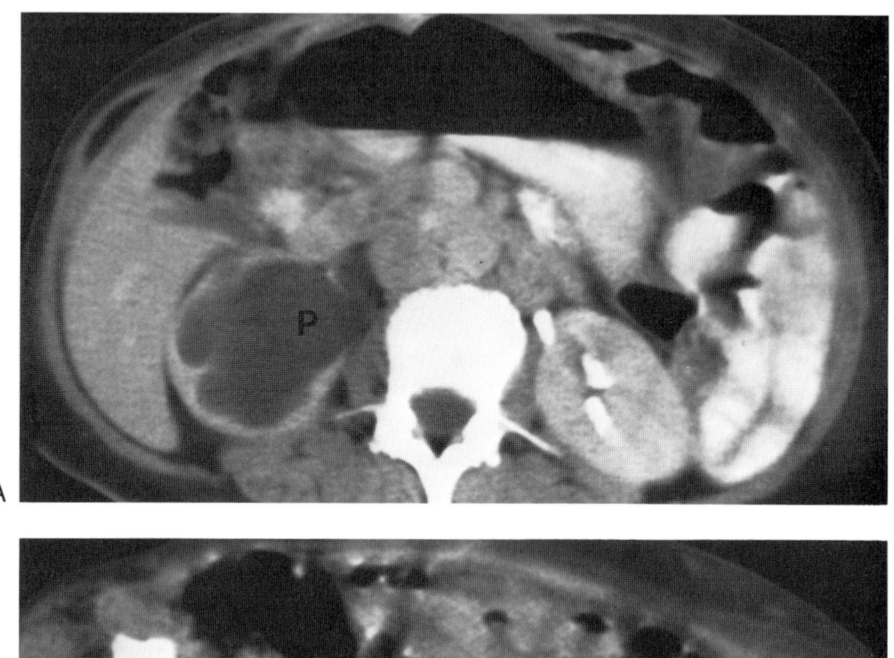

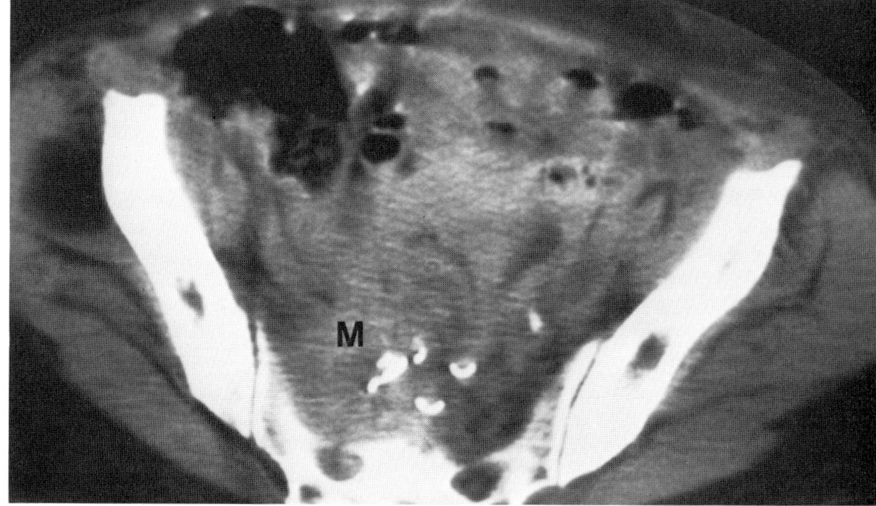

FIG. 6-9.   Carcinoma of the rectum had been resected surgically in the past in this 57-year-old woman. (A) Follow-up enhanced CT shows marked right hydronephrosis. p, pelvis. (B) The dilated right ureter extended into a presacral mass (M) (surgical clips present). *(Figure continues.)*

congenital or acquired. It is debatable whether confirmation by antegrade or retrograde pyelography is necessary. In some cases, this is valuable, since dilatation of the stricture may be done. However, if the kidney is not salvageable, nephrectomy may be performed directly.

Unfortunately, in patients with a history of previous malignancy and newly discovered ureteral obstruction, CT is unable to distinguish acquired stricture

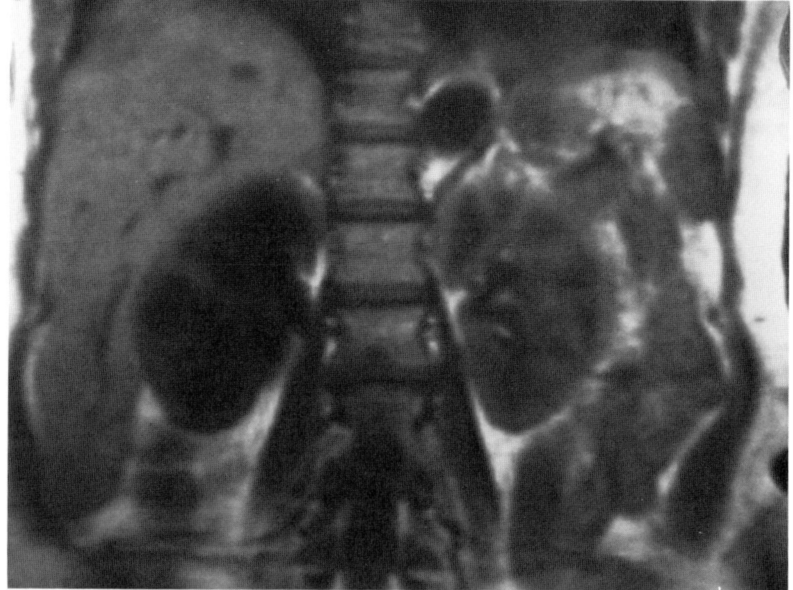

FIG. 6-9 *(Continued).* (C) Coronal T_1-weighted MRI also shows marked hydronephrosis, thinned parenchyma, and loss of corticomedullary junction on the right. *(Figure continues.)*

from neoplasm in all cases.[9] This difficulty arises most often when there has been previous treatment of retroperitoneal disease, such as radiation therapy. The point of obstruction can be recognized, often with some wispy changes around it but no discrete mass. Biopsy may reveal malignancy and should therefore be done if management will be changed by that result.

Congenital anomalies can cause upper urinary tract obstruction. The most common such lesion is congenital ureteropelvic junction obstruction. With this entity, CT will show a hydronephrotic kidney, but no dilated ureter. Obstructive anomalies are common in duplicated systems, particularly when one ureter has an ectopic distal end. Although there are a great variety of anomalies, upper pole hydronephrosis resulting from an obstructed ectopic ureter is the most common.[10] Most often the diagnosis is made using urography, voiding cystourethrograms, sonography, and radionuclide procedures. While urinary anomalies are usually discovered in childhood, they may present in adulthood. CT can be useful in selected circumstances, primarily because it can visualize the entire course of the dilated ureter better than sonography in adults[10] (Fig. 6-5). The site of insertion of the ectopic ureter may be identified. If a ureterocele is present, it can be seen directly. CT will rarely be necessary in children; in adults it can be an efficacious means of making the diagnosis, since many other etiologies of obstruction need to be excluded and CT may give all the relevant information, including parenchymal thickness.

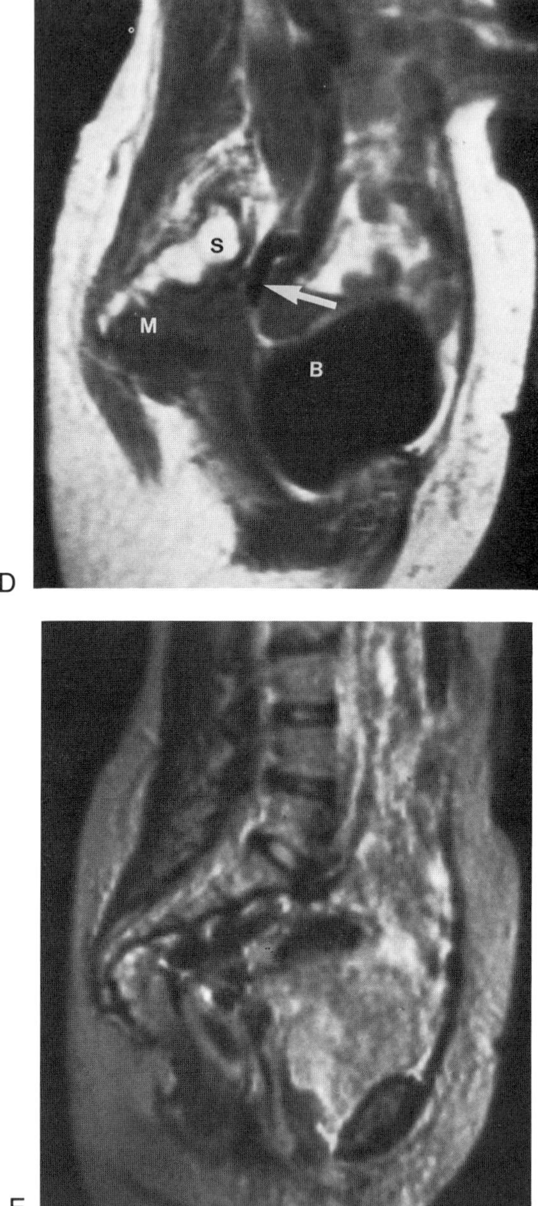

FIG 6-9 *(Continued).* (D) Sagittal T_1-weighted MRI shows the dilated urine filled ureter (arrow) extending to the mass (M). S, sacrum; B, bladder. (E) The mass of recurrent tumor is inhomogeneous and does not have the expected hyperintensity on this T_2-weighted (TR 1,500 ms, TE 80 ms) scan. The low signal is partly due to clip artifact.

Pitfalls

Despite the potential value of CT in evaluating obstruction, it is susceptible to certain errors. As with sonography, a dilated, nonobstructed system may be mistaken for an obstructed one; a nondilated obstructed system may be missed.[6,7] These errors are particularly likely if no contrast material is administered. Even with contrast enhancement, partial obstruction can be missed in the presence of minimal dilatation and good renal function. A more quantitative functional test such as diuretic renography is more accurate at detecting or excluding obstruction. Such a test should be used if determining whether or not obstruction is present is the primary clinical question. Functional impairment can be attributable to many causes, and a poorly functioning kidney due to end-stage papillary necrosis or chronic pyelonephritis could simulate hydronephrosis.

Technical errors can occur. If the obstructing lesion is small, it may be missed if it happens to lie in an interslice gap (Fig. 6-10). Both small tumors and small calculi can be obscured by contrast material and missed if precontrast images are not obtained. The most common error probably is the failure to identify a subtle abnormality because of failure to scrutinize the ureter on every slice.[12] When reading CT, the assumption is made that the ureter follows a straight course and will appear in nearly the same position on contiguous slices. Errors in interpretation can occur when a tortuous ureter passes around an extrinsic, nonobstructing lesion (Fig. 6-11).

MRI OF OBSTRUCTION

Limitation on the Role of MRI

The same factors that limit the utility of CT in evaluating upper urinary tract obstruction are even more significant in regard to MRI. MRI is even more expensive and less widely available than CT. With the availability of sonography and CT, virtually no cases could be said to require the use of MRI for diagnosis. Very ill patients make poor MRI subjects. Calculi are not readily apparent with most MRI techniques. Interpretation of MRI is complex, and many radiologists are inexperienced, especially in areas of limited use, such as the urinary tract.

Nonetheless, MRI can be diagnostic of urinary tract obstruction and has certain potential advantages. Avoidance of ionizing radiation and of potentially nephrotoxic contrast material is a limited advantage compared with CT. The ability to produce high-quality images comparable to that of axial CT in any plane can be helpful. More importantly, certain physiologic features of an obstructed kidney are apparent on MRI in addition to morphologic changes. MRI contrast material is much less toxic than iodinated contrast material. MRI characteristics of the obstructing lesion may be characteristic of a certain process (i.e., tumor versus fibrosis). Despite the fact that MRI is comparable to CT in

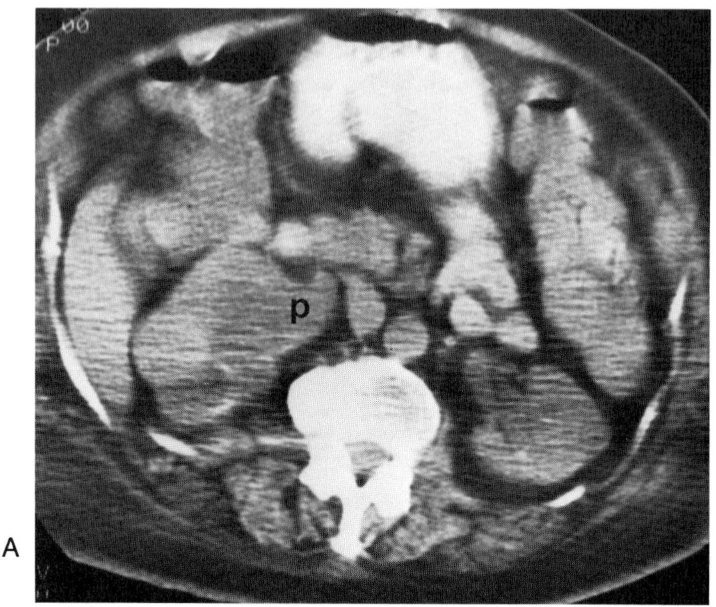

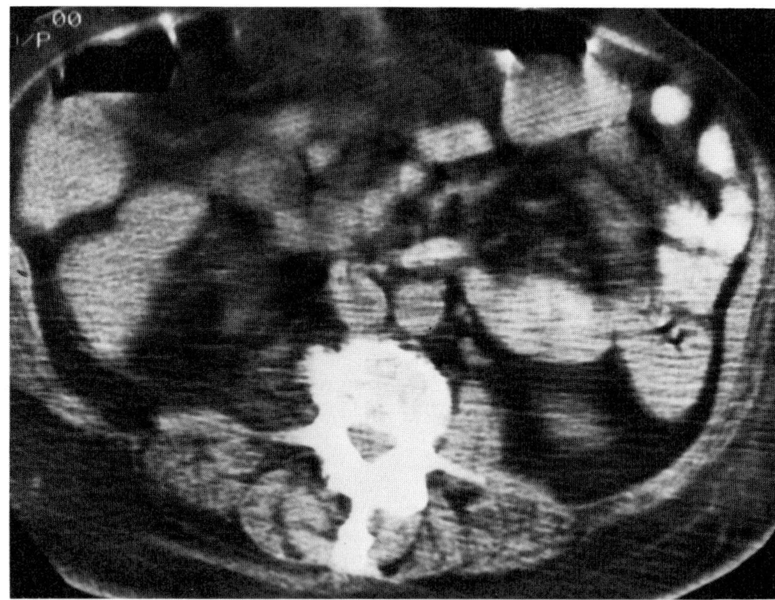

FIG. 6-10. CT was requested to rule out abscess in this 63-year-old woman with urosepsis. (A) Noncontrast scan shows right hydronephrosis. p, pelvis. (B) The scan was initially done with 10-mm gaps between 10-mm slices (alternate slices). No right ureteral lesion was seen. *(Figure continues.)*

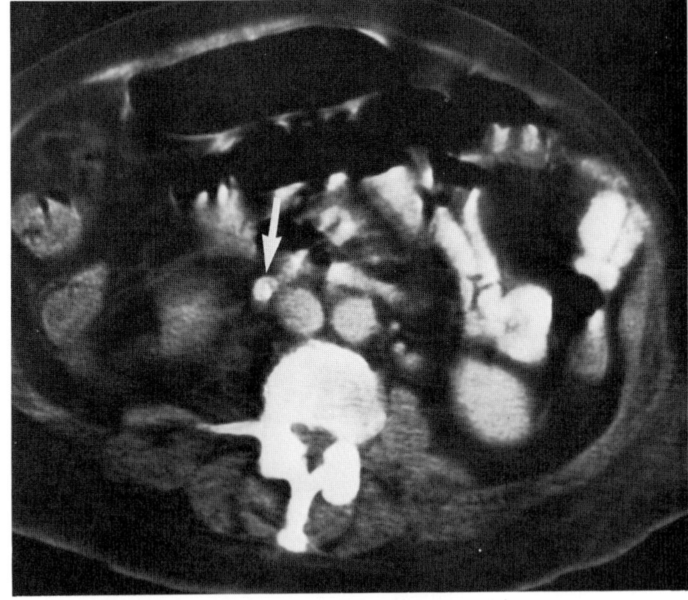

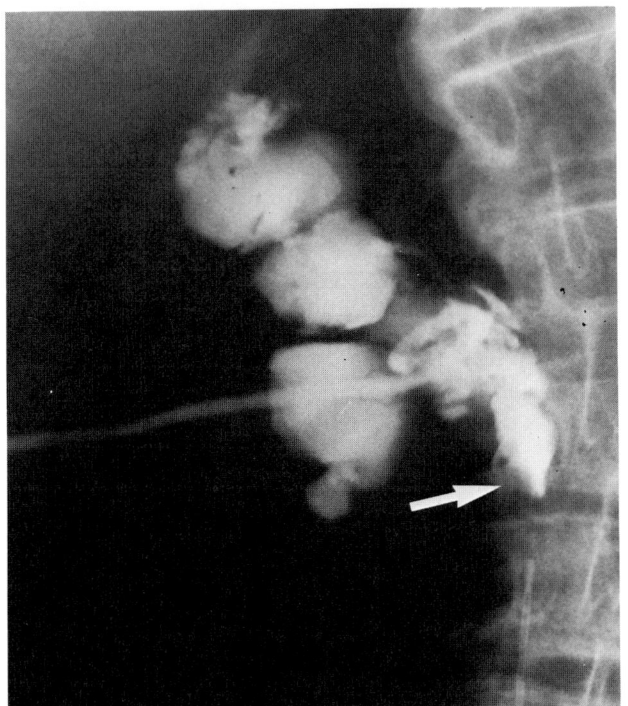

FIG. 6-10 *(Continued).*   (C) Repeat scan with contiguous images showed a dilated proximal ureter obstructed by a calculus (arrow). (D) Nephrostogram confirmed pyonephrosis with an obstructing calculus (arrow).

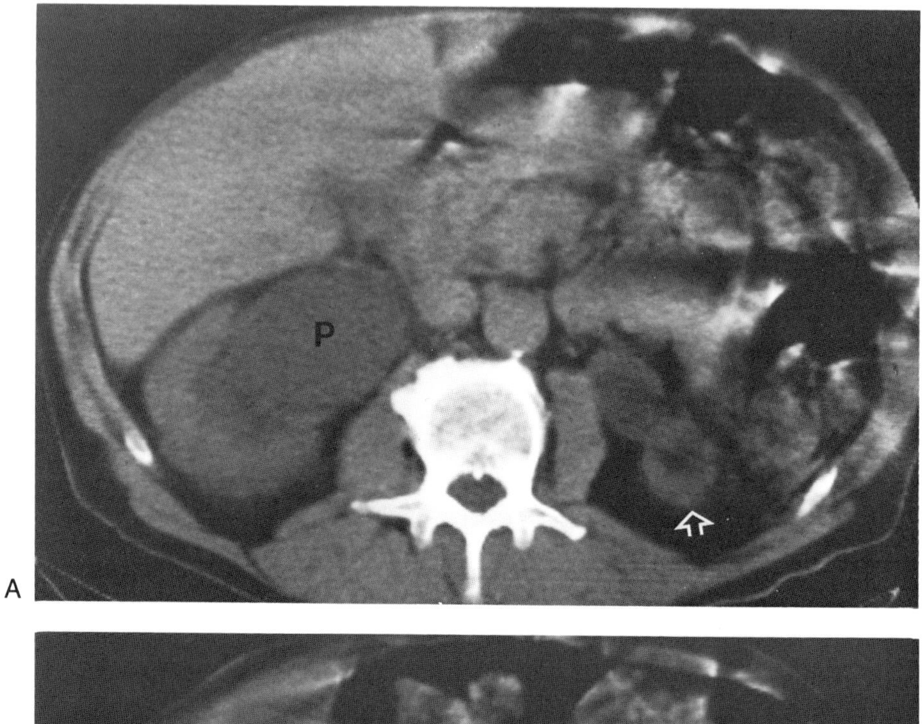

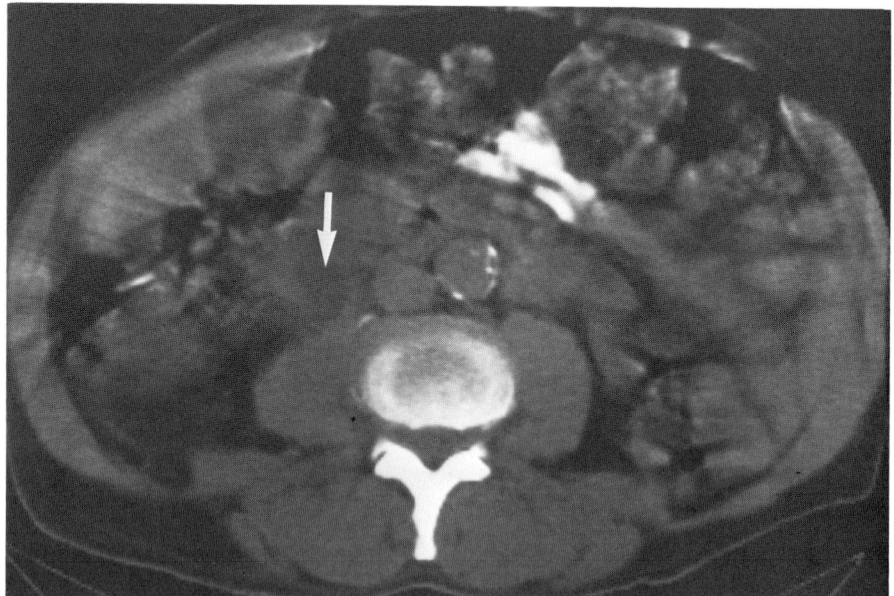

FIG. 6-11. This 76-year-old man presented with right flank pain and renal failure. Sonography showed right hydronephrosis of uncertain etiology and failed to visualize a left kidney. (A) Noncontrast CT shows dilated right pelvis (P) and atrophic left kidney (arrow). (B) The unopacified proximal right ureter (arrow) appears dilated. (*Figure continues.*)

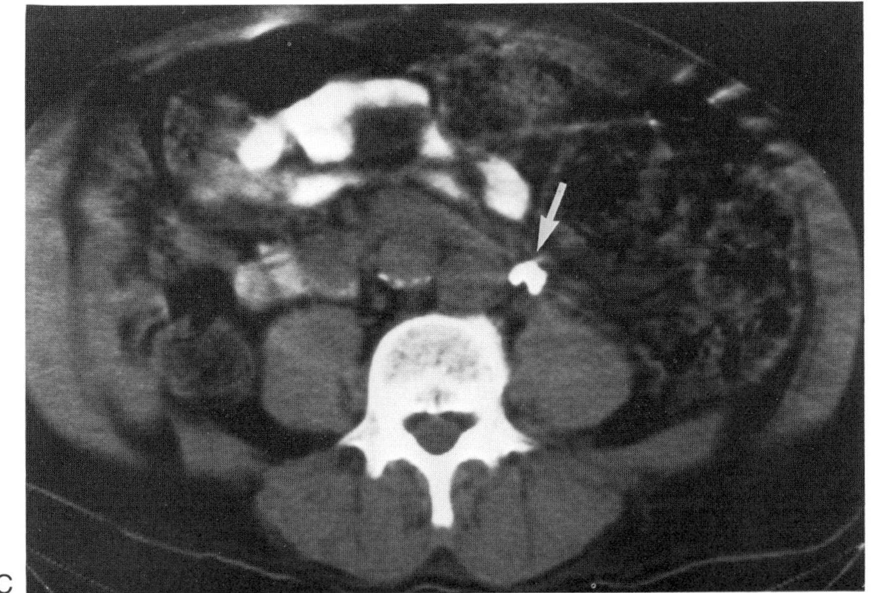

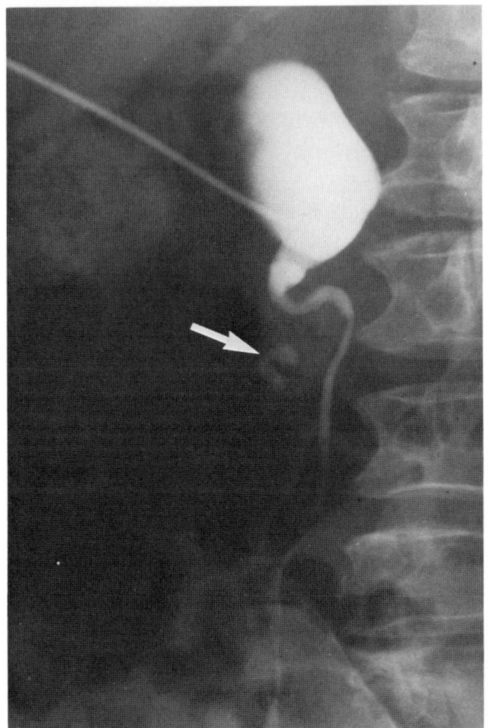

FIG. 6-11 *(Continued).*   (C) On the next slice, a calcification (arrow) is present; this was assumed to be an obstructing ureteral calculus. (D) Nephrostogram shows the calcification (arrow) is not in the ureter and probably is a calcified lymph node. A sloughed papilla apparently caused acute worsening of a chronic ureteropelvic junction obstruction.

many urinary tract disorders, its role is undefined and should be considered largely investigational. Its use is not cost-effective except in selected circumstances when other procedures have not been diagnostic.

MRI Findings

High-resolution images of the kidney are achievable with both high- and low-field-strength MRI.[24,25] Relatively T_1-weighted spin-echo images are most useful. Detailed anatomy can be seen with this technique (Fig. 6-12). The renal cortex is distinguishable as a peripheral, medium-intensity (isointense with liver) structure surrounding the lower-intensity medullary tissue. This distinct corticomedullary distinction is a result of the lower T_1 relaxation time of normal cortex compared with medulla. Renal sinus fat is bright. Urine in the collecting system is very dark. The pelvis can usually be identified; the normal ureter can sometimes be recognized, especially on coronal views (Fig. 6-12). T_2-weighted scans are less useful. Cortex and medulla are both bright, with no corticomedullary distinction. In addition, fat, urine, hematoma, and tumor give high-intensity signals on T_2-weighted scans. Consequently, there is little contrast between normal structures and abnormal tissues, leading to an inability to recognize and differentiate the two. The normal ureter cannot be easily recognized on T_2-weighted scans.

There are two categories of MRI findings in ureteral obstruction: morphologic and physiologic. With chronic obstruction, the expected morphologic changes of dilatation and renal parenchymal thinning are clearly shown on MRI[26] (Figs. 6-9 and 6-13). Dilated ureters can be followed to the point of obstruction, and the lesion identified, just as with CT. The physiologic changes that take place in the parenchyma of an obstructed kidney are reflected in changes in signal intensity. The water content of the cortex increases within a few hours of acute ureteral occlusion,[26] producing an increase in the effective T_1 value of the cortex. As a consequence, the normal corticomedullary distinction on T_1-weighted scans is lost (Fig. 6-13). Although these changes may be useful in making the diagnosis of obstruction, other renal diseases cause loss of corticomedullary distinction as well.

Renal excretion of paramagnetic contrast agents such as gadolinium diethylenetriaminepentaacetic acid (Gd-DTPA) causes changes in the signal intensity of renal parenchyma and urine filled structures.[27] These are best shown with fast scanning techniques such as gradient-recalled echo sequences. The acutal pattern is complex, since the relationship between signal intensity and concentration of Gd-DTPA is nonlinear. However, alteration of this pattern caused by ureteral obstruction has been described.[25] In the normal kidney, the medullary signal intensity showed a decrease as urine with highly concentrated Gd-DTPA is excreted; conversely, in obstructed kidneys, an increase in signal intensity was shown.[27] Further investigation may lead to contrast-enhanced MRI findings that are specific for obstruction. The results are preliminary.

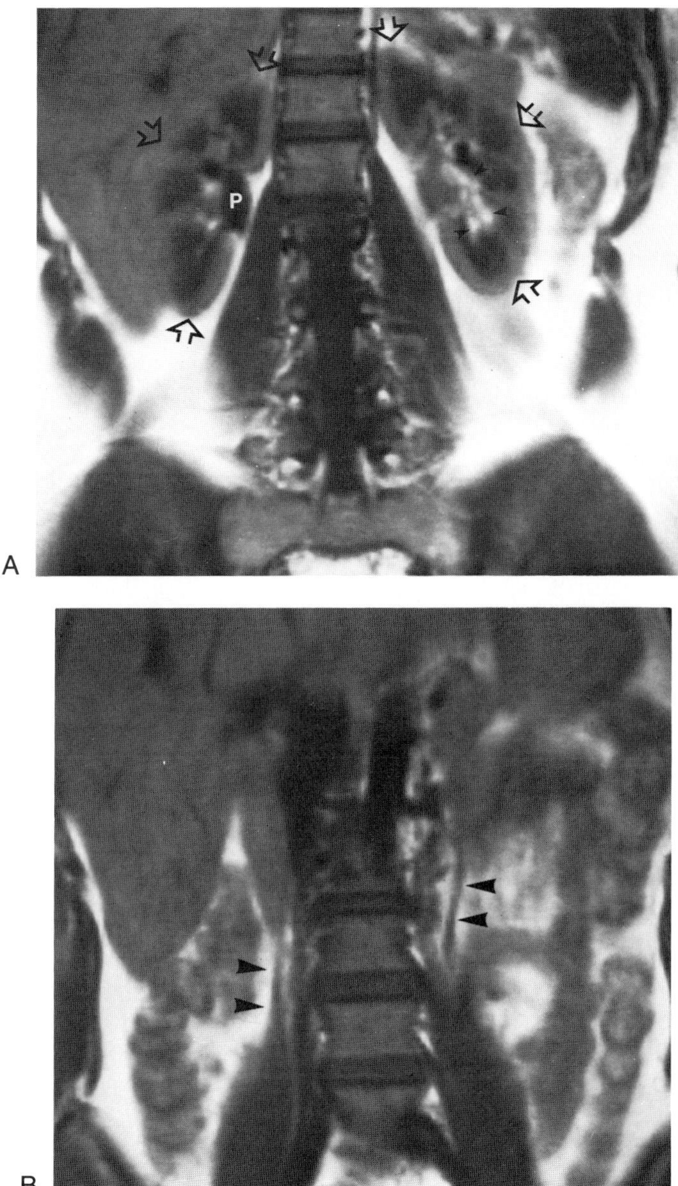

FIG. 6-12.   (A) Coronal T_1-weighted (TR 300 ms, TE 20 ms) spin-echo images show normal kidneys (open arrows). Note the clear corticomedullary distinction, the low-intensity right renal pelvis (P), and bright renal sinus fat (arrowheads). The left renal pelvis shows partial volume effect, artifactually increasing the apparent intensity. (B) A more anterior slice shows normal ureters (arrowheads) passing anterior to the psoas muscles.

MRI can detect both intrinsic and extrinsic tumors obstructing the ureter (Figs. 6-7 and 6-9). MRI has little advantage over CT in this regard. The tumor is recognizable on T_1-weighted scans, since it has a higher signal intensity than urine, which is very dark. On T_2-weighted images, the tumor is hyperintense, but may be more difficult to recognize, since urine and the surrounding fat are also very intense. MRI is less susceptible to artifacts from surgical clips than is CT (Fig. 6-7). However, paramagnetic metals do cause local artifacts because of distortion of the magnetic field. With lack of a bowel contrast agent, it may be difficult to distinguish tumor from bowel on MRI. As noted above, calcification is rarely discernible on MRI. MRI has some potential clinical value. Because of its advantages in staging pelvic malignancies, such as cervical and bladder cancer, MRI can be used at the same time to evaluate for ureteral obstruction.[28,29] Evaluating urinary anomalies may be easier with MRI than CT because of (1) the multiplanar imaging capability, (2) the superior depiction of pelvic anatomy by MRI, and (3) avoidance of ionizing radiation in patients who have not completed their childbearing years. MRI may be helpful in determining whether a mass obstructing a ureter is recurrent tumor or post-treatment fibrosis, since tumor typically has a high signal on T_2-weighted scans, while fibrosis typically has a low signal.[30,31]

Typical MRI features of retroperitoneal fibrosis (RPF) have also been de-

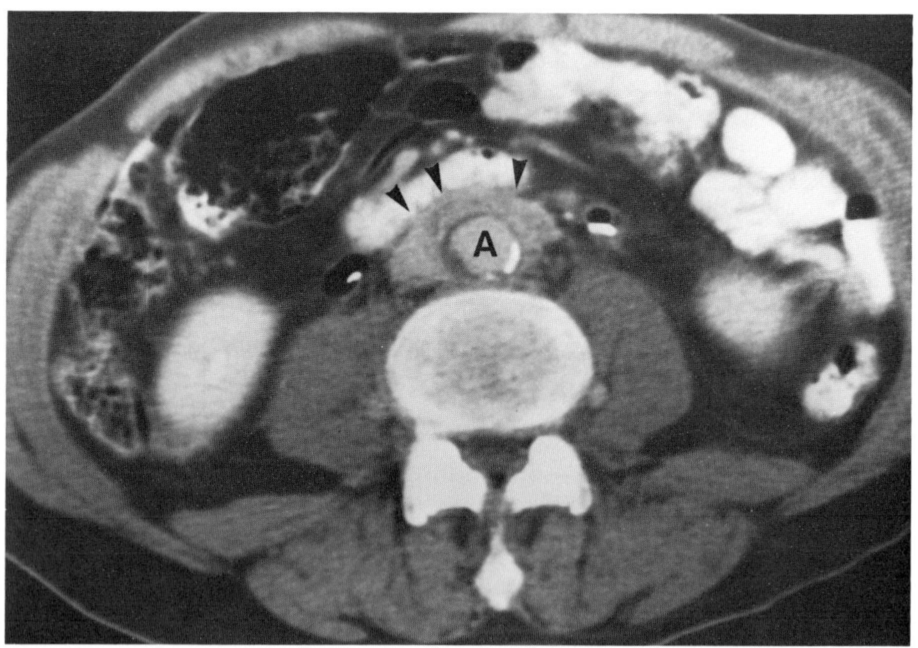

A

FIG. 6-13.   Renal failure was newly discovered in this 58-year-old man. Sonogram showed bilateral hydronephrosis. (A) CT was done after stent placement. A soft tissue mass (arrowheads) encases the aorta (A) without displacing it. (*Figure continues.*)

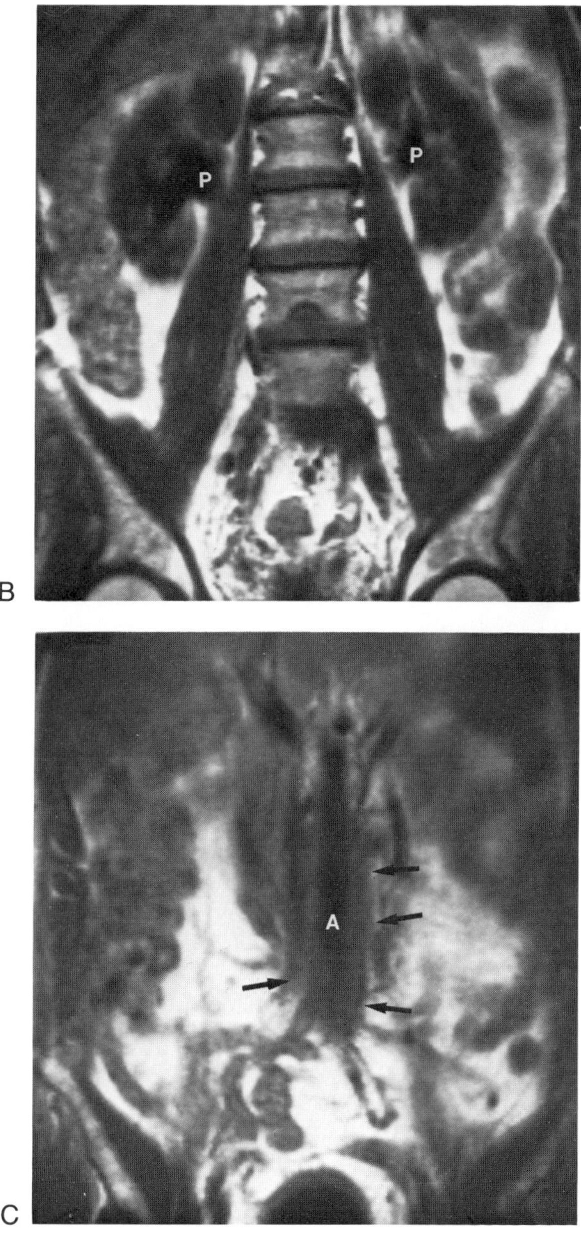

FIG. 6-13 *(Continued)*.   (B) Coronal T_1-weighted (TR 350 ms, TE 20 ms) MRI shows bilateral hydronephrosis. p, pelvis. Note absence of corticomedullary differentiation. (C) The aorta (A) is encased by abnormal tissue (arrows) that had medium intensity on both T_1- and T_2-weighted scans, typical of retroperitoneal fibrosis. The diagnosis was confirmed surgically.

scribed.[32] RPF is an uncommon cause of renal failure. Some historical, clinical, and urographic features may be suggestive, but often the diagnosis is not strongly suspected. CT is superior to sonography in detecting evidence of RPF.[33] On CT, a bulky soft tissue mass enveloping the retroperitoneal structures may be seen. Sometimes only a fibrous sheet is evident, and in some cases no fibrotic tissue is identified, especially if the process is limited to the pelvis.[34] While the density and extent overlap with that of malignant disease, some CT features can suggest the diagnosis. The anterior margin of RPF is often well demarcated, while it is indistinct posteriorly. The process rarely extends cephalad to the renal hilum. Most specific may be its tendency to envelop, but not displace, the retroperitoneal structures[35]; in particular, even with sizeable masses, the aorta tends not to be displaced away from the spine (Fig. 6-13). CT also can detect etiologic conditions such as aortic aneurysms. MRI has some potential advantages in evaluating patients with suspected RPF. Soft tissue masses can be distinguished from vessels without the need for iodinated contrast, which may be injurious in these patients, who often are in renal failure. The multiplanar imaging capability is useful. MRI signal characteristics may be helpful. Malignant masses usually have high signal intensity on T_2-weighted scans. RPF usually is of medium or low intensity[32] (Fig. 6-13). However, because there may be active inflammation, the signal intensity can be expected to be variable.

The specificity of MRI remains controversial, since only limited experience has been reported. Inaccuracies may occur because both inflammation and neoplasia cause an increase in T_2 relaxation time, and microscopic tumor deposits surrounded by fibrotic tissue will likely have a low signal.[36]

SUMMARY

CT represents a useful but expensive tool in diagnosis of upper urinary tract obstruction. Proper and cost-effective use of it depends on an understanding of when and how to use it in relationship to other diagnostic methods. In limited circumstances, it may be the best method to make the correct diagnosis. The findings of obstruction must be known because of the possibility of serendipitous discovery on a scan done for other reasons.

The role of MRI remains undefined. While it has capabilities and advantages in diagnosing obstruction, its expense, the lack of definitive research, and the excellent capabilities of sonography and CT limit its utility. The potential of MRI to detect physiologic changes by alteration of T_1 or T_2 values, altered excretion of MRI contrast agents, or spectroscopic changes hold the possibility of specific findings of obstruction, and perhaps even predictability of recovery.

REFERENCES

1. Sherman RL, Schneider M: Obstructive uropathy as seen by the internist: The role of ultrasound and CT scanning. Dis Mon 12:1, 1984
2. Jeffrey RB, Federle MP: CT and ultrasonography of acute renal abnormalities. Radiol Clin North Am 21:515, 1983

3. Arafa NM, Fathi MM, Safwat M, et al: Accuracy of ultrasound in the diagnosis of non-functioning kidneys. J Urol 128:1165, 1982

4. Talner LB, Scheible W, Ellenbogen PH, et al: How accurate is ultrasonography in detecting hydronephrosis in azotemic patients? Urol Radiol 3:1, 1981

5. Curry NS, Gobien RP, Schabel SI: Minimal-dilatation obstructive nephropathy. Radiology 143:531, 1982

6. Maillet PJ, Pelle-Francoz D, Laville M, et al: Nondilated obstructive acute renal failure: Diagnostic procedures and therapeutic management. Radiology 160:659, 1986

7. O'Reilly PH, Lupton EW, Testa HJ, et al: The dilated nonobstructed renal pelvis. Br J Urol 53:205, 1981

8. Forbes WSC, Isherwood I, Fawcitt RA: Computed tomography in the evaluation of the solitary or unilateral nonfunctioning kidney. J Comput Assist Tomogr 2:389, 1978

9. Bosniak MA, Megibow AJ, Ambos MA, et al: Computed tomography of ureteral obstruction. AJR 138:1107, 1982

10. Cronan JJ, Amis ES, Zeman RK, Dorfman GS: Obstruction of the upper-pole moiety in renal duplication in adults: CT evaluation. Radiology 161:17, 1986

11. Parienty RA, Ducellier R, Pradel J, et al: Diagnostic value of CT numbers in pelvocalyceal filling defects. Radiology 145:743, 1982

12. Kenney PJ, Stanley RJ: Computed tomography of ureteral tumors. J Comput Assist Tomogr 11:102, 1987

13. Neal DE, Simpson W, Bartholomew P, Keavey PM: Comparison of dynamic computed tomography, diuresis renography and DTPA parenchymal transit time in the assessment of dilatation of the upper urinary tract. Br J Urol 57:515, 1985

14. Pollack HM, Arger PH, Banner MP, et al: Computed tomography of renal pelvic filling defects. Radiology 138:645, 1981

15. Hillman BJ, Drach GW, Tracey P, Gaines JA: Computed tomographic analysis of renal calculi. AJR 142:549, 1984

16. Newhouse JH, Prien EL, Amis ES, et al: Computed tomographic analysis of urinary calculi. AJR 142:545, 1984

17. Gatewood OMB, Goldman SM, Marshall FF, Siegelman SS: CT in the diagnosis of transitional cell carcinoma of the kidney. J Urol 127:876, 1982

18. Gill WB, Lu CT, Bibbo M: Retrograde brush biopsy of the ureter and pelvis. Urol Clin North Am 6:577, 1979

19. Booth CM, Cameron KM, Pugh RC: Urothelial carcinoma of the kidney and ureter. Br J Urol 52:430, 1980

20. Geerdsen J: Tumors of the renal pelvis and ureter. Scand J Urol Nephrol 13:287, 1979

21. Baron RL, McClennan BL, Lee JKT, Lawson TL: Computed tomography of transitional-cell carcinoma of the renal pelvis and ureter. Radiology 144:125, 1982

22. Lee JKT: Retroperitoneum. p. 707. In Lee JKT, Sagel SS, Stanley RJ (eds): Computed Body Tomography with MRI Correlation. 2nd Ed. Raven Press, New York, 1989

23. Lee JKT, Marx MV: Pelvis. p. 851. In Lee JKT, Sagel SS, Stanley RJ (eds): Computed Body Tomography with MRI Correlation. 2nd Ed. Raven Press, New York, 1989

24. Kenney PJ: Magnetic resonance imaging of the abdomen and pelvis: Report of the council on scientific affairs. JAMA 261:420, 1989

25. Newhouse JH, Markisz JA, Kazam E: Magnetic resonance imaging of the kidneys. Cardiovasc Intervent Radiol 8:351, 1986

26. Thickman D, Kundel H, Biery D: Magnetic resonance evaluation of hydronephrosis in the dog. Radiology 152:113, 1984

27. Kikinis R, von Schulthess GK, Jager P, et al: Normal and hydronephrotic kidney: Evaluation of renal function with contrast-enhanced MR imaging. Radiology 165:834, 1987

28. Hricak H, Stern JL, Fisher MR, et al: Endometrial carcinoma staging by MR imaging. Radiology 162:297, 1987

29. Rholl KS, Lee JKT, Heiken JP, et al: Primary bladder carcinoma: Evaluation with MR imaging. Radiology 163:117, 1987

30. Krestin GP, Steinbrich W, Friedmann G: Recurrent rectal cancer: Diagnosis with MR imaging versus CT. Radiology 168:307, 1988

31. Ebner F, Kressel HY, Mintz MC, et al: Tumor recurrence versus fibrosis in the female pelvis: Differentiation with MR imaging at 1.5T. Radiology 166:333, 1988

32. Mulligan SA, Holley HC, Koehler RE, et al: CT and MRI in the evaluation of retroperitoneal fibrosis. J Comput Assist Tomogr 13:277, 1989

33. Feinstein RS, Gatewood OMB, Goldman SM, et al: Computed tomography in the diagnosis of retroperitoneal fibrosis. J Urol 126:255, 1981

34. Brun B, Laursen K, Sorensen IN, et al: CT in retroperitoneal fibrosis. AJR 137:535, 1981

35. Degesys GE, Dunnick NR, Silverman PM, et al: Retroperitoneal fibrosis: Use of CT in distinguishing among possible causes. AJR 146:57, 1986

36. de Lange EE, Fechner RE, Wanebo HJ: Suspected recurrent rectosigmoid carcinoma after abdominoperineal resection: MR imaging and histopathologic findings. Radiology 170:323, 1989

7 Cancer of the Prostate

RAY E. STUTZMAN

Adenocarcinoma of the prostate is the second most common carcinoma in males in the United States and the third leading cause of male deaths from neoplastic disease. The reported incidence is second only to lung cancer in the male population; however, the true incidence is probably much higher but is frequently not the cause of death or may never have been diagnosed before the patient's death. The true prevalence of prostatic carcinoma is unknown but, considering autopsy data and data from surgical specimens, it is probably the most prevalent neoplasm in man. Epidemiologic surveys suggest that the incidence of prostatic cancer has increased over the years; however, this may also be correlated with improved methods in diagnosis and an aging population. The incidence of unsuspected or incidental carcinoma of the prostate found at transurethral resection of the prostate (TURP) ranges from 4 percent in the fourth decade of life to 80 percent in the ninth decade of life. The incidence at autopsy has somewhat higher figures as many cancers begin in the outer periphery of the prostate gland and are missed by incomplete transurethral resection.[1]

The etiology of prostatic carcinoma is unknown. The growth and function of a normal prostate is dependent on testosterone and dihydrotestosterone. Castration prior to puberty would prevent prostatic carcinoma. There are also data to suggest increased incidence of prostatic cancer in relatives of prostate cancer patients. There are some racial, national, and regional differences in the disease; however, populations migrating from low- to high-incidence areas gradually tend to assume the risks in the new geographic location. The role of infectious agents is unknown. There has been no direct cause or relationship of prostatic cancer and various viral infections. There has been a reported increased incidence of carcinoma of the uterine cervix among the wives of prostate cancer patients. Industrial and environmental exposure have been implicated, but studies have not been able to confirm this.

SIGNS AND SYMPTOMS

The most frequent sign leading to the diagnosis of adenocarcinoma of the prostate is that of a prostatic nodule or induration discovered on a routine examination. This will usually lead to a biopsy of the prostate; approximately

30 to 40 percent of prostatic nodules or indurations in the prostate will be positive for adenocarcinoma. Other lesions causing induration can be localized benign prostatic hyperplasia, granulomatous disease including tuberculosis, chronic prostatitis, calcifications within the prostate, and postsurgical induration. Other signs and symptoms of prostatic carcinoma can include bladder outlet obstruction although this is more common with benign prostatic hyperplasia. Bone pain or bone lesions found on routine radiography can suggest metastatic or stage D2 disease. Ureteral obstruction would suggest significant localized disease. Hematuria can occur in cancer of the prostate but is more common with benign prostatic hyperplasia.

GRADING

Several grading systems have been devised, including well-differentiated, moderately differentiated, and poorly differentiated. The Gleason system, however, is the most commonly used and is based on glandular differentiation.[2] Five different patterns are described. Grade 1 is well differentiated, grade 5 is poorly differentiated. Two patterns within the biopsy specimen are added together with a total score ranging from 2 to 10.

Diagnosis and Staging

Digital rectal examination continues to be the most reliable way to diagnose prostatic cancer. There are no reliable, cost-effective biochemical or imaging studies that can routinely be used to screen a large population for prostate cancer. Transrectal ultrasound has been an excellent adjunct in screening patients with benign prostatic hyperplasia scheduled for surgery and for patients with suspected carcinoma. Transrectal ultrasound, however, is not reliable or cost-effective for routine screening as yet. There are too many false-positive findings to warrant its routine use. The diagnosis of adenocarcinoma can be confirmed by needle biopsy or aspiration biopsy or may be an incidental finding at either transurethral resection or open prostatectomy.

Digital rectal examination is still reliable in ascertaining whether the neoplasm is confined to the prostate gland. Rectal ultrasound is sensitive in assessing prostatic size and can demonstrate capsular and seminal vesicle involvement. It is not accurate in determining microscopic and even occasional gross invasion. Transrectal prostatic ultrasonography is useful as an aid in placement of the biopsy needle within a suspicious area.

Studies have shown that the obturator and iliac nodes are usually the first site of metastases; these structures will be positive on pathologic examination in 5 to 50 percent of patients with prostatic cancer. There is a direct correlation and higher incidence of nodal metastases in patients with increased tumor volume in the prostate, higher Gleason grade of neoplasm, and/or higher levels of preoperative prostatic specific antigen (PSA). Current imaging techniques are not always reliable in picking up early or microscopic lymph node metastases. Assessment of the pelvic nodes by MRI and CT scan has not been reliable unless there is lymph node enlargement. If the enlargement of the nodes is secondary to metastases, the acid phosphatase and/or prostatic specific antigen (PSA) is usually already elevated. Bone metastases are commonly associated with extensive nodal disease.

The most commonly used staging system is the Whitmore/Jewett system (Table 7-1). Stage A adenocarcinoma of the prostate is pathologically proved carcinoma in tissue removed during a prostatectomy, either open or TURP for preoperative diagnosis of benign prostatic hyperplasia. Stage A is further subdivided into stage A1 disease, carcinoma in less than 5 percent of resected tissue and consisting of a well-differentiated neoplasm. All other incidentally discovered carcinomas are stage A2 and are considered potentially more aggressive.

Stage B carcinoma of the prostate refers to disease confined within the prostatic capsule on rectal examination and current imaging techniques, with no evidence of any systemic metastases. This is further subdivided into stage B1, which represents tumor occupying less than one entire lobe of the prostate, often a solitary nodule, and stage B2, which represents tumor occupying one complete lobe or both lobes of the prostate.

Stage C carcinoma is based on rectal examination or imaging techniques that show the disease confined to the area of the prostate with extension outside the prostatic capsule, possible fixation within the rectal fossa, and/or extension of the carcinoma into the seminal vesicles. Not infrequently, a pathologic stage C carcinoma will be found following a radical prostatectomy for what was thought to be stage B disease, the surgical margins are found not to be free of tumor, and/or there is extension of neoplasm into the seminal vesicles.

Stage D carcinoma implies metastases outside the area of the prostate. It is

TABLE 7-1   Staging of prostatic carcinoma

Stage	Description
A	Clinically undetectable; found on pathologic examination after prostatectomy
A1	Focal; well differentiated
A2	Diffuse; poorly differentiated
B	Confined to prostate
B1	Solitary nodule; <1.5 cm; one lobe
B2	One whole lobe or both lobes
C	Locally extending outside of prostatic capsule or into seminal vesicles
D	Metastatic disease
D1	Pelvic lymph node metastases
D2	Distant metastases, usually bone

further subdivided into D1 carcinoma of the prostate, in which positive pelvic lymph nodes are found in a patient with a negative bone scan. This is discovered at either elective pelvic lymphadenectomy for staging or at radical prostatectomy. D2 adenocarcinoma of the prostate implies extranodal metastases, usually bone. These metastases are delineated by a positive bone scan and may be demonstrated radiographically. Most of these patients will have elevated biologic markers, PSA and acid phosphatase.

Serologic markers of prostate cancer, such as PSA and prostatic acid phosphatase, are not reliable for screening in early or localized disease but are usually elevated in metastatic disease. PSA is an excellent marker to follow in patients who have had a radical prostatectomy.[3] Any elevation implies that disease persists. This elevation usually precedes any other signs of metastases, such as a positive bone scan or palpable local recurrence.

The results of both MRI and CT scan in accurately staging early invasive disease have been disappointing to us and others.[4,5] Pollack[6] has recently described the development of a surface coil placed rectally using a 1.5 Tesla MRI unit. Early results suggest excellent local staging. The prostatic capsule cannot be consistently visualized even in normal subjects.[7] Normal-sized lymph nodes that are partially or totally replaced by tumors can go undetected with currently available MRI technology. For advanced disease, CT and MRI are quite accurate and correlate with digital examination and PSA. MRI has the advantage over CT in having the ability to image directly in all three orthogonal planes and to enhance soft-tissue contrast with a combination of T_1- and T_2-weighted images.[8]

Treatment

The therapy of prostatic carcinoma is somewhat controversial but may be approached on the basis of the stage of disease (Table 7-2). If the neoplasm is limited to the prostate (no evidence of local spread or metastatic disease) and the patient is under 75 years of age, has an anticipated 10-year survival, and has no contraindicating medical diseases, he is a candidate for a curative treatment. Radiation therapy and radical prostatectomy are the primary modes of treatment. Radical prostatectomy appears to provide slightly less morbidity and long-term survival. In the hands of a urologist experienced in this type of surgery, the complications are minimal, and less than 2 percent of patients develop incontinence. A modification of the traditional radical prostatectomy permits the removal of all cancerous tissue yet spares the pelvic nerves that control erection; there is preservation of pre-existing potency in greater than 80 percent of patients.[9]

The management in stage A disease is controversial. In a younger (e.g., <65 years) man with A1 disease who is at higher risk of recurrence because of his expected longevity, radical prostatectomy is recommended. For the older patient (e.g., >65 years) observation is usually recommended.[10] The patient

TABLE 7-2   Management of prostate carcinoma

Clinical Stage	Treatment Options
A1	Observation
	Radical prostatectomy
	Radiation therapy
A2	Radical prostatectomy
	Radiation therapy
B	Radical prostatectomy
	Radiation therapy
C	Radiation therapy
	Androgen suppression
D	Observation
	Androgen suppression
	Chemotherapy

with A2 disease is at considerable risk of developing metastases; radical prostatectomy is recommended.

Most patients with extensive localized prostatic cancer, stage C, are best treated by definitive radiotherapy. If significant bladder outlet obstruction is present, the patient may also need a TURP; this combination of treatment does result in an increased incidence of urinary incontinence.

Metastatic or stage D prostatic cancer is best managed by hormonal therapy or androgen suppression (castration or drug therapy). Studies have shown that hormonal therapy initiated at the time of diagnosis does not prolong survival but may delay the onset of symptomatic metastases compared with hormonal therapy initiated only in response to symptoms (such as bone pain).[11] Diethylstilbestrol (DES) (3 mg/day) and orchiectomy give similar results, producing an 85 to 90 percent partial symptomatic response rate in previously untreated patients. The duration of response is on the average 18 months, although prolonged remissions have been documented. There is no advantage to combining orchiectomy and estrogen therapy. Generally, estrogen therapy, which causes salt and water retention, should be avoided in patients who also have an edema-forming illness (such as severe congestive heart failure or nephrotic syndrome) not controlled by diuretics.[12] With newer medications, DES is not as commonly used. Luteinizing hormone/releasing hormone (LH/RH) analogues (Luprolide, Zoladex) have proved just as effective as castration or estrogens, with fewer side effects.[13] These analogues in combination with Flutamide, a potent antiandrogen, provide total androgen blockade and appear to be more effective than Luprolide alone. There have been a number of investigational trials using cytotoxic chemotherapy in all stages of prostatic carcinoma, but none are as effective as androgen deprivation and are only

TABLE 7-3   Survival with appropriately managed prostatic carcinoma

Stage	5 yr	10 yr	15 yr
A1	Normal life expectancy		
A2	50–80	40–70	15–35
B	50–90	40–70	15–40
C	15–70	5–60	0–30
D	5–30	3–10	0–3

(% Survival header spans the 5 yr, 10 yr, 15 yr columns)

partially effective in patients who fail hormonal therapy and have extensive metastatic disease.[14]

Much of the controversy in the diagnosis and management of prostatic cancer results from the inability to assess accurately the influence of prostate cancer on longevity.[15] Prostate cancer occurs in older men who often have coexisting diseases that influence longevity. Also, the natural history of the disease is not well understood. The best estimates for survival of patients with various stages of prostatic cancer with the treatments discussed above are listed in Table 7-3.

REFERENCES

1. Stamey TA: Cancer of the prostate. In Stamey TA (ed): Monographs in Urology 3:67, 1982

2. Gleason DF: Histologic grading and clinical staging of prostatic carcinoma. p. 171. In Tannenbaum M (ed): Urological Pathology: The Prostate. Lea & Febiger, Philadelphia, 1977

3. Oesterling JE, Chan DW, Epstein JI, et al: Prostate specific antigen in the preoperative and postoperative evaluation of localized prostatic cancer treated with radical prostatectomy. J Urol 139:766, 1988

4. Hricak H, Dooms GC, Jeffrey RB, et al: Prostatic carcinoma: Staging by clinical assessment, CT, and MR imaging. Radiology 162:331, 1987

5. Platt JF, Bree RL, Schwab RE: The accuracy of CT in staging of carcinoma of the prostate. AJR 149:315, 1987

6. Pollack HM: Recent advances in prostatic imaging. p. 494. Abstract of the Seventeenth International Congress of Radiology, Paris, July 7, 1989

7. Biondetta PR, Lee JKT, Ling D, Catalona WJ: Clinical stage B prostate carcinoma: Staging with MR imaging. Radiology 162:325, 1987

8. Kwon ED, Williams RD: Magnetic resonance imaging in evaluation of prostatic cancer. World J Urol 7:17, 1989

9. Walsh PC, Lepor H, Eggleston JC: Radical prostatectomy with preservation of sexual function: Anatomical and pathological considerations. Prostate 4:473, 1983

10. Epstein JI, Oesterling JE, Walsh PC: The volume and anatomical location of residual tumor in radical prostatectomy specimens removed for stage A1 prostate cancer. J Urol 139:975, 1988

11. Trachtenberg J: Hormonal management of stage D carcinoma of the prostate. Urol Clin North Am 14:685, 1987

12. Veterans Administration Cooperative Urological Research Group: Treatment and survival of patients with cancer of the prostate. Surg Gynecol Obstet 124:1011, 1967

13. Smith JA Jr: New methods of endocrine management of prostatic cancer. J Urol 137:1, 1987

14. Sogani PC, Fair WR: Treatment of advanced prostatic cancer. Urol Clin North Am 14:353, 1987

15. Catalona WJ, Miller DR, Kavoussi LR: Intermediate-term survival in clinically understaged prostate cancer patients following radical prostatectomy. J Urol 140:540, 1988

8 MRI and CT of the Prostate Gland

ANDREW YANG
SHIRLEY YANG

APPLICATIONS OF MRI IN EVALUATING THE PROSTATE GLAND

MRI is superior to CT in its ability to define the zonal anatomy of the prostate. Because benign adenomas are common and arise primarily in the central zone and cancer of the prostate arises primarily in the peripheral zone, definition of the zonal anatomy is critical. Additional pulse sequences are then used for further tissue characterization.

Compared with transrectal ultrasound, MRI has the following distinct advantages: (1) a much larger field of view in order to identify adenopathy; (2) relatively operator-independent reproducibility of imaging plane and image quality on follow-up studies; and (3) better tissue characterization, especially for complex lesions such as postoperative studies or bleeding adenomas. Transrectal ultrasound on the other hand, can be used for guided biopsy of suspicious hypoechoic lesions[1] and is less expensive.

Imaging Techniques

The exact pulse-sequence parameters depend on the type of scanner and software available. The key features of optimal MRI of the prostate gland are the use of small pixels for anatomic definition, reduction of respiratory motion, and maximizing water/fat contrast.

The patient is placed supine with ideally a half- to three-quarter-full bladder. If the patient is small, a foam mat is used to place him in the center of the body coil, where the field is most homogeneous. Abdominal compression will reduce respiratory motion in the pelvis. If the patient is already known to have prostate cancer and is having MRI done for staging, the upper abdomen is also scanned with T_2-weighted pulse sequences using respiratory compen-

TABLE 8-1 MR pulse sequences as used on 1.5-T Signa scanner

Sequence Spin Echo	1 T_1 Coronal	2 T_2 Axial	3 T_1 Axial	4 T_2 Sagittal	5 T_2 Axial
TR (ms)	600	2,500	600	2,500	2,700
TE (ms)	20	(20, 80)	20	(20, 80)	(20, 80)
Slice width (mm)	5	5	5	5	10
Slice gap (mm)	1.5	0.5	0.5	0.5	2
Field of view (cm)	48	28	28	28	Patient's width
Matrix averages	(128 × 256) 2	(192 × 256) 2	(256 × 256) 1	(128 × 256) 1	(128 × 256) 2
Start	S/I joints anteriorly	Symphysis cranially	Symphysis cranially	Center on prostate	Sacrum cranially
Frequency centering	Midpoint	Water	Midpoint	Water	Water
Images	14	(22 × 2)	24	(22 × 2)	(24 × 2)
Data base		CSMEMP Classic	CSMEMP Presaturation	CSMEMP	Respiratory compensation

sation. It is rare to find disease in the upper abdomen if pelvic lymph nodes are normal. The patient is positioned such that the center of the field of view is 15 cm above the pubic symphysis. In order to minimize artifact from bowel peristalsis, glucagon 1 mg IM may be used, but is not routinely necessary.

The parameters we use on our 1.5 Signa (General Electric, Milwaukee, WI) for routine evaluation of the prostate gland are listed in Table 8-1. The rationale for each pulse sequence is listed below.

1. *T_1-weighted coronal scout film* (Fig. 8-1). Besides localizing the prostate and looking for para-aortic nodes, this scout film affords a quick look at the vertebral bodies of the lumbar spine for metastatic disease and the kidneys for obstructive hydronephroses secondary to prostate enlargement.

2. *Spin-density and T_2-weighted axial images* (Fig. 8-2). This T_2-weighted pulse sequence provides the contrast necessary to separate the central zone from the peripheral zone and to permit the detection of prostate cancer that most commonly arises in the peripheral zone of the gland.

   Use of Classic and water frequency centering increases fat-water contrast. In other scanners, T_2-weighted inversion recovery or fat-suppressed spoiled gradient-echo technique may give even better fat-water contrast. A thin slice with small slice gap is essential and can be achieved either by interleaving, which will double the acquisition time, or by using a slice pulse profile which has low cross-talk such as the Frodo pulse on Siemen scanners and CSMEMP on GE scanners.

3. *T_1-weighted axial image through pelvis* (Fig. 8-3). The purpose of this sequence is to better define the neurovascular bundle, the periprostatic fat, the prostate contours, and the separation of the periprostatic venous plexus from the peripheral zone. The contour changes permit detection of minimal periprostatic extension of prostate cancer. This enables the surgeon to consider a neurovascular bundle-sparing operation (and, hopefully, preserve potency). The better definition of the vessels also allows detection of small lymph nodes in the pelvis.

4. *Spin-density and T_2-weighted sagittal image* (Fig. 8-4). This sagittal imaging plane defines the relationship of the median lobe to the base of the bladder. This also provides another look at the seminal vesicles for invasion in patients with cancer. The sagittal plane also defines the relationship of the urethra to the adenoma in patients pre- and post-transurethral prostatectomy.

5. *T_2-weighted pulse sequence through upper abdomen.* With staging of known prostate cancer, we recommend this pulse sequence to image the abdomen from the diaphragm to the upper pelvis. Respiratory compensation and spatial presaturation in the superior inferior plane for better vessel definition is recommended. The purpose is to look for nodal involvement. The metastatic lymph nodes are medium to high in signal on T_2-weighted images, whereas scar tissue will be low in signal postradiation.

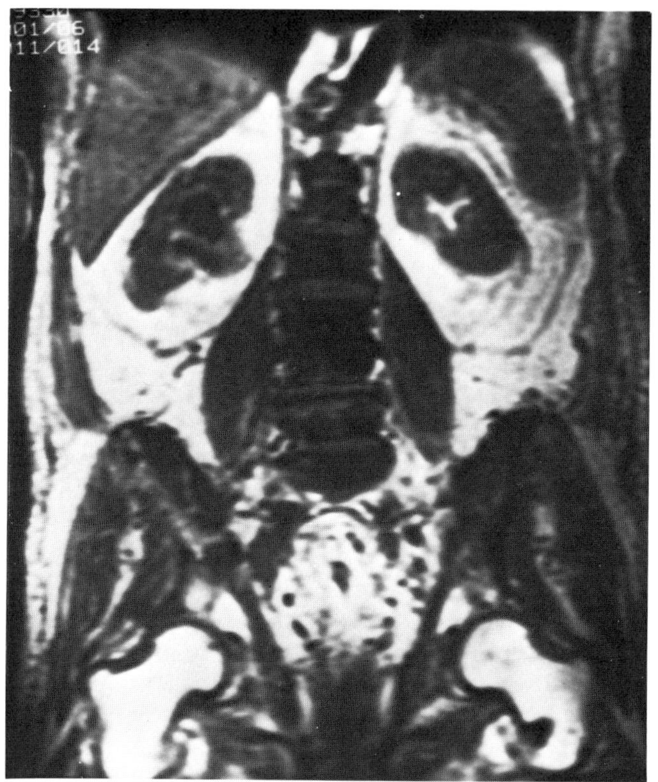

FIG. 8-1.   Stage D prostatic cancer. Coronal T_1-weighted localizer image showing stage D prostate cancer with osteoblastic metastases to lumbar spine, ilium, and pelvic adenopathy.

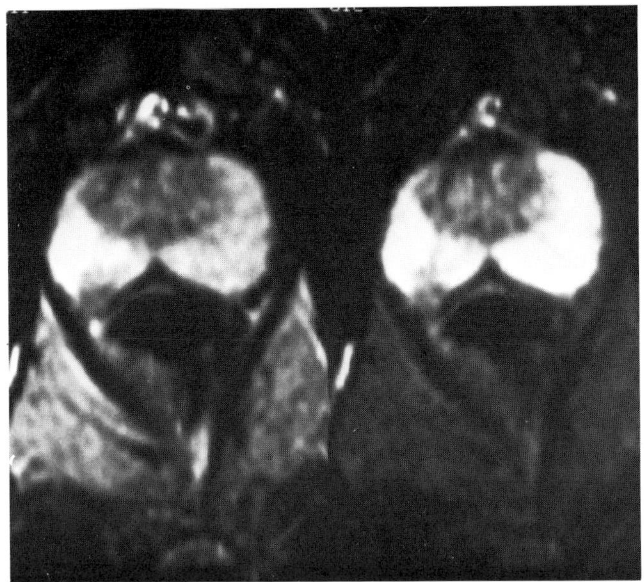

FIG. 8-2. Prostatic cancer with invasion of the right neurovascular bundle. Axial spin density (left) and T_2 (right) images (magnified) showing zonal anatomy. Low-signal focal surgically proven prostate cancer is seen with invasion of the right neurovascular bundle. Contralateral neurovascular bundle spared with retention of potency.

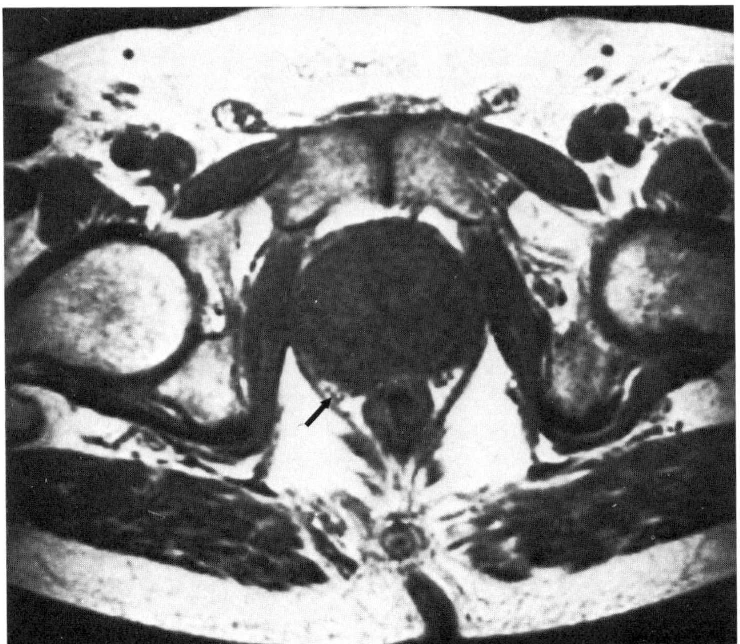

FIG. 8-3. Normal axial T_1-weighted image. Neurovascular bundle (arrow) and prostate contour well defined against periprostatic fat.

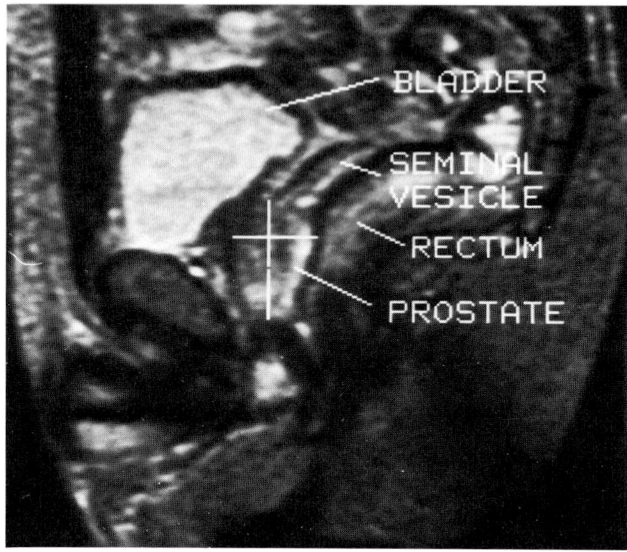

FIG. 8-4.   Normal sagittal T_2-weighted image showing prostate zonal anatomy and relationships of seminal vesicles. Prostate dimension illustrated for volumetric estimate by three-axis method.

High-Resolution Imaging with Surface Coil

High-resolution imaging of the prostate gland requires the use of local receivers or surface coils. Surface coils placed in the anterior or posterior pelvis will only enhance the signal minimally, as the prostate is in the middle of the pelvis, relatively far from the surface. Even a double coil in the Helmholtz configuration is not perfect. Recently, several institutions have been experimenting with intrarectal surface coils specifically designed for prostate imaging.[2,3] Basically, a flexible wire loop surface coil is constructed inside an inflatable device. The inflation allows snug fit of the surface coil against the anterior surface of the rectal wall and the posterior surface of the prostate gland and diminishes motion from normal rectal peristalsis. Insertion requires only lubricant and, except for the largest models, topical anesthetics are not necessary (Fig. 8-5). Very high-resolution images, with pixel sizes of 0.35 to 0.40 mm, are obtainable with one or two averages. The seminal vesicle, posterior peripheral zone, and neurovascular bundle are well demonstrated. However, the areas far from the coil (e.g., the anterior zone of the prostate, the urethra, and the anterior peripheral zone near the apex) may be less optimally defined (Fig. 8-6). It is believed that such coils will soon be commercially available.

The high signal obtained is ideal for spectroscopy of the prostate gland. Natural abundance ^{13}C-spectroscopy shows promise in research but is still limited in clinical practice due to poor localization of the spectra relative to the small size (1 to 2 mm) of early-stage prostate cancer.[4] Comparison of

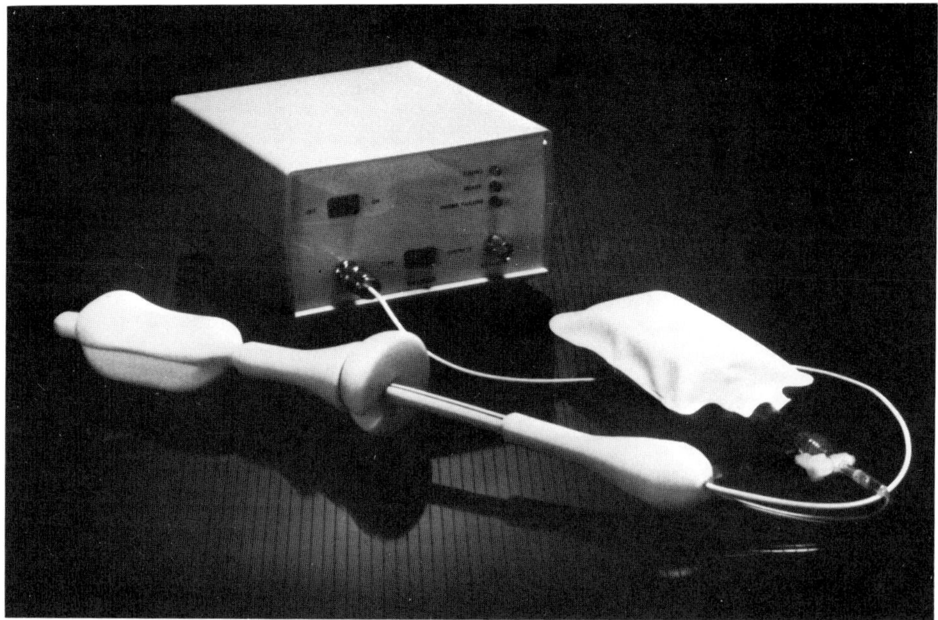

FIG. 8-5.   Endorectal MRI coil. System consists of a Silastic introducer with a coil molded into an inflatable rubber balloon. The endorectal component is disposable. Box contains tuning electronics. (Courtesy of Jonathan Read, Medrad, Pittsburgh, PA.)

prostatic carcinoma with adjacent benign prostatic hypertrophy (BPH) using natural-abundance ^{13}C-spectroscopy shows that the cancers contained larger amounts of triacylglycerols and smaller amounts of citrate and acidic mucins, thought to be due to alterations in ATP-citrate lyase.

The small field of view of the intrarectal coil mandates that additional imaging be done with the body coil to look for adenopathy in the pelvis in patients with cancer. This may be done with the intrarectal coil in place.

CT OF THE PROSTATE GLAND

Preoperative CT of the pelvis to look for enlarged lymph nodes is still the standard of care, especially in institutions where MRI is not available. Optimal results require thorough opacification of bowel loops with oral contrast (supplemented by rectal contrast if there is slow transit). Eight- to 10-mm-thick contiguous slices are taken from the diaphragm to the midbladder after intravenous contrast injection. Where available, this is best done with a power injector and dynamic (or rapid) image mode. This is followed by 4- to 5-mm-thick contiguous slices through the prostate gland to the symphysis. The purpose of IV contrast is to define the bladder wall and to differentiate pelvic vessels from small nodes. The thinner slices permit evaluation of prostatic contour, prostate-rectal interface, and seminal vesicle contour (Fig. 8-7).

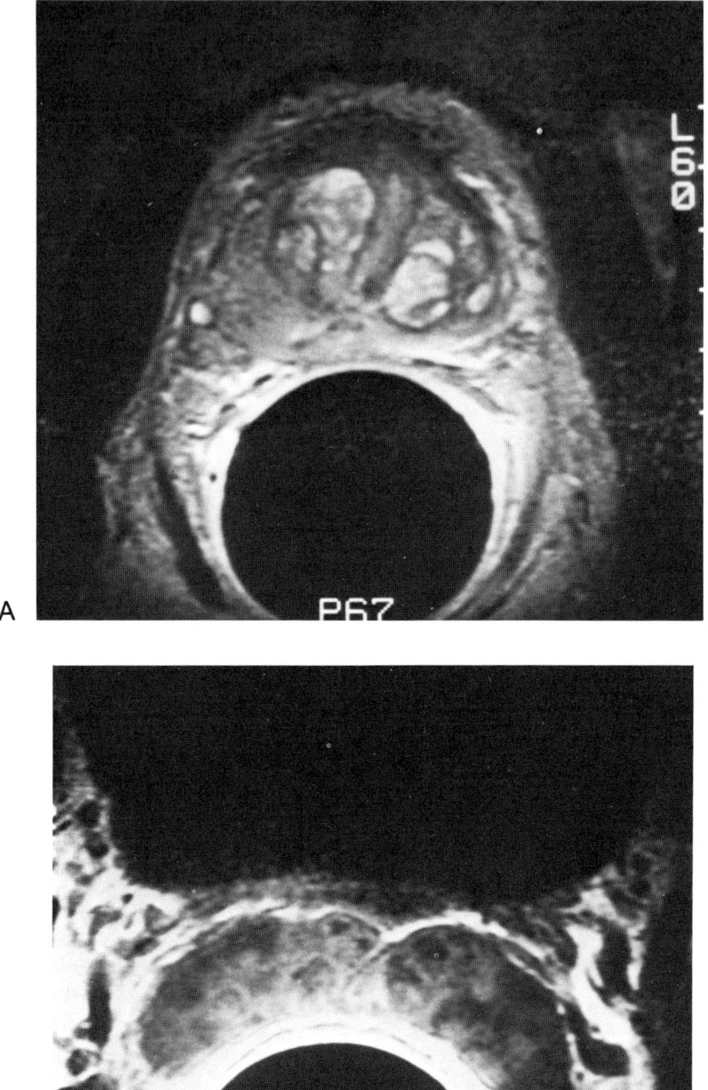

FIG. 8-6. Prostatic carcinoma invading the neurovascular bundle demonstrated by high-resolution MRI obtained with endorectal surface coil. (A) T_2-weighted axial image (12-cm field of view, 3 mm thick) demonstrating the carcinoma invading neurovascular bundle. (B) T_1-weighted (10-cm field of view, 3 mm thick) demonstrating details of the seminal vesicles. (Figs. A & B courtesy of Dr. Herbert Kressel, University of Pennsylvania Medical Center, Philadelphia, PA.)

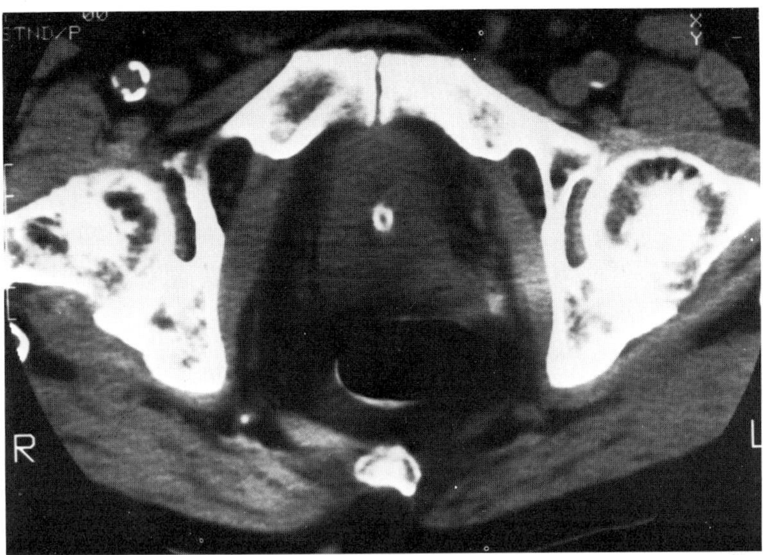

FIG. 8-7.   Invasive prostatic cancer. Axial 5-mm-thick CT image showing contour deformity with cancer extending into the left posterior periprostatic fat. Foley catheter marks location of urethra.

The images should be filmed with soft-tissue window settings and in cases with advanced disease with bone window settings as well. Plesnicar[5] found that osteoblastic bone metastases are more amenable to hormonal therapy, while mixed osteolytic changes are suggestive of recurrence of primary tumor or concomitant metastases in nonosseous sites such as lung and lymph nodes. Mixed osteolytic metastases are thought to be more resistant to hormonal therapy.

Percutaneous biopsy of suspicous enlarged pelvic lymph nodes may be done under CT guidance. For advanced disease that is to be treated by radiation therapy, reference markers should be placed on the patient's skin delineating the superior to inferior as well as the anterior to posterior extent of the suspected disease areas defined for radiation planning.

ZONAL ANATOMY OF THE PROSTATE GLAND

McNeal and co-workers defined the prostate as four zones.[6-9] The sagittal and axial anatomy as defined by McNeal are illustrated in Figures 8-8 and 8-9. The MRI axial anatomy is illustrated in Figure 8-10.[6,7,10]

1. *The peripheral zone.* This zone contains 70 percent of the normal-sized glandular prostate. The posterior peripheral zone is the only part that is palpable by digital rectal examination. The anterior portion of the peripheral zone is not accessible by rectal examination and is an area in which MRI may be most helpful. The peripheral zone is an area of

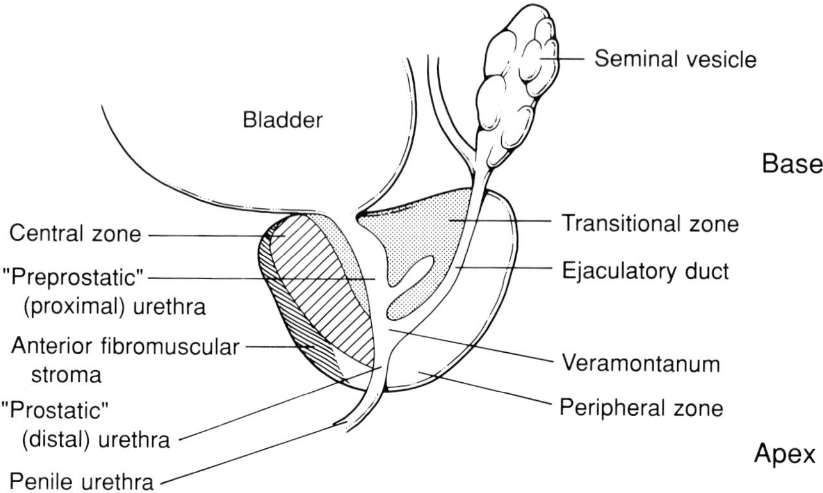

FIG. 8-8.   Sagittal zonal anatomy of the prostate gland. Note that the transitional zone and central zone are indistinguishable on MRI. (Schematic drawn from data in Hricak et al.[6] and Sommer et al.[7])

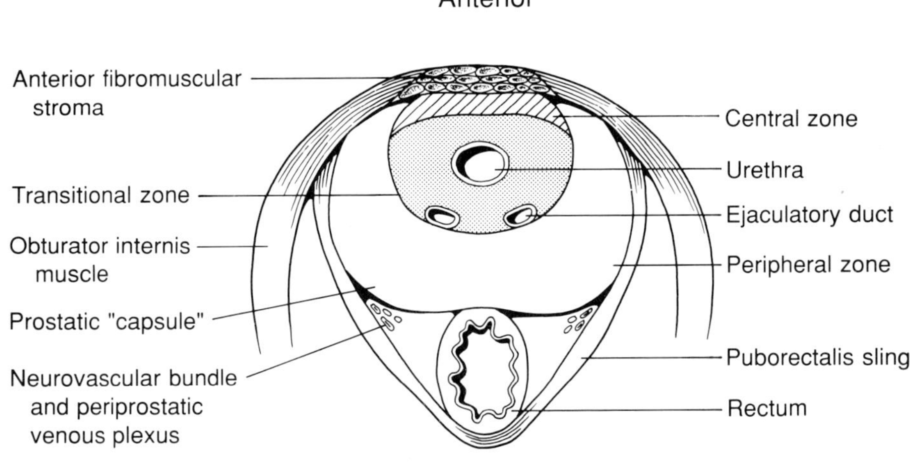

FIG. 8-9.   Axial zonal anatomy of the prostate gland. Proportions illustrated for gland with mild benign prostatic hyperplasia.

very high signal intensity on T_2-weighted images. The peripheral zone is the dominant zone in the most caudal portion, the apex of the gland (Fig. 8-11). On T_1-weighted images, the peripheral zone is of low signal intensity, inseparable from the central zone.

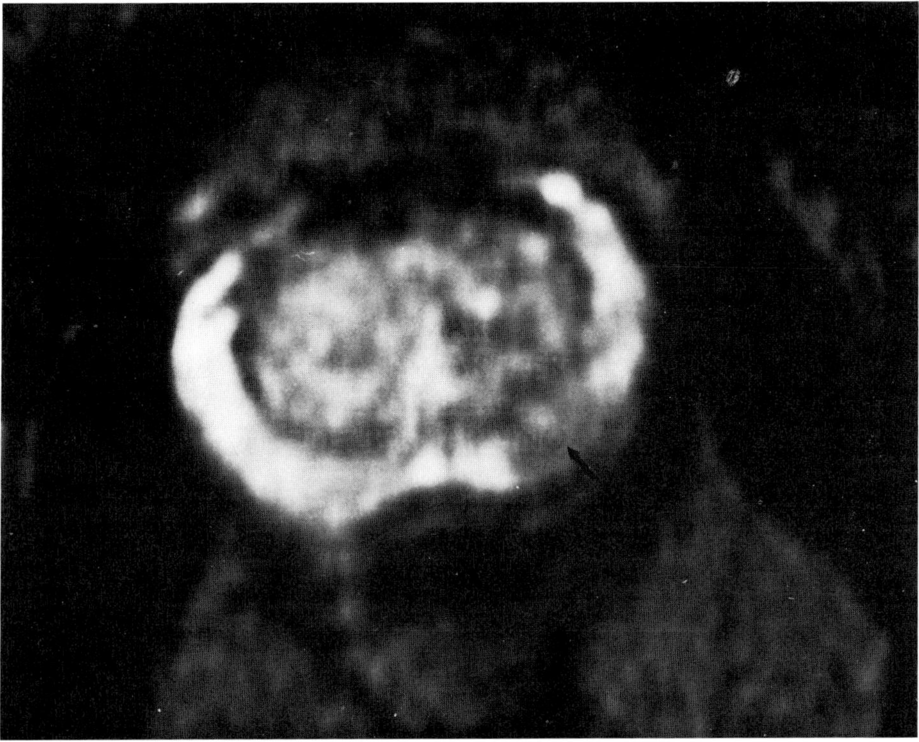

FIG. 8-10.   Axial T$_2$-weighted image showing zonal anatomy. Stage B2 cancer is seen in the left posterior peripheral zone (arrow).

2. *The central zone.* This zone has more stroma and constitutes about 25 percent of the gland in normal-sized prostates. This is the median signal area on T$_2$-weighted MRI.

3. *The transition zone.* Also called the preprostatic area, or the prostatic urethral segment, this zone is the area of benign prostatic hyperplasia, which arises primarily in the median lobe at the base of the bladder.

4. *An anterior fibromuscular stroma.* This zone, forming the anterior boundary, is contiguous with the puboprostatic ligament. There is no definite capsule around the prostate gland, especially the posterolateral portion of the peripheral zone, so there is no boundary to the extension of neoplasm from the prostate gland to the neurovascular bundle. The anterior fibromuscular stroma is clearly visible as a low-signal band anteriorly on T$_2$-weighted images. Some fibromuscular stroma occurs in the posterolateral portion but is usually so thin that it is not visible on routine MRI. The asymmetric dark band on T$_2$-weighted images seen at the lateral edge of the prostate gland is due to a chemical shift artifact and *is not* the capsule.

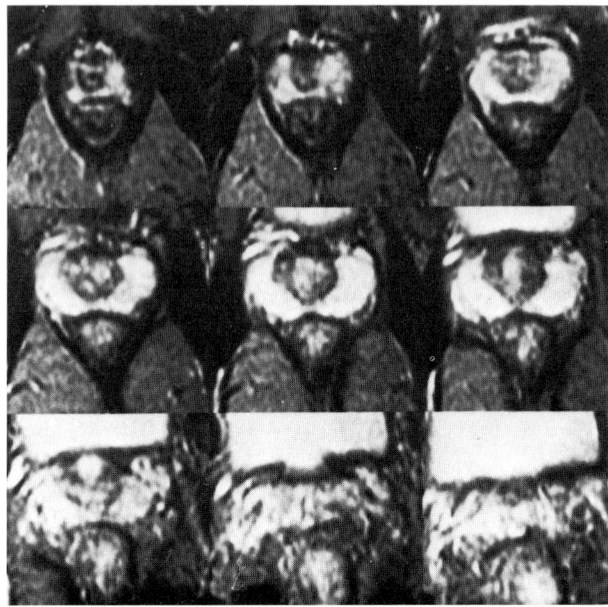

FIG. 8-11.   Sequential T_2-weighted axial images demonstrating relative proportions of central and peripheral zone. Left uppermost: caudal, primarily urethra and peripheral zone. Right lower: seminal vesicle with normal high signal intensity posterior to bladder.

The nomenclature of the gland as defined by McNeal needs to be clarified. The McNeal "transitional" zone is inseparable from the central zone on MRI. In the MRI literature, the medium signal central zone on MRI includes the McNeal "central zone," the McNeal "transitional zone," the anterior fibromuscular stroma, and the periurethral muscle sphincter.

APPEARANCE OF PROSTATIC PATHOLOGY ON MRI

With BPH, the transition zone, which normally occupies only about 5 percent of the gland, enlarges and dominates the MRI central zone. Prostate cancers have low-signal areas in T_2-weighted images. The high-signal areas correspond to dilated glandular elements (cystic ectasia), while the low-signal areas usually represent collagen (scar) and fibromuscular stroma.[11,12] The ejaculatory duct and prostatic secretions empty into the distal urethra. The ridge of the verumontanum separates the McNeal "preprostatic urethra" from the "prostatic urethra." Benign hypertrophic changes occur in the stromal tissue (the McNeal "transitional zone"), which surrounds the preprostatic urethra, and in the smooth muscle sheaths of the internal urethral sphincter. Thus, BPH changes involve the base of the bladder rather than the apex of the gland.[9]

On the other hand, McNeal[8] found that 66 percent of cancers arose within the peripheral zone. Mostofi and Price[13] found cancers only in the peripheral zone in about one-half of cases and in both the central zone and peripheral zone in about one-half of cases. In only about 0.5 percent of cases was the cancer found to be limited to the central zone. This suggests that evaluation of only the peripheral zone should permit the diagnosis of most of the carcinomas. Breslow[15] found that 64 percent of prostate cancers involve the apical portion of the peripheral zone. The exact extent needs to be defined by imaging to allow preservation of the external sphincter during surgery without compromising surgical margins, important for postoperative continence.

The cancer is identified as a medium- to low-signal area within the normally high signal of the peripheral zone on T_2-weighted images. On the spin-density image (20-ms echo), the cancer is lower in signal than both the peripheral zone and the periprostatic fat. On T_1-weighted images, the carcinoma is not separable from the peripheral zone except when central necrosis (signal intensity lowers even more) or hemorrhage (T_1 shortening increases signal) has occurred. Leiomyomas of the prostate are also low in signal on T_2-weighted sequences but are quite rare. Scars in the peripheral zone are also low in signal and are often indistinguishable from carcinoma. Unfortunately, in our experience, MRI has a high sensitivity but relatively low specificity in detection of early prostatic cancer. Gadolinium contrast injection has not yet been shown to be helpful in increasing specificity.

On T_2-weighted images, the ejaculatory ducts are the paired symmetric low-signal paracentral structures in the junction between the central zone and the peripheral zone and may occasionally be mistaken for carcinoma by the unwary. Asymmetric contour changes in this area, however, are sometimes due to cancer and may imply anterior rectal wall involvement.

One should also look for the periprostatic venous plexus and the neurovascular bundle tucked in medial to the puborectalis sling. The prostate is attached anteriorly by the puboprostatic ligament to the symphysis and separated posteriorly from the rectum by Denonvillier's fascia. These attachments decrease but do not prevent, direct invasion by prostate cancer.

The overwhelming majority of tumors of the prostate gland are adenocarcinomas. Other tumors that may arise in the prostate gland include periurethral duct carcinomas (transitional cells), leiomyomas,[16] sarcomas such as leiomyosarcomas, rhabdomyosarcomas[17] and fibrosarcomas, endometrioid tumors, and adenocystic carcinomas. Cancer of the bladder or rectum can secondarily invade the prostate gland by direct extension (Fig. 8-12). These have high signal on T_2-weighted images, extending into the central zone.

STAGING OF PROSTATE CANCER

The present staging scheme of prostate cancer is a combination of digital examinations and surgical findings. The scheme demonstrated in Table 8-2 presents information from cross-sectional imaging. One should be aware, however, that nonenlarged lymph nodes may contain disease and there may be microscopic extensions into adjacent periprostatic soft tissue that will upstage the tumor during surgery.

Management of different stages is discussed in detail in Chapter 7. Generally, stage A1 lesions (depending on age) are managed by repeat examinations or

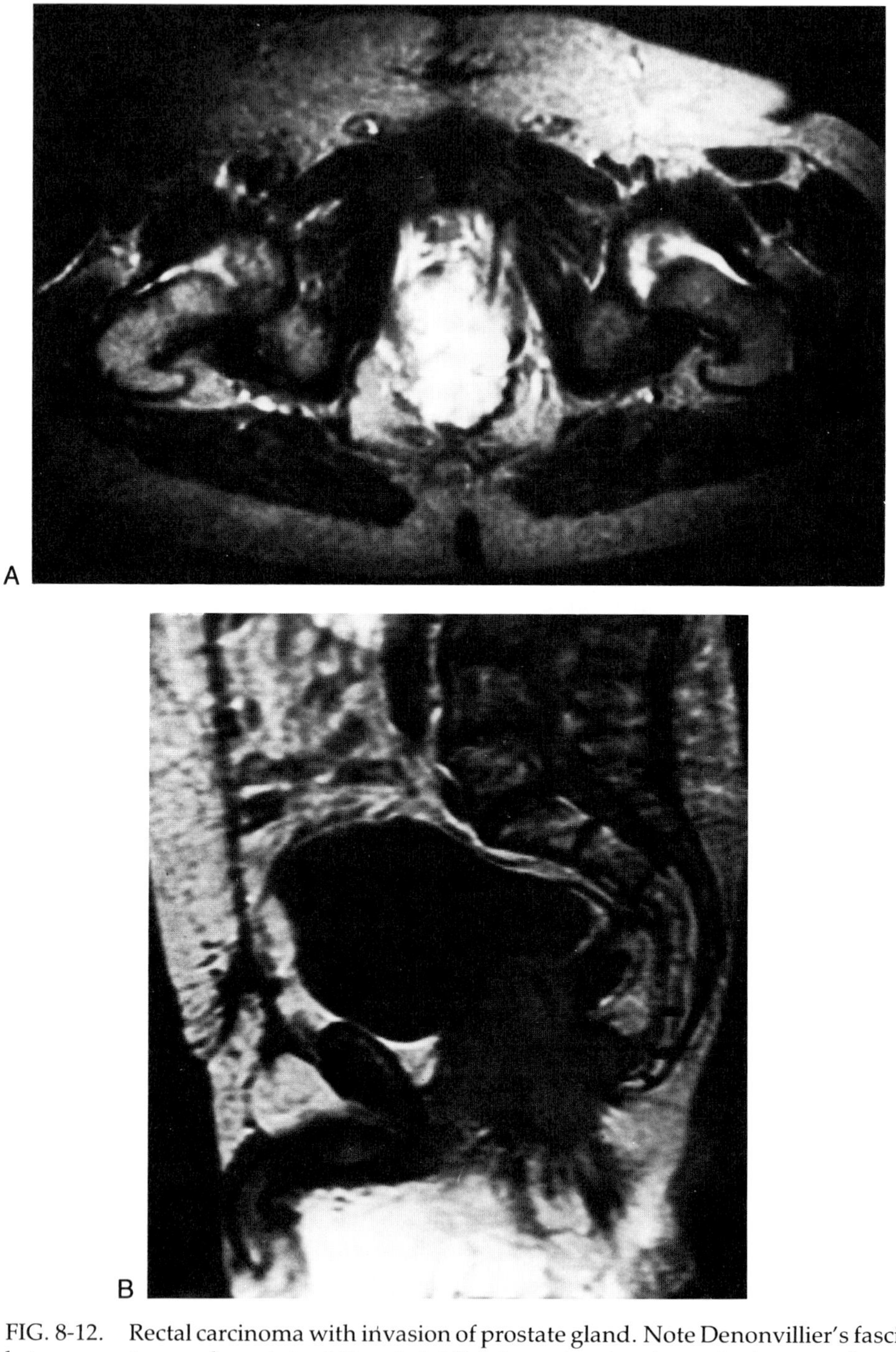

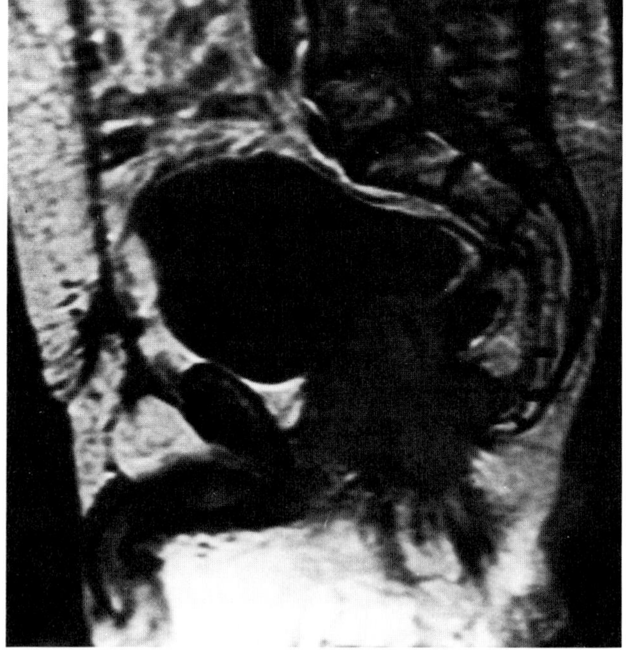

FIG. 8-12.   Rectal carcinoma with invasion of prostate gland. Note Denonvillier's fascia between rectum and prostate obliterated. High irregular signal seen in the central zone of prostate. (A) Axial T_2-weighted MRI scan. (B) Sagittal spin-density weighted MRI scan.

TABLE 8-2   Modified clinical/MRI staging scheme for Prostatic cancer[a]

Stage	Description
A(T1)	Tumor not clinically palpable
A1	Focal
A2	Diffuse or multifocal
B(T2)	Tumor palpable but confined to prostate gland
B1	Tumor <1.5 cm in diameter
B2	Tumor >1.5 cm in diameter
B3	Tumor occupying more than one lobe
C(T3)	Tumor extension into extracapsular perioprostatic tissue: seminal vesicle, perioprostatic fat, urinary bladder, urethra, levator ani
D(T4)	Metastatic disease
D1 (N1–N3)	Pelvic lymph nodes involved (enlarged >1.5 cm)
D2 (N4)	Bony metastases or other distant metastases

[a]Acid phosphatase should be normal in stage A and B lesions. Bone scan should be negative in stage A, B, C, and D1, lesions.

biopsies at 6-month intervals and occasionally by surgery. Stage A2 and B lesions are managed by radical (or Walsh's modified radical[18,19] prostatectomy), and limited lymph node dissection[20] or ^{125}I-intracavitary or external beam radiation. Stage C tumors are treated by external beam radiation to the regions involved. Stage D tumors are treated hormonally, with diethylstilbestrol (DES), orchiectomy, or antiandrogens.[21] Metastatic disease to the lumbar spine is best imaged with MRI to look for spinal cord compression and, if present, is treated with local external beam radiation. If unavailable, CT myelography (or, less satisfactorily, routine myelography) can be substituted.

In our experience, patients are referred for MRI of the prostate gland for the following reasons: (1) high Gleason grading on biopsy, (2) abnormal digital rectal examination, (3) elevated PSA or prostatic acid phosphatase (PAP), and (4) cancer discovered incidentally on transurethral resection in younger patients. *Detailed understanding of the clinical and epidemiologic implications of each of these indications is critical to image interpretation and determining when a study is appropriate in an environment in which not all clinicians have as yet a clear understanding of the limitations and applications of MRI in prostatic cancer.* Each of these indications is discussed below.

High Gleason Grading on Biopsy

Many histologic grading patterns are available. The Gleason grade is relatively reproducible and has prognostic value in the biologic potential of the tumor. Cantrell et al.[22] reported that the size of incidental carcinomas is related to progression. Only 2 percent with 5 percent or less of the gland involved progressed, whereas 30 percent with more extensive tumor progressed. No patient with Gleason grade 4 or less progressed, while 11 percent of Gleason grade 5 to 6 and 33 percent of Gleason grade 7 to 9 progressed. Similar findings are reported by Sagalowsky et al.[23] and by Kramer et al.[24]

The Gleason grade is based on the worst component present in at least one-third of the specimen. Catalona et al.[25] reported that the needle biopsies undergraded the tumor in about 33 percent and was correct in about 60 percent. Gleason grade tumors higher than 5 are usually stage B and C tumors and have a higher incidence of positive pelvic nodes. High Gleason grades correlated well with capsular penetration, involvement of the seminal vesicle, and lymph node metastasis. If clinical information of the Gleason grade of the tumor is available, incorporation of that information into the receiver operator characteristic will enhance overall diagnostic accuracy.

The Abnormal Digital Rectal Examination

Rectal examination is about 80 percent sensitive and 50 percent specific in experienced hands. Much data on its reliability predate the availability of MRI and ultrasound. In our series of 53 patients with a unilaterally palpable prostate nodule, 22 of 53 (42 percent) had nonpalpable cancer in the contralateral lobe on step-sectioned pathologic specimens after radical prostatectomy. Causes of induration include infection, granulomatous prostatis, prostate abscess (see Fig. 8-16), benign prostatic hyperplasia, and prostate infarction. The limitations of the digital examination were demonstrated by a study by Hodge et al.[1] comparing digital examination and ultrasound-guided biopsy of prostatic lesions. A mean of 6.2 biopsies per patient using a spring-loaded biopsy gun was performed; 36 percent of palpably firm prostates had cancer. Random biopsy of the contralateral lobe in 56 men showed cancer in 42 percent (stage B1) to 60 percent (stage B2). In 53 percent (23 of 43) of patients with negative digitally guided biopsy, ultrasound-guided biopsy diagnosed cancer.

Jewett[26] found that 50 percent of palpated nodules are benign; 84 percent of the small nodules (confined to one lobe) are localized on surgical pathology. However, 50 percent of the larger tumors are upstaged at surgery. One role of MRI is to improve preoperative staging to eliminate unnecessary surgery.

Prostatic Specific Antigen and Prostatic Acid Phosphatase

Knowledge of the implications of high serum markers will enable radiologists to suggest adjunct tests such as bone scan when the MRI findings do not correlate with the high serum markers. In a study of 2,200 serum samples,[27] PSA was elevated in 122 of 127 patients with newly diagnosed cancer. PAP was elevated in only 57 of 127 patients. However, PSA was elevated in 86 percent with benign prostatic hyperplasia and PAP in 14 percent in patients with BPH. After radical prostatectomy for cancer, PSA fell to undetectable levels with a half-life of 2.2 days. PAP fell to normal limits within 24 hours but remained detectable. Prostatic massage, needle biopsy, and transurethral resection transiently increased the PSA and PAP. Stamey et al. concluded that PSA was more sensitive, but neither is specific for prostate cancer. However, PSA is useful in monitoring tumor post-therapy or in patients without evidence of BPH or prostatitis.

A serum PSA level of more than 50 ng/ml is not seen in BPH.[28] Using a PSA normal limit of 2.7 ng/ml, PSA and PAP were elevated in 3 to 4 percent in noncomplicated BPH and chronic prostatis. In complicated BPH and acute prostatitis, PSA was elevated in 65 percent and 24 percent, respectively, and PAP in 20 percent and 16 percent, respectively.[29] PSA was elevated in 98 percent of 86 men with active stage D2 disease. In stage A or B disease, PSA was greater than 10 ng/ml in 59 percent with extracapsular disease and only 7 percent without extracapsular disease.[30,31] Prostate specific antigen was correlated with volume of prostate cancer (r = 0.7), with approximately 3.5 ng/ml serum level for every cc of cancer, about 10 times that of BPH. As no patients with lymph node metastasis had serum levels of less than 10 ng/ml, it is useful as a preoperative marker[32] and as an indicator of suspicion prior to performing MRI.

Incidental Cancers Detected on Transurethral Resection for BPH

Epidemiologic data suggest that incidentally diagnosed A1 prostate cancers with low Gleason grade (2 to 4) usually do not progress and probably do not have to be treated. Whether higher Gleason scores need to be treated remains controversial. Cantrell et al.[22] showed that the size of the tumor is also a good predictor of progression. It is here that the size estimate gained from MRI may be useful in determining whether further therapy is indicated. However, size estimates are difficult in diffuse cancer, and MRI tends to underestimate the larger tumors and to overestimate the smaller tumors.[33]

The disease has a worse prognosis in younger patients. In the patient over 70 years of age with early carcinoma (stage A or B) of the prostate, conservative treatment usually results in a normal life expectancy. Unfortunately, this is not true for those under 70.[14]

A study of 158 step-sectioned autopsy prostate specimens showed a 41 percent incidence of carcinoma in men aged 70 to 80 years and a 57 percent incidence in men over 80 years of age.[34] The high incidence of prostate cancer in autopsy specimens in patients of the seventh and eighth decades suggests that many prostate cancers go undetected and are not the cause of mortality in most of these patients.

The incidence of atypical hyperplasia in prostatic glands without carcinoma was 3 percent but 49 percent in patients with carcinoma. Hence, the finding of severe dysplasia on prostatectomy or transrectal ultrasound (TUR) specimen should alert the radiologist to the high probability that malignant transformation had occurred or that carcinoma is already present in parts of the gland not sampled.[35]

MRI IN STAGING OF EARLY PROSTATIC CARCINOMA

At present, the primary role of MRI in prostate cancer is not in diagnosis or screening but in preoperative staging. Postoperative follow-up may be performed with either CT or MRI. The relative merits of TRU and MRI in the staging of A2, B, and C tumors are yet to be resolved. A four-center study comparing MRI with TRU using surgical pathologic correlation is ongoing at Johns Hopkins Medical School, Thomas Jefferson School of Medicine, University of Michigan Medical School, and University of California, San Francisco, School of Medicine. It is an area with such rapid technologic advances that the results may be outdated even as the data are being collated. Many reports[36,37] of accuracy of MRI in staging prostate cancer are invalid because of suboptimal imaging techniques (poor-quality scanners, large pixel size, suboptimal pulse parameters) and lack of direct pathologic correlation. It is difficult for mid- and low-field machines to achieve the necessary signal-to-noise (S/N) ratio for the 4- to 5-mm-thick small field of view sections necessary for prostate imaging and still maintain a long enough TR ($>2,500$ ms) for the high-T_2 contrast. No data are yet available on the accuracy of MRI in the screening mode in the elderly general population.

Lytton[38] states that pelvic lymph node dissection is not therapeutic. It should be used only for prognosis and to assess the need for radiotherapy as an adjunct to radical prostatectomy. To minimize such complications as lymphocele and deep venous thrombosis, dissection is limited to the distal common iliac, internal iliac, obturator, and proximal external iliac nodes. The presacral, presciatic, para-aortic, and deep inguinal nodes may also be involved, but removal requires marked extension of the operative field. It is in these nodal areas that staging CT or MRI can play an important role. Prout et al.[39] found 10 percent of patients with negative surgical lymph nodes progressing to bony metastasis versus 60 percent for patients with positive lymph nodes.

The involvement of seminal vesicles has traditionally been considered a contraindication to radical prostatectomy. Detection of seminal vesicle invasion by imaging is important but is not as yet very accurate. The difficulty lies in the fact that the most medial inferior portion of the seminal vesicle inserts deep into the prostate gland. Invasion of the seminal vesicle usually occurs via extracapsular invasion and appears as low-signal areas against the high-signal seminal vesicles on T_2-weighted images.[10] The middle portion of the gland may have a low signal due to insertion of the ductus deferens.

Stamey et al.[20] found penetration of the cancer into the periprostatic fat to be common, occurring in 33 percent of patients with preoperative stage A or B disease; the most common location for capsular penetration is in the area of the neurovascular bundle. Recently, Walsh and co-workers[18,19] developed a potency-sparing radical prostatectomy surgical technique that preserves the neurovascular bundle at least unilaterally if it does not compromise surgical margins. Their rate of positive margins of 10 percent is similar to that achieved with older techniques. Hence, prediction of neurovascular invasion by MRI preoperatively will be extremely useful in deciding which neurovascular bundle(s) to sacrifice. Tempany et al.[40] found larger tumor volume and higher Gleason grade to correlate with the incidence of capsular invasion. MRI using body coil was 68 percent sensitive and 69 percent specific in predicting extracapsular penetration in the region of the neurovascular bundle. Tumor size greater than 2 ml near the neurovascular bundle, change in contour of the prostrate gland locally, and loss of fat planes at the neurovascular bundle are all risk factors for extracapsular penetration. Greater accuracy may be achieved in the equivocal cases by slightly overestimating capsular penetration in patients with larger tumors and high Gleason grade. The use of surface coils (Figs. 8-5 and 8-6) offer promise of more accurate staging for early disease. Special attention should be paid to the peripheral zone anteriorly near the apex of the gland, where the neurovascular bundle is not well visualized.

Treatment of early stage C disease is controversial. Some would advocate glandular removal; others prefer radiation therapy. The prognostic data are based on clinical staging. Hricak[41] found that 62 percent of patients clinically determined to have stage B2 disease were surgically revised to stage C. MRI staging was 83 percent accurate versus 65 percent for CT. The areas of difficulty for CT are in the bladder base and the levator ani sling and in differentiating small vessels from lymph nodes.[42] Using multiple criteria, MRI had a sensitivity of 72 percent, a specificity of 84 percent, and an accuracy of 78 percent in the differentiation of stage A or B from stage C or D disease. In the detection of lymph node metastasis, the sensitivity was 69 percent, specificity 95 percent, and accuracy 88 percent.[43] In another study, extraglandular spread of cancer of the prostate was diagnosed with an accuracy rate of 79 percent by MRI and 46 percent by CT.[44]

POSSIBLE FUTURE APPLICATION OF MRI IN BENIGN PROSTATIC HYPERTROPHY

Several potential applications of MRI have arisen due to recent nonsurgical therapy for benign prostatic hyperplasia. However, its high cost and relatively low specificity at present preclude its use in routine mass screening for prostate cancer.

With approximately 8 to 10 percent of incidental cancers found during transurethral resection for BPH, widespread use of medical therapy will decrease cancer detection rate. MRI provides a means of screening for suspicious cancers in selected cases. As scars may mimic cancer in the peripheral zone, MRI is sensitive, although not specific. In a large prospective multi-institutional study involving 234 patients with radical prostatectomy with preoperative intrarectal ultrasound and MRI, accuracy of clinical staging on a lesion by lesion basis was 44 percent (by ultrasound 58 percent; by MRI 69 percent).[49]

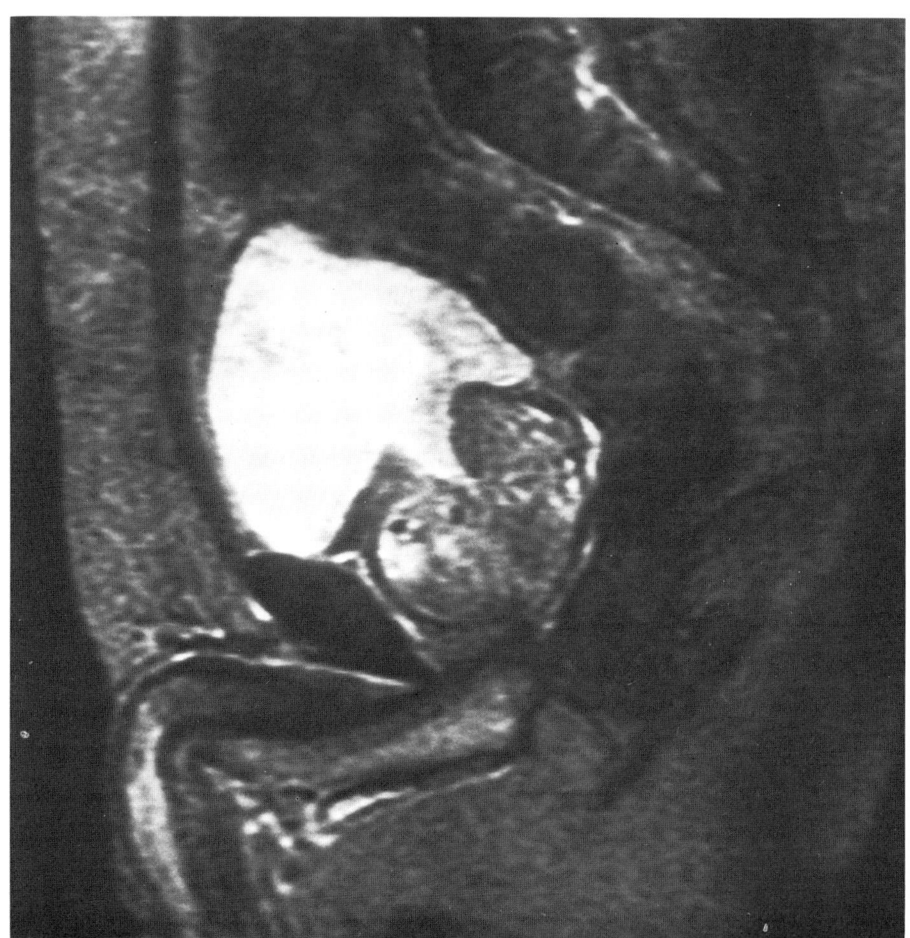

FIG. 8-13.   Recurrent benign prostatic hypertrophy after transurethral resection (TUR). Sagittal T$_2$-weighted images. (A) Recurrence of obstruction 3 years post-TUR. Proximal urethra deviated posteriorly by adenoma, preventing urethral catheterization. (*Figure continues.*)

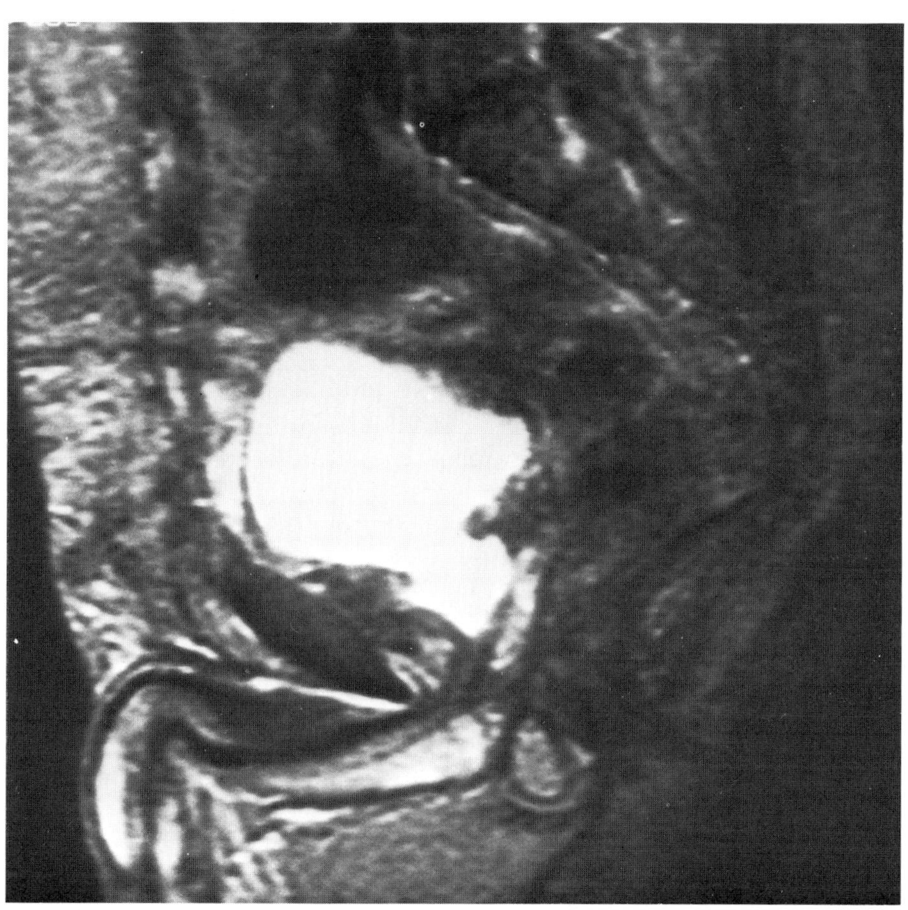

FIG. 8-13 *(Continued)*.   (B) After suprapubic subtotal prostatectomy, central adenoma removed, leaving peripheral zone.

TABLE 8-3 Normal size of prostate and seminal vesicles

Structure	Size (cm)
Prostate	
Anteroposterior	3.0 ± 0.6
Transverse	3.6 ± 0.8
Craniocaudal	3.2 ± 0.8
Seminal vesicle	
Length	3.1 ± 0.7
Width	1.4 ± 0.4

(Data from Phillip et al.[10])

After androgen deprivation therapy, the prostate size should be monitored. As MRI is more accurate and less operator dependent than ultrasound for prostate size measurement[45] and the expected change is small, serial follow-up evaluation is done more accurately with contoured volumetric estimations from MRI than with the three axis methods. The general estimation of prostate size is adequate with ultrasound, CT, or MRI. The formula is 0.525 × transverse diameter × anteroposterior diameter × craniocaudal length, for volume (in ml), and multiplied by a specific weight of 1.05 g/ml for weight. The normal size of the prostate and seminal vesicles is shown in Table 8-3.[10]

Normal prostate glands weigh 20 g plus or minus 6 in young men of the third decade. Hyperplasia is only 4 percent in the fourth decade and 50 percent in the fifth decade. However, in patients without hyperplasia, mean prostatic weight actually starts to decline in the fifth decade, reaching a mean of about 12 g by the seventh decade. There is a diurnal variation of about 20 percent in some patients. After castration and estrogen therapy, prostatic size decreases exponentially, reaching a plateau approximately 1 to 6 months later.[15] Most urologists will perform transurethral prostatectomy for glands weighing up to 60 g and retropubic or suprapubic prostatectomy for larger glands.

In complicated BPH (Fig. 8-13) with urinary obstruction or hematuria post-transurethral resection, MRI may be used in surgical planning and in the identification of bleeding adenomas as shown by high-signal T_1-weighted images (Fig. 8-14). About 2 to 3 percent of all transurethral resections will require a second operation. After transurethral resection, a fluid-filled defect is seen in the transition zone adjacent to the proximal urethra. Radiographically apparent prostatic calculi are seen in 14 percent of men. The relationship to infection is unclear.[37] Infection of the seminal vesicles is manifested by an increase in signal on T_1-weighted and spin-density images with maintenance of high-signal T_2-weighted images (Fig. 8-15). Acute prostatitis is manifested with high signal in the central zone on T_2-weighted images[46] (Fig. 8-16). It is difficult to distinguish chronic prostatitis in the peripheral zone from cancer.

Another way to improve urodynamics in BPH uses transurethral balloon dilation or stent placement.[47] However, the method is suboptimal when the

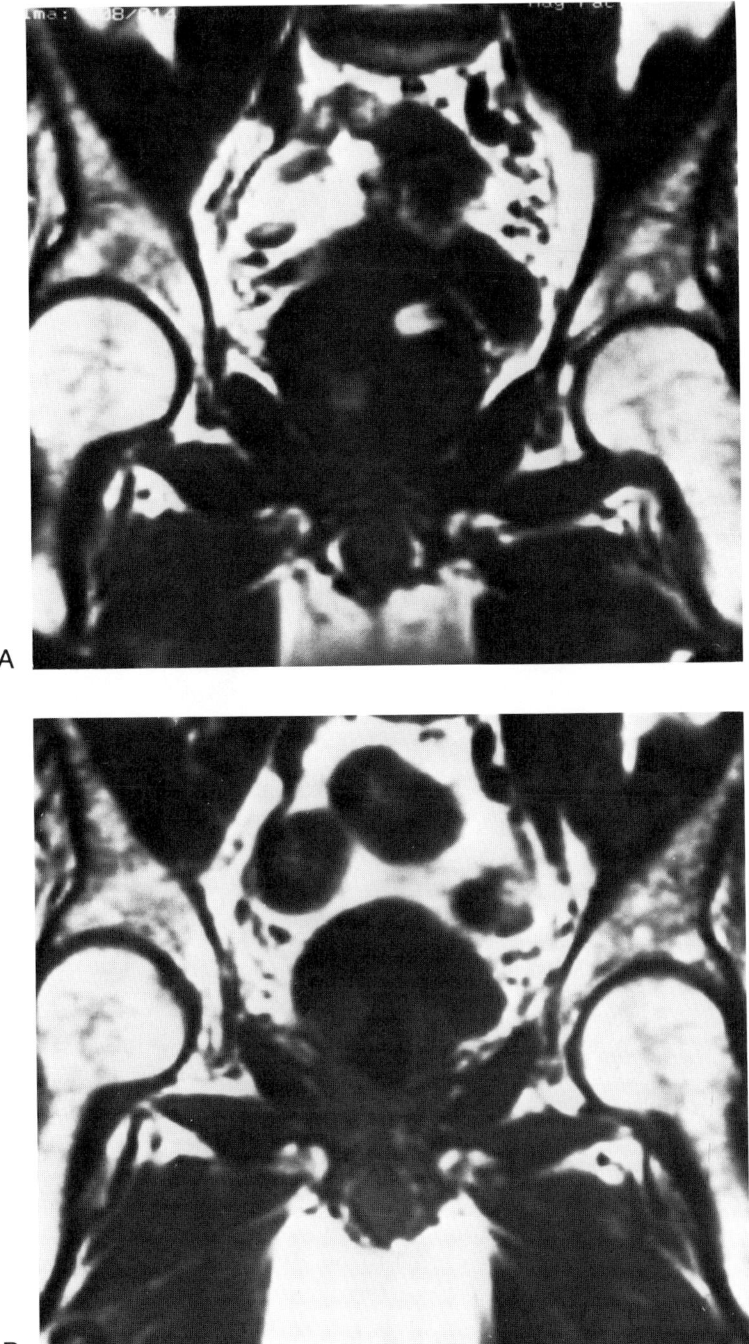

FIG. 8-14.   Intraprostatic bleeding 3 years after transurethral resection (TUR). (A) Coronal T_1-weighted MRI scan illustrating source of gross hematuria post-TUR. (B) Relationship of bladder neck relative to prostate gland illustrated after subtotal prostatectomy. Patient now asymptomatic.

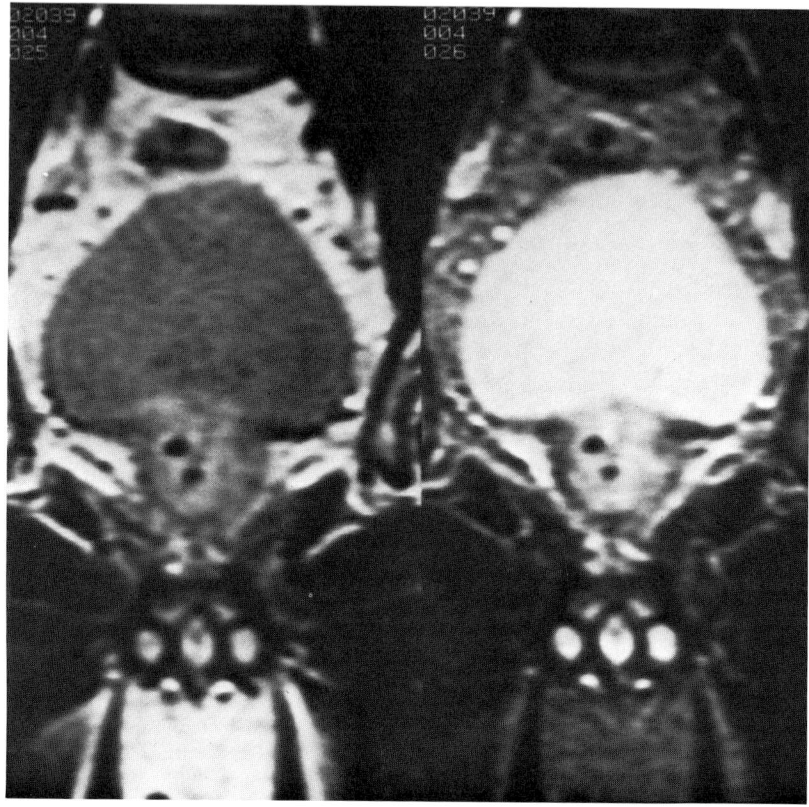

FIG. 8-15.   Acute prostatitis with incidental calcifications. Note high signal intensity in central zone in spin-density (left) and T_2- (right) weighted coronal MRI scans.

hyperplasia is predominantly in the middle lobe.[48] Imaging may be helpful in identifying the location and morphometry of the hyperplastic nodules.

CONCLUSION

MRI of the prostate gland is superior to CT and is more reproducible than transrectal ultrasound. Its wide application is limited at present by its relatively high cost. Its most promising application is in preoperative planning for potency-saving radical prostatectomies in patients with early-stage prostate cancer and in the planning and follow-up evaluation of patients with more advanced neoplasms. Accuracy in diagnosis is best increased by adjusting receiver operating characteristics to known clinical information.

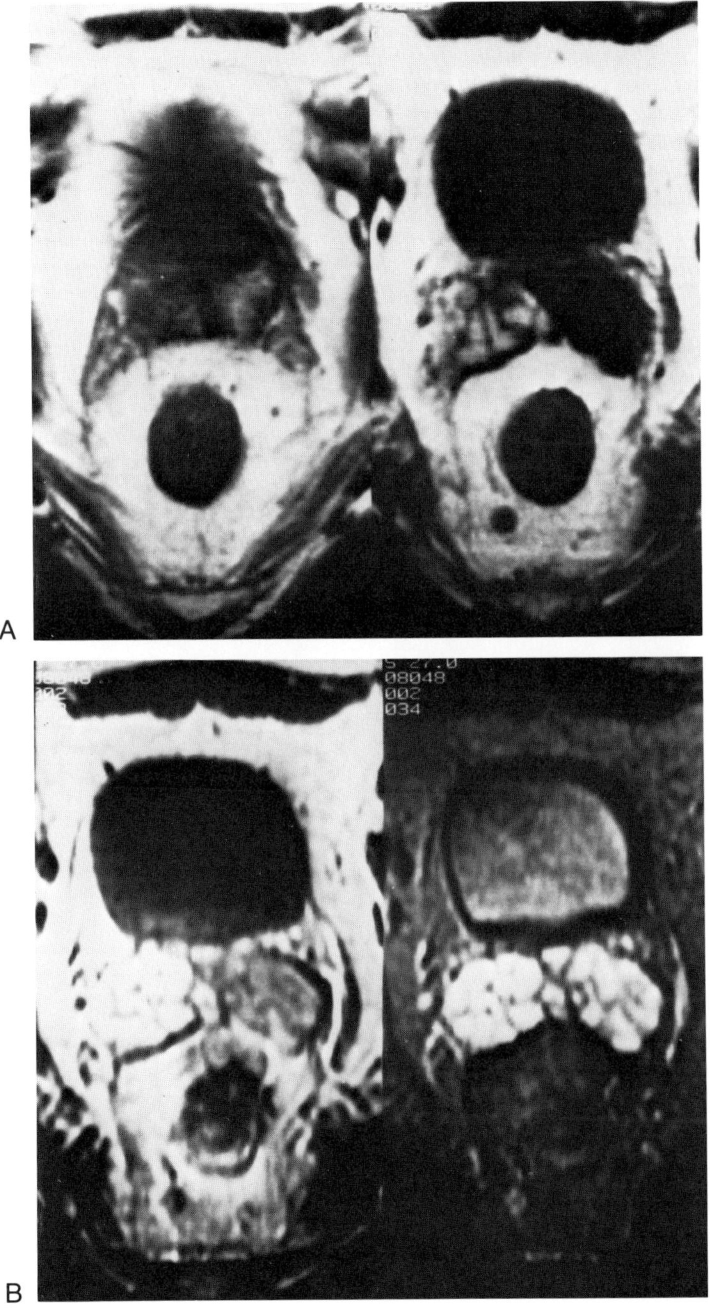

FIG. 8-16.   Infection of the seminal vesicles. (A) T_1-weighted images show increased signal in the right seminal vesicle with a normal left seminal vesicle. (B) Spin-density images show increased signal in the infected seminal vesicle. T_2-weighted images on the right do not distinguish the normal from the inflamed seminal vesicle because of normally high fluid content.

REFERENCES

1. Hodge KK, McNeal JE, Stamey TA: Ultrasound guided transrectal core biopsies of the palpably abnormal prostate. J Urol 142:66, 1989
2. Schnall MD, Lenkinski RE, Pollack HM, et al: Prostate: MR imaging with an endorectal surface coil. Radiology 172:570, 1989
3. Martin JF, Hajek P, Baker L, et al: Inflatable surface coil for MR imaging of the prostate. Radiology 167:268, 1988
4. Halliday KR, Fenoglio PC, Sillerud LO: Differentiation of human tumors from nonmalignant tissue by natural abundance ^{13}C NMR spectroscopy. Magnetic Resonance Med 7:384, 1988
5. Plesnicar S: The course of metastatic disease originating from the carcinoma of the prostate. Clin Exp Metast 3:103, 1985
6. Hricak H, Dooms GC, McNeal JE, et al: MR imaging of the prostate gland: Normal anatomy. AJR 148:51, 1987
7. Sommer FG, McNeal JE, Carrol CL: MR depiction of zonal anatomy of the prostate at 1.5T. J Comput Assist Tomogr 10:983, 1986
8. McNeal JE: Origin and development of carcinoma in the prostate. Cancer 23:24, 1969
9. McNeal JE: Origin and evolution of benign prostatic enlargement. Invest Urol 15:340, 1978
10. Phillip, ME, Kressel HY, Spritzer CE, et al: Normal prostate and adjacent structures. MR at 1.5T. Radiology 164:381, 1987
11. Hruban, RH, Zerhouni EA, Dagher AP, et al: Morphologic basis of MR imaging of benign prostatic hyperplasia. J Comput Assist Tomogr 11:1035, 1987
12. Schiebler ML, Tomoszczewski JE, Bezzi M, et al: Prostatic carcinoma and benign prostatic hyperplasia: Correlation with high resolution MR and histopathological findings. Radiology 172:131, 1989
13. Mostofi FK, Price EB Jr: Tumors of the Male Genital System. Atlas of Tumor Pathology. 2nd series, fascicle 8. Ch. 9, p. 94. Armed Forces Institute of Pathology, Washington, DC.
14. Chisolm, GD: Natural history of prostate cancer. p. 94. In Blandy JP, Lytton B (eds): The Prostate. Butterworth, London, 1986
15. Breslow N, Chan CW, Dhom G, et al: Latent carcinoma of prostate at autopsy in seven areas. Int J Cancer 20:680, 1977
16. Genenois PA, Gysels M, Corbusier A, et al: Leiomyoma of the prostate. Appearance on MRI. Apropos of 2 cases. J Radiol 68:631, 1987
17. Bartologzzi C, Selli C, Olmastroni M, et al: Rhabdomyosarcoma of the prostate gland: MR findings. AJR 150:1333, 1988
18. Walsh PC: Radical prostatectomy, preservation of sexual function and cancer control. The controversy. Urol Clin North Am 14:663, 1987
19. Walsh PC, Lepor H, Eggleston JC: Radical prostatectomy with preservation of sexual functions: Anatomical and pathological considerations. Prostate 4:473, 1983
20. Stamey TA, McNeal JE, Freiha FS, et al: Morphometric and clinical studies on 68 consecutive radical prostatectomies. J Urol 139:1235, 1988
21. Lee JK, Marx MV: Pelvis. p. 859. In Lee JK, Sagel SS, Stanley RJ (eds): Computed Tomography with MRI Correlation. Raven Press, New York, 1989
22. Cantrell BB, Deklerk DP, Eggleston JC, et al: Pathological factors that influence prognosis in stage A prostatic cancer: Influence of extent versus grade. J Urol 125:516, 1981
23. Sagalowsky AI, Milam H, Reveley R, et al: Prediction of lymphatic metastases by Gleason histological grading in prostate cancer. J Urol 128:951, 1982

24. Kramer SA, Spahr J, Brendler CB, et al: Experience with Gleason's histopathological grading in prostate cancer. J Urol 124:223, 1980

25. Catalona WJ, Stein AJ, Fair WR: Grading errors in prostatic needle biopsy relation to the accuracy of tumor grade in predicting pelvic lymph node metastasis. J Urol 127:919, 1982

26. Jewett HJ: The present status of radical prostatectomies for stage A and B cancer. Urol Clin North Am 2:105, 1975

27. Stamey TA, Yang N, Hay AR, et al: Prostate specific antigen as a serum marker for adenocarcinoma of the prostate. N Engl J Med 317:909, 1987

28. Baron JC, Peyret C, Leroy M, et al: Prostatic specific antigen in prostatic cancer. Am J Clin Oncol 11(suppl 2):S75, 1988

29. Daver A, Soret JY, Coblentz Y, et al: The usefulness of prostate specific antigen and prostatic acid phosphotase in clinical practice. Am J Clin Oncol 11(suppl 2):S53, 1988

30. Ercole CJ, Lange PH, Mathisen M, et al: Prostatic specific antigen and prostatic acid phosphatase in the monitoring and staging of patients with prostate cancer. J Urol 138:1181, 1987

31. Lange PH, Brawer MK: Serum prostate specific antigen: Its use in diagnosis and management of prostate cancer. Urology 33(suppl 6):13, 1989

32. Stamey, TA, Kabalin JN, McNeal JE, et al: Prostate specific antigen in the diagnosis and treatment of adenocarcinoma of the prostate gland. II. Radical prostatectomy treated patients. J Urol 141:1076, 1989

33. Carrol CL, Sommer FG, McNeal JE, Stamey TA: The abnormal prostate: MR imaging at 1.5T with histopathological correlation. Radiology 163:521, 1987

34. Scott R Jr, Mutchnik DL, Laskowski TZ, et al: Carcinoma of the prostate in elderly man: Incidence, growth characteristics, and clinical significance. J Urol 101:602, 1969

35. Helpap B: The biological significance of atypical hyperplasia of prostate. Virchows Arch [A] 387:307, 1980

36. Ling D, Lee, JK, Heiken JP, et al: Prostatic carcinoma and benign prostatic hyperplasia: Inability of MR to distinguish between the two diseases. Radiology 158:103, 1986

37. Friedman, AC, Seidmon, EJ, Radecki, PD, et al: Relative merits of MRI, transrectal endosonography, and CT in diagnosis and staging of carcinoma of the prostate. Urology 31:530, 1988

38. Lytton B: Early prostatic cancer. p. 163. In Blandy JP, Lytton B (eds): The Prostate. Butterworth, London, 1986

39. Prout GR, Heaney, JA, Griffin PP, et al: Nodal involvement as a prognostic indicator in patients with prostatic carcinoma. J Urol 124:226, 1980

40. Tempany CM, Rahmouni A, Zerhouni EA, et al: Evaluation of the role of MRI in predicting invasion of the neurovascular bundle by prostate cancer. p. 129. Presented at the Annual Meeting of the Society of Magnetic Resonance in Medicine, August 12, 1989, Amsterdam, 1989 (abst)

41. Hricak H: Imaging prostate carcinoma. Radiology 169:569, 1988

42. Bryan PJ, Butler HE, Nelson, AD, et al: Magnetic resonance imaging of the prostate. AJR 146:543, 1986

43. Bezzi M, Kressel HY, Allen KS: Prostatic carcinoma, staging with MR imaging at 1.5T. Radiology 169:339, 1988

44. Beer M, Schmidt H, Riedl R: The clinical value of preoperative staging of bladder and prostatic cancer with nuclear magnetic resonance imaging and computed tomography. Urologe 28:65, 1989

45. Hricak H, Jeffrey RB, Dooms GC: Evaluation of prostate size. A comparison of ultrasound and MRI. Urol Radiol 9:1, 1987

46. Papanicolaou N, Pfister RC, Stafford SA, Parkhurst EC: Prostatic abscess. Imaging with transrectal sonography and MR. AJR 149:981, 1987

47. Reddy PK, Wasserman N, Castaneda F, et al: Balloon dilation of the prostate for treatment of benign hyperplasia. Urol Clin North Am 15:529, 1988

48. Castaneda F, Reddy P, Wasserman N, et al: Benign prostatic hypertrophy: Retrograde transurethral dilation of the prostatic urethra in humans. Work in progress. Radiology 163:649, 1987

49. Rifkins MD, Gatsonis CA, Zerhouni EA, et al: Endorectal US and MR imaging: Accuracy for staging prostate cancer. Abstract, RSNA 1989, Scientific Meeting, Chicago, Illinois. Radiology 173(p):143, 1989

9 Carcinoma of the Bladder

CHARLES B. BRENDLER

EPIDEMIOLOGY

Incidence and Mortality

Carcinoma of the bladder is the second most common genitourinary malignancy behind carcinoma of the prostate. It is estimated that in 1989 in the United States more than 47,000 new cases of bladder cancer will be diagnosed and that more than 10,000 people will die of this disease. The disease has a 3 to 1 male prevalence, and occurs more frequently in whites than in blacks.[1]

Risk Factors

In 1895 Rehn observed that aniline dye manufacturers were at risk of the development of bladder cancer. This was one of the first associations made between an industrial carcinogen and malignancy. Similar associations with a variety of aromatic amines were subsequently reported. Epidemiologists have estimated that 18 to 34 percent of male bladder cancer cases result from occupational exposure.[2]

Cigarette smoking is today the most significant risk factor for the development of bladder cancer with 30 to 40 percent of cases attributable to smoking. Men who smoke between $\frac{1}{2}$ and 2 packs per day have double the risk of bladder cancer, while men who smoke more than 2 packs per day triple their risk. Similar observations have been made in women.[3]

Artificial sweeteners including sodium cyclamate and sodium saccharin have also been linked to bladder cancer because of their carcinogenic effect in laboratory animals. Cyclamates were withdrawn from the market in 1969; to date, there have been no clinical studies linking saccharin to human bladder cancer.[4]

Schistosomiasis infection is associated with an increased incidence in bladder cancer, usually of the squamous cell type. Other risk factors for bladder cancer include chronic irritation and infection, previous exposure to cyclophosphamide (Cytoxan), which is known to produce an acute hemorrhagic cystitis, and previous pelvic irradiation. An association between coffee drinking and bladder cancer has been made, but the evidence is inconclusive.[5]

BIOLOGIC BEHAVIOR

Most bladder cancers begin as superficial lesions in the mucosa. Bladder cancer develops, however, in two forms. The first is a papillary lesion that tends to grow into the bladder lumen on a stalk and presents as a well-defined lesion within the bladder. The second type of tumor develops as a flat, "ink-stain" type of lesion that spreads insidiously across the bladder surface and presents as a lesion that may be difficult to distinguish from benign inflammation.

It is now well recognized that the papillary form of tumor is, in general, a slow growing lesion that, unless associated with flat carcinoma, rarely invades the bladder wall and rarely metastasizes.[6] Thus, unless papillary tumors present with muscle invasion at their initial diagnosis, these lesions seldom result in patient mortality. They may cause hematuria and irritative bladder symptoms, but they can usually be controlled with transurethral resection and topical chemotherapy.

In contrast, flat carcinoma tends to involve multiple areas within the bladder and invades the bladder muscle early on in the disease. Melamed et al.[7] first recognized the grave biologic significance of flat carcinoma and reported that 9 of 12 patients treated with transurethral resection and radiation progressed to invasive cancer. Utz et al.[8] reported that 40 percent of patients with flat carcinoma died of their disease within 5 years.

Flat carcinoma may exist simultaneously with papillary lesions. Since flat carcinoma may be difficult to detect cystoscopically, it is important to determine its presence by obtaining urine for cytology and by performing random bladder biopsies from suspicious areas.

HISTOLOGY

Ninety percent of bladder tumors are transitional cell carcinomas, with the remainder being mainly squamous cell carcinomas and adenocarcinomas. Squamous cell carcinoma is often associated with chronic infection and inflammation and is the type of tumor seen in patients with schistosomiasis. Squamous cell carcinoma tends to behave more aggressively than transitional cell carcinoma but, stage for stage, it appears to have about the same prognosis.[9]

Adenocarcinoma accounts for only 1 to 2 percent of bladder tumors. These tumors usually develop either on the dome of the bladder in association with the urachus or on the trigone of the bladder. Adenocarcinomas are also seen in patients with bladder exstrophy. Adenocarcinomas generally behave aggressively and have a poor prognosis.[10]

STAGING

The staging systems of bladder cancer are shown in Table 9-1. These fall mainly into two categories, the Jewett-Marshall system which uses stages A to D, and the International Union Against Cancer (UICC) TNM system. Regardless

TABLE 9-1   Staging systems of bladder cancer

Jewett	Marshall	Bladder Cancer Staging (Clinical-Pathologic)	American Joint Committee UICC (1974) Clinical	Pathologic
	0	No tumor—definitive specimen	T0	P0
		Carcinoma in situ	TIS	PIS
A		Papillary tumor—no invasion	TA	PA
	A	Papillary tumor—lamina propria invasion	T1	P1
B1	B1	Superficial ⎱ muscle invasion	T2	P2
B2	B2	Deep ⎰	T3A	P3A
C	C	Invasion of perivesical fat	T3B	P3B
	D1	Invasion of contiguous viscera	T4	P4
		Involvement of pelvic nodes		N1–3
	D2	Involvement of juxtaregional nodes		N4
		Distant metastases		M1

of the classification system used, it is important to recognize that the biologic potential of a tumor changes significantly once it has penetrated the basement membrane of the lamina propria and invades the muscle wall of the bladder. Jewett and Strong demonstrated the clinical significance of this event in 1946. Their observations, based initially on autopsy findings, were that tumors confined to the mucosa and lamina propria were 100 percent curable, whereas tumors that had invaded the muscle wall were only 86 percent curable, and tumors extending into perivesical fat were only 26 percent potentially curable.[11] Subsequent studies have shown that the prognosis for patients with bladder cancer becomes progressively poorer as tumors extend from superficial through deep muscle and into perivesical fat. Thus, in general, topical therapy is appropriate only for patients with tumors confined to the mucosa or lamina propria. More aggressive therapy is generally indicated in patients with muscle invasive disease.

GRADE

The grade of bladder tumors also significantly affects prognosis. Tumors are usually graded from I through III depending on their cytologic appearance. In one series, only 19 percent of grade I tumors progressed to muscle invasion, whereas 69 percent of grade III tumors progressed to muscle invasion, one-half of them within 6 months.[12] Grade III flat carcinoma has a particularly ominous prognosis and often progresses despite aggressive topical therapy.

DIAGNOSIS

Symptoms

Hematuria, either gross or microscopic, is the most common symptom of bladder cancer, occurring in about 85 percent of patients.[13] Irritative symptoms, including frequency, urgency, and strangury, can also occur and are frequently associated with flat carcinoma. Unfortunately, patients with irritative symptoms are frequently followed and treated for other conditions for a lengthy period of time before the actual diagnosis is established. This can have tragic consequences because flat carcinoma often behaves aggressively and may present with muscle invasion at the time of initial diagnosis.

Signs

The physical findings in bladder cancer are usually nonexistent except with advanced disease. In this setting, a mass may be felt in the posterior aspect of the bladder on rectal examination. Bimanual examination under anesthesia is more accurate in detecting induration. The only other physical finding is abnormal lymphadenopathy due to metastatic disease.

Diagnostic Procedures

The diagnosis of bladder cancer is usually made on cystoscopy. An intravenous pyelogram (IVP) will detect most papillary tumors, but will not detect flat, noninvasive lesions. Cystoscopy will detect almost all papillary tumors and will reveal suspicious areas that may represent flat carcinoma. Transurethral resection of obvious tumors and biopsies of suspicious areas with cold cup forceps will establish the diagnosis.

In addition to cystoscopy and biopsy, urinary cytology can be extremely helpful, particularly in high-grade flat lesions. Whereas urinary cytology will be positive in only 3 percent of low-grade papillary tumors, it will be positive in more than 50 percent of grade II and III tumors.[14] Urinary cytology is more sensitive when bladder washings rather than voided specimens are obtained, since this allows for better cellular yield, better preservation of cells, and better representation of the bladder epithelium. In addition to urinary cytology, flow cytometry is being used to analyze nuclear shape and DNA histograms of malignant cells in urine in order to predict more accurately the biologic potential of a tumor.

RADIOGRAPHIC EVALUATION

Excretory Urography

Intravenous pyelography is essential in evaluating patients with bladder cancer, since it will detect 75 percent of bladder tumors greater than 1 cm in diameter. More importantly, IVP will also detect urothelial tumors in the upper tracts, which may occur in 5 to 8 percent of patients with bladder cancer. In addition, IVP is a useful screen for other upper tract abnormalities including renal masses and calculi.[15]

CT Scanning

CT with enhancement with intravesical contrast and air is useful in detecting bladder wall thickening, perivesical extension of tumor, and pelvic lymphadenopathy. *Ideally, CT should be done before transurethral biopsy and resection,* since diathermy may cause induration of the bladder wall, which may be mistaken for tumor. Unfortunately, many patients have had previous superficial tumors resected when first evaluated by CT, thus, the finding of bladder wall thickening is often nonspecific and should never be regarded as definitive evidence for muscle invasion.

CT is more accurate in detecting perivesical extension and pelvic lymphadenopathy. In a recent study of 60 patients, perivesical tumor growth or extension to neighboring organs was detected correctly in 68 percent of cases, with overstaging observed in 25 percent and understaging in 8 percent of cases.[16] Most of the problems encountered concerned assessment of tumors in the anterior bladder wall and identification of the plane between the bladder and seminal vesicles. CT is very accurate in detecting involvement of pelvic lymph nodes, with accuracy in reported series varying from 87 to 99 percent.[17]

Sonography

Diagnostic evaluation of bladder tumors with sonography has been done mainly in Japan, and experience in the United States is limited. It appears that the most sensitive approach with this modality is through a transurethral route.[18] Further experience is needed comparing sonography with CT to establish its value.

MRI

Early experience with MRI suggested that it might be more useful than CT in staging bladder carcinoma. In a recent study of 34 patients, however, the accuracy of MRI compared with final pathologic stage in patients undergoing radical cystectomy was only 50 percent. Twenty-nine percent of patients were understaged and 21 percent overstaged. In addition, MRI detected metastatic nodal disease in only two of five patients.[19] This may be a somewhat pessimistic report, whereas initial papers tended to be overly optimistic. Although the final staging accuracy of MRI is unknown, it probably will be in the 75 to 85 percent range. The major advantage of MRI over CT is the ability to perform multiplanar imaging, which may be helpful in determining operability of large, bulky tumors.

Section Summary

At the Johns Hopkins Hospital, we rely on transurethral resection of the primary tumor to determine the depth of local invasion. We use CT to evaluate for extravesical extension of disease and pelvic lymphadenopathy. We have found pelvic MRI to be equivalent but not superior in this regard. Evaluation for distant metastatic disease includes abdominal and chest CT and a radionuclide bone scan.

TREATMENT OF SUPERFICIAL BLADDER CANCER

Transurethral resection is the initial treatment for patients with bladder tumors. In general, tumors should be resected rather than fulgurated in order to obtain tissue for staging. In resecting bladder tumors, it is important to obtain muscle beneath the tumor to evaluate for invasion. In patients with known superficial, low-grade tumors, it may be reasonable to fulgurate these tumors with either electrocautery or a YAG laser to reduce the risks of hemorrhage and bladder perforation.

At the time of resection, random biopsies should be taken adjacent to the tumor and from other quadrants within the bladder as well as the prostatic urethra to rule out the presence of flat carcinoma. It is also important to obtain a bladder washing for cytology.

Intravesical Chemotherapy

Patients at increased risk of either recurrent disease or disease progression should receive adjuvant intravesical therapy following transurethral resection. Patients with rapid tumor recurrence, high-grade lesions, flat carcinoma, or a positive urine cytologic examination are good candidates for topical chemotherapy. The intravesical agents used are shown in Table 9-2. Thiotepa is an alkylating agent that was introduced during the early 1960s. Until the introduction of Calmette-Guérin bacillus (BCG), Thiotepa was the most common agent used. It appears more effective in the prophylactic treatment of papillary tumors than in the treatment of flat carcinoma. The major toxicity

TABLE 9-2   Intravesical therapy for superficial bladder cancer

Agent	Dosage (mg)	Regimen	Complete Response Rate (%)
Thiotepa	30–60	weekly × 4–6, then monthly	30
Mitomycin C	40	weekly × 8, then monthly	45
Adriamycin	40–50	weekly × 4, then monthly	40
BCG	60–120	weekly × 6–12	60–80

of Thiotepa is myelosuppression, which may occur if the drug is absorbed systemically.[20]

Mitomycin C and Adriamycin are both expensive agents whose use in the United States has generally been restricted to patients who have failed primary therapy with Thiotepa or, more recently, BCG. Both have similar complete response rates to Thiotepa.[21] The major side effect of these agents is chemical cystitis. Mitomycin C infrequently causes myelosuppression, but its use sometimes produces a rash, usually over the palmar surface of the hand and genitalia, but occasionally covering the whole body. Mitomycin C also produces dense pale scars in the bladder sometimes associated with calcification and bladder contracture. Adriamycin, like mitomycin C, is associated with a relatively high incidence of chemical cystitis, but it is not absorbed through the bladder wall; systemic toxicity is therefore minimal.

Calmette-Guérin bacillus is a vaccine made from attenuated *Mycobacterium bovis* that was first demonstrated to have antineoplastic activity against bladder tumors by Morales et al. in 1976.[22] Subsequent randomized trials have shown that this agent has a complete response rate of 60 to 80 percent in both the prophylactic treatment of recurrent bladder tumors and, more importantly, in the treatment of flat carcinoma in situ.[23] Several strains of BCG are available; the most commonly used strains in the United States are Tice and Pasteur. Although there is evidence to suggest a direct immunologic effect on the bladder, the mechanism of action of this agent remains unclear. The major side effect of BCG is vesical irritability with usually mild urinary frequency and urgency that resolves within 24 hours after each dose. Systemic absorption can result in severe toxicity and, occasionally, fatality. Systemic tuberculosis infections are unusual but have been reported.

Despite its potential toxicity, BCG is usually associated with only mild local irritative symptoms. BCG is generally regarded as the most effective topical agent against superficial bladder cancer. Since 1984 we have used BCG at the Johns Hopkins Hospital as a first-line agent and have used mitomycin C as a secondary agent for treating BCG failures.

Photodynamic therapy (PDT) is an experimental modality that holds promise in the treatment of superficial bladder cancer, particularly flat carcinoma in situ (CIS). PDT involves the administration of a photosensitizing agent that is selectively retained by malignant cells. The photosensitizing agent most commonly used has been hematoporphyrin derivative (HpD). HpD is injected intravenously; 48 to 72 hours later, the bladder is illuminated with a laser of an appropriate wavelength that is absorbed by the photosensitizer. The malignant cells that have retained the HpD are selectively destroyed by a photochemical reaction that appears to involve liberation of singlet oxygen and disruption of mitochondrial function.[24]

PDT has been tested and found effective against a wide variety of tumors that can be illuminated, in particular, superficial bladder cancer.[25] Local toxicity can be severe with marked vesical irritability and, occasionally, bladder contracture. In addition, small amounts of the photosensitizer remain in the skin for up to three months after treatment, necessitating extreme precautions to prevent sunburn. PDT must be regarded as a last resort prior to cystectomy, but its application may increase as new photosensitizers and lasers are developed.

TREATMENT OF MUSCLE INVASIVE BLADDER CANCER

Treatment options for muscle invasive bladder cancer include partial cystectomy, cystectomy, radiotherapy, or a combination of surgery and radiotherapy. Partial cystectomy is infrequently indicated in the treatment of invasive bladder cancer because of the multifocal nature of this disease. Partial cystectomy should be reserved for initial, solitary tumors located away from the bladder neck and measuring less than 5 cm in diameter. If one observes proper indications, the results of partial cystectomy are equivalent to those achieved with total cystectomy.[26]

Radical cystectomy involves in men the removal of the bladder and prostate and in women the removal of the bladder, urethra, and female genital organs, including the anterior wall of the vagina, as well as the pelvic lymph nodes in both sexes. Survival statistics after radical cystectomy have improved dramatically in the past 40 years, in large part due to better patient selection and improvements in perioperative care. A recent series reported a 5-year survival of 73 percent in pathologic stage B2 disease and 57 percent in pathologic stage C disease.[27]

External beam radiotherapy was used in this country for many years as the sole treatment for bladder cancer, and remains popular in some European centers. Data from the United States are generally disappointing and far less satisfactory than the results achieved with surgery. It is difficult to compare the results of radiotherapy versus surgery because of the lack of comparative pathologic staging, but, in general, 5-year survival figures with radiotherapy vary from 20 to 35 percent.[28]

When radiotherapy was more popular, there was enthusiasm for combining radiotherapy with surgery. Early reports suggested that radiotherapy resulted in tumor downstaging in a significant proportion of patients and was associated with decreased rates of local recurrence. Unfortunately, these observations were made by comparing historical series rather than by controlled trials. Thus, the results of integrated radiotherapy and cystectomy were compared with earlier trials, when the mortality of cystectomy was much higher. Pelvic recurrence and survival rates with contemporary cystectomy series are equivalent to those achieved with combined radiotherapy and surgery, casting doubt on the value of radiation. At the Johns Hopkins Hospital, we abandoned preoperative radiotherapy in 1984 and now rely on radical cystectomy alone as the primary treatment for muscle invasive bladder cancer, administering systemic chemotherapy postoperatively to those patients with unfavorable pathology.

TREATMENT OF ADVANCED DISEASE

Until several years ago, there was no effective treatment for patients with advanced or metastatic carcinoma of the bladder. More recently, encouraging results have been obtained using a variety of regimens that all combine cis-platinum with other agents. The combination most frequently used at present is M-VAC (methotrexate, vinblastine, Adriamycin, and cis-platinum), which was initially developed at Memorial Sloan-Kettering Cancer Center (MSKCC) in New York City. Other combination regimens include CMV (M-VAC without Adriamycin) and intra-arterial CISCA (cis-platinum, Cytoxan, and Adriamycin).

Sternberg and associates from MSKCC initially reported a 69 percent response rate and 37 percent rate of complete remission in 83 patients with advanced bladder cancer.[29] Results from other series, however, have not been as favorable. Tannock and associates recently reported a 40 percent response rate with M-VAC and only a 13 percent complete response rate with a median duration of response of only 8 months.[30] A large international trial is being conducted comparing M-VAC with cis-platinum alone in patients with advanced bladder cancer. Previous randomized prospective trials have failed to demonstrate any benefit in terms of tumor response or survival for patients treated with other drug combinations compared with cis-platinum alone.

M-VAC is also being evaluated in a neoadjuvant trial comparing preoperative M-VAC followed by cystectomy versus cystectomy alone in patients with muscle invasive bladder cancer. We have been reluctant to treat patients preoperatively with M-VAC because of the uncertain efficacy and marked toxicity of this regimen. Therefore, our current approach at the Johns Hopkins Hospital to patients with muscle-invasive but organ-confined disease is to perform cystectomy first and to offer chemotherapy subsequently to patients with unfavorable pathology. Ultimately, the use of M-VAC and other combination regimens in either a metastatic or adjuvant setting can be justified only by the demonstration of improved survival in well-designed, randomized, controlled clinical trials.

REFERENCES

1. Soloway MS: Current concepts in the diagnosis and management of bladder cancer. Astra Urol June, 1989
2. Cole P: A population-based study of bladder cancer. p. 83. In Doll R, Vodopija I (eds): Host Environment Interactions in the Etiology of Cancer in Man. IARC, Lyon, 1973

3. Cole P, Monson RR, Haning H, et al: Smoking and cancer of the lower urinary tract. N Engl J Med 284:129, 1971

4. Wynder EL, Stellman SD: Artificial sweetener use and bladder cancer: A case-control study. Science 207:1214, 1980

5. Marrett LD, Walter SD, Miegs JW: Coffee drinking and bladder cancer in Connecticut. Am J Epidemiol 117:113, 1983

6. Cutler SJ, Heney NM, Friedell GH: Longitudinal study of patients with bladder cancer: Factors associated with disease recurrence and progression. p. 35. In Bonney W, Prout G (eds): AUA Monographs. Vol. I: Bladder Cancer. William & Wilkins, Baltimore, 1982

7. Melamed MR, Voutsa NG, Grabstald H: Natural history and clinical behavior of in situ carcinoma of the human urinary bladder. Cancer 17:1533, 1964

8. Utz DC, Schmitz SE, Fugelso PD, Farrow GM: A clinicopathologic evaluation of partial cystectomy for carcinoma of the urinary bladder. Cancer 32:1075, 1973

9. Richie JP, Waisman J, Skinner DG, et al: Squamous carcinoma of the bladder: Treatment by radical cystectomy. J Urol 115:670, 1976

10. Jacobo E, Loening S, Schmidt JD, et al: Primary adenocarcinoma of the bladder: A retrospective study of 20 patients. J Urol 117:54, 1977

11. Jewett HJ, Strong GH: Infiltrating carcinoma of the bladder: Relation of depth of penetration of the bladder wall to incidence of local extension and metastases. J Urol 55:366, 1946

12. Limas C, Lange PH, Fraley EE, et al: A, B, H antigens in transitional cell tumors of the urinary bladder: Correlation with the clinical course. Cancer 44:2099, 1979

13. Varkarakis MJ, Gaeta J, Moore RH, et al: Superficial bladder tumor: Aspects of clinical progression. Urology 4:414, 1974

14. Esposti PL, Zajicek J: Grading of transitional cell neoplasms of the urinary bladder from smears of bladder washings: A critical review of 326 tumors. Acta Cytol 16:529, 1972

15. Friedland GW, Filly R, Goris ML, et al: Uroradiology: An integrated approach. Churchill Livingstone, London, 1983

16. Nurmi M, Katevuo K, Puntala P: Reliability of CT in preoperative evaluation of bladder carcinoma. Scand J Urol Nephrol 22:125, 1988

17. Salo JO, Kivisaari L, Rannikko S, Lehtonen T: The value of CT in detecting pelvic lymph node metastases in cases of bladder and prostate carcinoma. Scand J Urol Nephrol 20:261, 1986

18. Nakamura S, Nijuma T: Staging of bladder cancer by ultrasonography: A new technique by transurethral intravesical scanning. J Urol 124:341, 1980

19. Wood DP, Lorig R, Pontes JE, Montie JE: The role of magnetic resonance imaging in the staging of bladder carcinoma. J Urol 140:741, 1988

20. Soloway MS, Ford KS: Thiotepa induced myelosuppression: Review of 670 bladder instillations. J Urol 130:889, 1983

21. Soloway MS: Intravesical therapy for bladder cancer. Urol Clin North Am 5:661, 1988

22. Morales A, Eidinger D, Bruce AW: Intracavitary bacillus Calmette-Guérin in the treatment of superficial bladder tumors. J Urol 115:180, 1976

23. Herr HW, Pinsky CM, Whitmore WF Jr, et al: Effect of intravesical BCG on carcinoma in situ of the bladder. Cancer 51:1323, 1983

24. Dougherty TJ, Kaufman JE, Goldfarb A, et al: Photoradiation therapy for the treatment of malignant tumors. Cancer Res 38:2628, 1978

25. Benson RC Jr, Kinsey JH, Cortese DA, et al: Treatment of transitional cell carcinoma of bladder with hematoporphyrin derivative phototherapy. J Urol 130:109, 1983

26. Merrell RW, Brown HE, Rose JF: Bladder carcinoma treated by partial cystectomy: A review of 54 cases. J Urol 122:471, 1979

27. Montie JR, Straffon RA, Stewart BH: Radical cystectomy without radiation therapy for carcinoma of the bladder. J Urol 131:477, 1984

28. Wallace DM, Bloom HJG: The management of deeply infiltrating (T_3) bladder carcinoma: Controlled trial of radical radiotherapy versus preoperative radiotherapy and radical cystectomy (first report). Br J Urol 48:587, 1976

29. Sternberg CN, Yagoda A, Scher HI, et al: Preliminary results of M-VAC (methotrexate, vinblastine, doxorubicin and cisplatin) for transitional cell carcinoma of the urothelium. J Urol 133:403, 1985

30. Tannock I, Gospodarowicz M, Connolly J, Jewett M: M-VAC (methotrexate, vinblastine, doxorubicin and cisplatin) chemotherapy for transitional cell carcinoma: The Princess Margaret Hospital experience. J Urol 142:289, 1989

10 CT and MRI of the Bladder

MARCO A. AMENDOLA
HOWARD M. POLLACK

CT OF THE BLADDER

Technique

The normal bladder distended with urine is well demonstrated in cross-sectional CT as a round or ovoid midline pelvic structure with a thin smooth wall outlined peripherally by perivesical fat and internally by near-water density urine. In children the thickness of the normal bladder wall is independent of gender, but men generally have a thicker bladder wall than do women. The thickness of the wall varies significantly (and inversely) with the degree of bladder filling. Data obtained from sonographic measurements obtained primarily from children and adolescents indicate that in this group, the wall of a normal empty bladder should measure less than 5 mm, while with full distention the bladder wall should be less than 3 mm thick.[1] However, at CT, when the bladder is filled with urographic contrast material, its wall is fairly imperceptible due to partial volume effects at the interface between the contrast material and the bladder mucosa. Streak artifacts may also occur when scanning the bladder distended with high-attenuation iodinated contrast. Because of these problems, the use of negative contrast agents, such as air and carbon dioxide, and of fatty agents, such as oil or fatty emulsions, has been advocated for better identification of the bladder and improved tumor delineation in patients with bladder carcinoma.[2–4] Another approach has been the use of a low-density opacification technique, wherein a controlled volume of dilute iodinated contrast agent is instilled into the bladder via an indwelling Foley catheter.[5] The same catheter may be used to insufflate gas and then obtain double-contrast scans with the patient in the supine, prone, and/or decubitus positions. While these technical refinements may be useful in selected cases, their main strength is the demonstration of intraluminal components of a lesion that in most cases would be better examined by cystoscopy. In addition, with state-of-the-art CT equipment and appropriate technical parameters, the incidence of scanning artifacts can be minimized. Thus, our current preference when performing CT for staging of bladder carcinoma is initially to obtain scans of the pelvis with a urine-filled bladder, followed by CT of the entire abdomen and pelvis after the administration of standard intravenous (IV) urographic contrast material and oral contrast for bowel opacification. This is complemented with rapid-sequence CT of the pelvis using 5-mm-slice thickness and 5-mm table increments during a bolus injection of 30 ml of urographic contrast to help in the differentiation of pelvic lymph nodes from blood vessels and other normal pelvic structures.[6]

Conventional axial transverse CT images usually provide an adequate anatomic display of lesion site and extent in the anteroposterior and transverse dimensions. Reformatted CT images in the sagittal and coronal planes have been advocated to delineate the craniocaudad extension of a tumor and to better examine difficult-to-see areas such as the dome and base of the bladder.[7,8] However, small lesions are frequently difficult to evaluate in the reformatted sagittal and coronal planes due to blurring, and the patient must be fully cooperative, not moving during the entire scanning procedure. Another approach is obtaining direct sagittal and coronal CT, which is feasible in most modern CT scanners with a gantry opening large enough to scan adults in these positions. These studies may be useful in selected patients, especially in demonstrating or excluding invasion of perivesical organs and pelvic walls in cases of extensive bladder carcinoma.[9]

CT of Bladder Rupture

The most common cause of bladder rupture is blunt pelvic trauma. This injury occurs in about 10 percent of patients sustaining fractures of the bony pelvis and may be associated with significant morbidity and mortality.[10] Currently, the most reliable radiologic test is retrograde cystography, with an accuracy rate of 85 to 100 percent when performed with adequate distention of the bladder with contrast medium and the performance of postdrainage films.[11] However, if an intra-abdominal injury is suspected in a patient with hematuria and pelvic fractures, CT of the abdomen and pelvis is often the first diagnostic test. CT is useful in confirming the presence and extent of extravasated contrast from the bladder[12] (Fig. 10-1). CT can depict complex extraperitoneal bladder rupture with extravasation of contrast beyond the perivesical space upward into the retroperitoneum and can differentiate it from intraperitoneal bladder rupture.[13] It must be emphasized that during routine abdominopelvic CT, IV administration of contrast material cannot be relied on to distend the bladder fully to demonstrate extravasation, a limitation analogous to that of excretory urography. Two instances of false-negative CT examinations in patients in whom subsequent retrograde cystograms showed gross intraperitoneal extravasation of opacified urine have recently been reported.[14] The tendency of

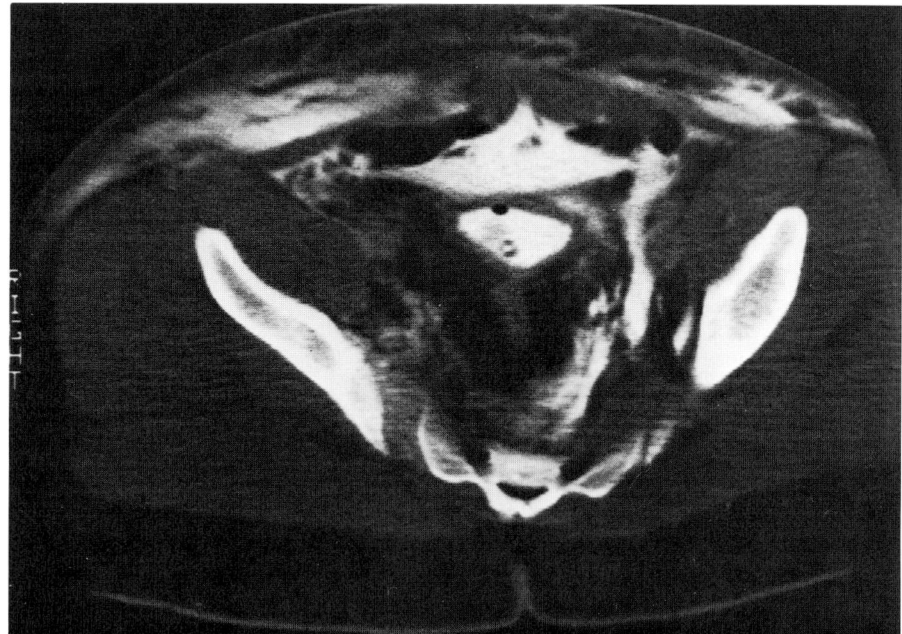

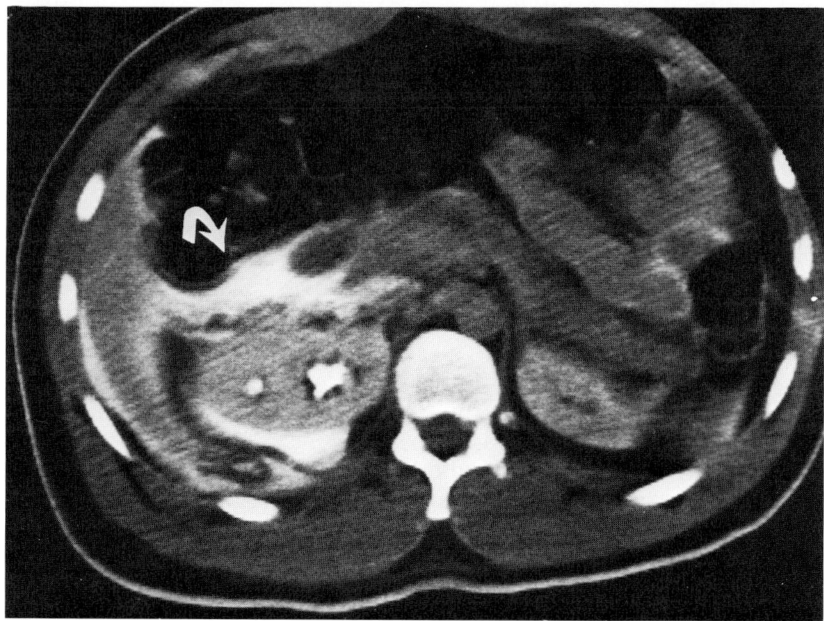

FIG. 10-1.   CT scans of the pelvis in a patient with a complex extraperitoneal bladder rupture. (A) Contrast material extends into the space of Retzius and anterior abdominal wall as well as into the perivesical space. (B) CT section through the level of the kidneys demonstrates contrast material in the anterior paranephric space surrounding the duodenum (arrow) and head of the pancreas, in the perinephric space, and in the posterior paranephric space. (From Sandler et al.,[10] with permission.)

the bladder detrusor to contract and temporarily seal off a rupture may explain why IV contrast material given at the time of CT does not distend the bladder enough to unmask these occult ruptures. It has been recommended that the routine CT technique for the investigation of bladder rupture be modified to include retrograde bladder filling with contrast material through a urethral catheter to distend the bladder more fully and thereby enhance the ability of CT to demonstrate the extravasation.[14] A potential pitfall that can produce a false-positive CT impression of bladder rupture occurs when contrast leaks from the bladder around a Foley catheter and pools in the most dependent portion of the vagina, the posterior fornix.[15]

Abnormalities in Position and Shape of the Bladder

Abnormalities in bladder position may occur secondary to herniation into the inguinal ring (predominantly in males) and into the femoral ring (especially in females). It has been stated that in elderly men with large hernias, the incidence of bladder herniation may be as high as 10 percent.[16] If the condition is not recognized preoperatively, inadvertent bladder injury may occur during herniorraphy. While CT is not the primary method of diagnosis of bladder hernia, clinically unrecognized cases may be scanned during an investigation of urologic or gastrointestinal (GI) complaints. The CT findings of bladder hernia include anterolateral and inferior angulation of the bladder base over the pubic bone.[17] CT scans of the pelvis that demonstrate anterolateral "pointing" of the urinary bladder should be scrutinized for signs of contrast or increased tissue within the inguinal ring. Additional caudal scans will confirm the presence of a possibly unsuspected and clinically relevant bladder herniation. In children, knuckles of the urinary bladder may normally protrude into the external inguinal rings prior to complete closure of the procesus vaginalis ("bladder ears").[18]

Pear-Shaped Bladder

CT is an effective method for evaluation of patients presenting with the multiple caused "pear-shaped" or "teardrop" bladder deformity; it usually obviates the need for more invasive diagnostic procedures. CT can confirm a suspected diagnosis of pelvic lipomatosis in a patient with or without increased radiolucency on conventional radiographic studies of the pelvis, excluding other more ominous diagnoses such as pelvic adenopathy, diffuse pelvic neoplasm, and inferior caval obstruction[19,20] (Figs. 10-2 and 10-3). Lymphoceles, abscesses, and pelvic hematomas causing the pear-shaped appearance of the bladder can also be excluded and the normal variant of teardrop bladder secondary to ileopsoas muscle hypertrophy in males with a narrow bony pelvis can be easily recognized[21] (Fig. 10-4).

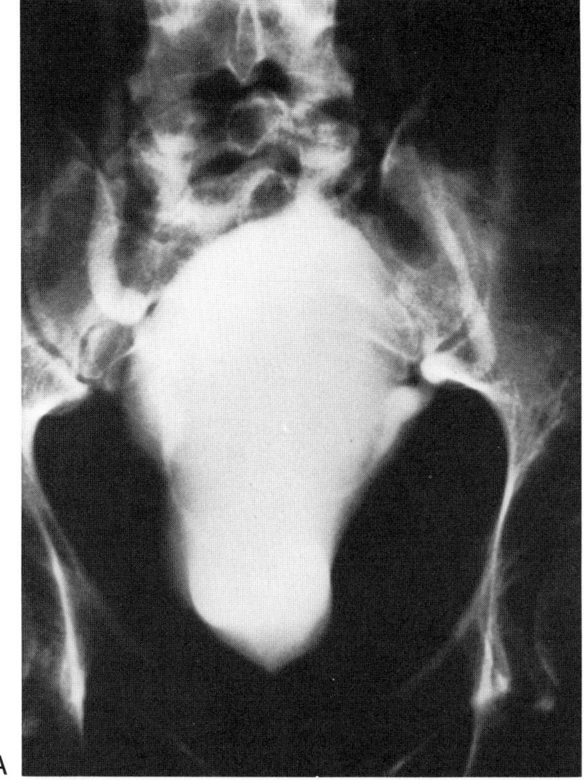

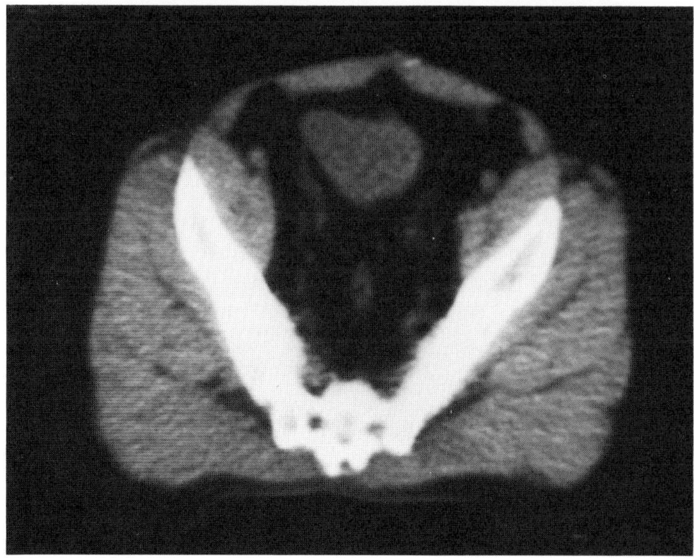

FIG. 10-2. (A) Pear-shaped bladder in a middle-aged black man with pelvic lipomatosis. (B) Pelvic CT scan demonstrates the typical appearance of increased fat deposition deforming and elevating the bladder as well as causing straightening and narrowing of the rectosigmoid colon.

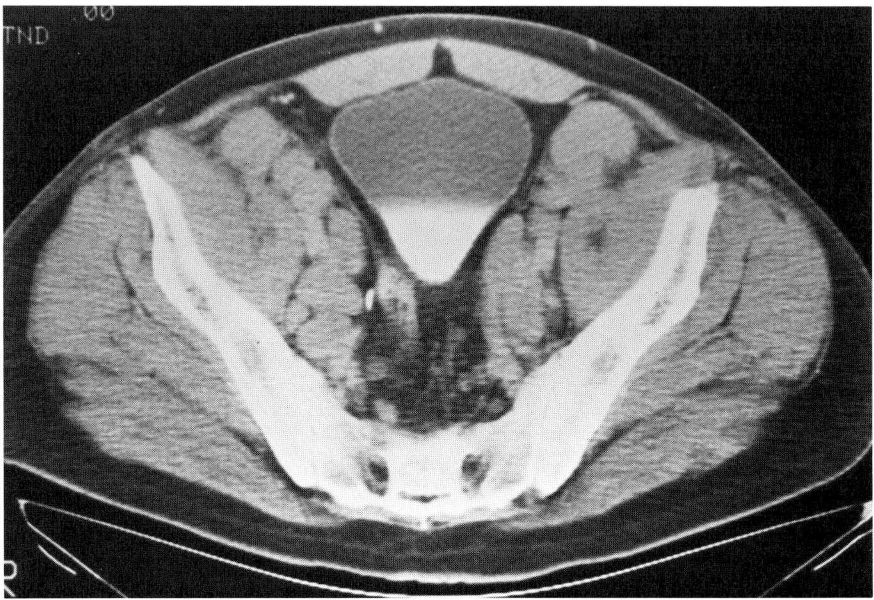

FIG. 10-3.   Pear-shaped bladder secondary to marked bilateral pelvic node enlargement in a patient with non-Hodgkin's lymphoma.

CT of Bladder Calcifications

CT is extremely sensitive in demonstrating bladder calcifications and in delineating their precise location. It frequently depicts calcifications not observable on plain radiographs. Worldwide, *Schistosoma hematobium* infestation (bilharziasis) is the most common cause of bladder wall calcification.[22] In a series of 20 patients with schistosomiasis studied by Jorulf and Lindstedt,[23] calcifications in the bladder wall were recorded in all cases on CT, but only in 13 cases on plain films. Bladder calcifications caused by schistosomiasis are characteristically linear, coarse, or flocculent and occasionally may be difficult to differentiate from other types of calcifications on plain films. The different radiologic appearances are at least in part related to the degree of bladder distention with urine.[24] The bilharzial bladder is usually quite distensible until the late stages of the disease (Fig. 10-5). Since CT examination after injection of IV urographic contrast may mask the calcifications, noncontrast CT should be performed first. Associated distal ureteral calcification found in up to 30 percent of patients can also be elegantly depicted by CT[25] (Fig. 10-5). Other causes of bladder wall calcifications, most of which have been reported to be well demonstrated by CT, include both transitional and squamous cell carcinomas, mesenchymal tumors, tuberculosis (Fig. 10-6), alkaline encrustation cystitis, cyclophosphamide-induced cystitis, and amyloidosis.[26–28] The shape or distribution of the calcification cannot be used to differentiate benign from

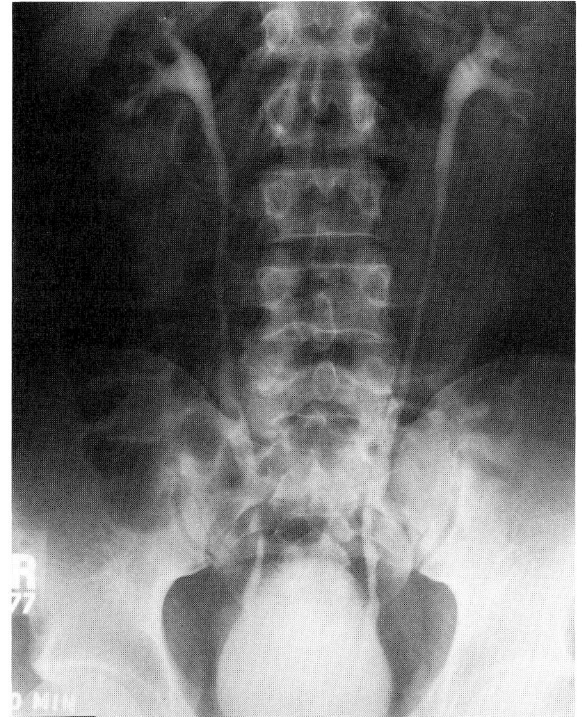

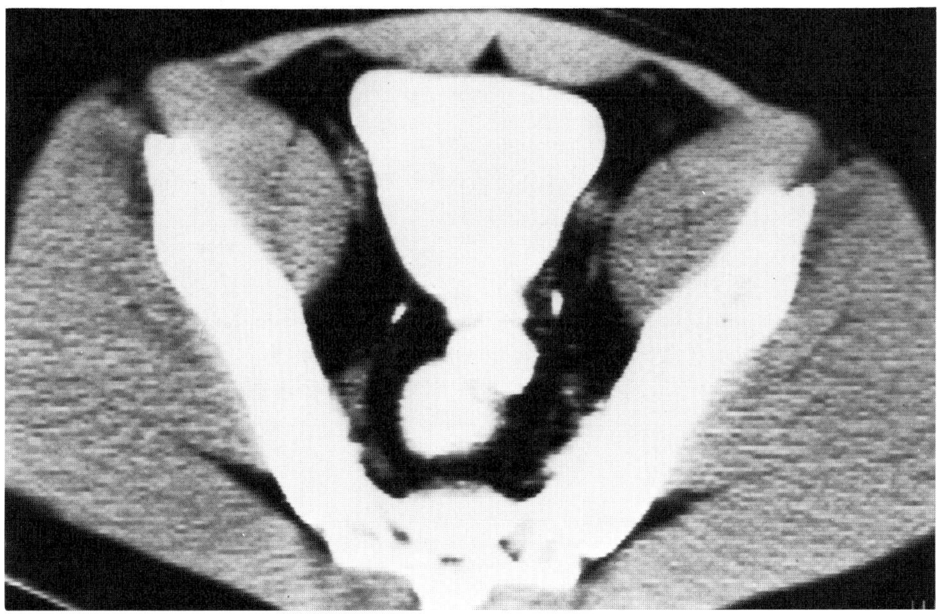

FIG. 10-4. (A) Excretory urogram in a muscular 26-year-old man with a history of blunt abdominal trauma demonstrates a pear-shaped bladder and medial deviation of the distal ureters. (B) CT of the pelvis documents the encroachment in the bladder by the hypertrophied psoas muscles in the same patient, who has a relatively narrow bony pelvis. (From Amendola,[85] with permission.)

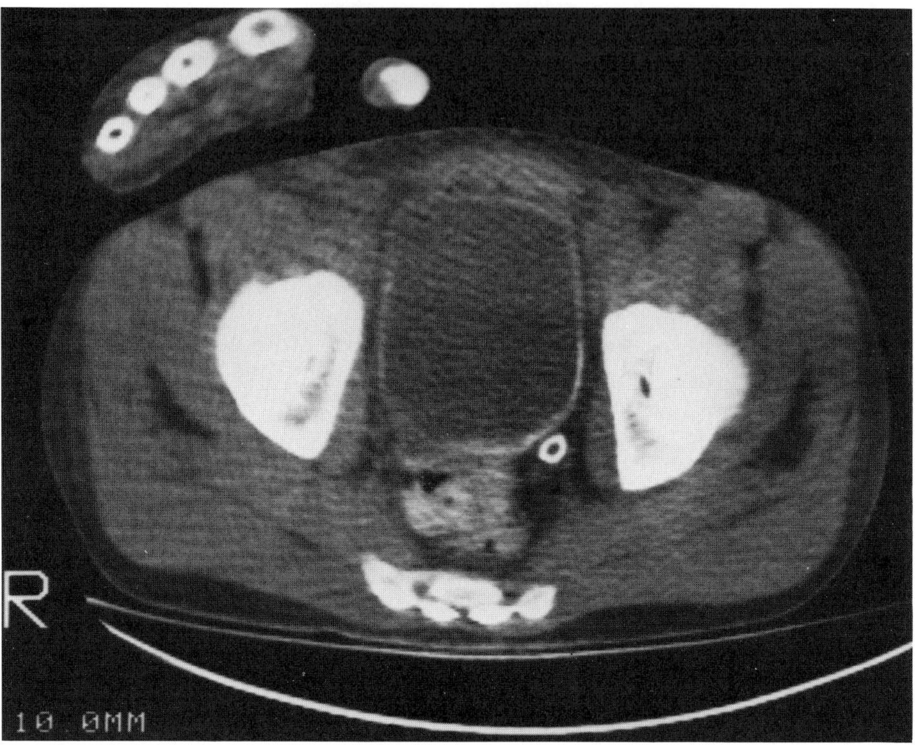

FIG. 10-5. CT scan after oral but not intravenous contrast administration demonstrating calcification in the bladder wall and circumferential calcification of the left ureter in a 19-year-old man with previously unsuspected schistosomiasis of the urinary tract. Note normal bladder distensibility. (From Aisen et al.,[25] with permission.)

malignant lesions.[28] However, the demonstration of associated bladder and ureteral mural calcification effectively narrows the differential diagnosis to schistosomiasis, tuberculosis, and amyloidosis.

Uric acid bladder calculi are nonopaque or poorly opaque and may also be overlooked on plain radiographs. On contrast studies, they occasionally mimic a blood clot or a tumor; however, they exhibit greater attenuation than does tumor or blood clot at CT.[29] Because of its excellent tissue density differentiation, CT may be useful in detecting radiolucent or poorly opaque intravesical foreign bodies when more conventional imaging modalities are nondiagnostic (Fig. 10-7).

CT of Enterovesical Fistulas

CT is a noninvasive and effective method for diagnosing the presence of a suspected enterovesical fistula. Gas in the bladder in the absence of recent catheterization or an infection with a gas-forming organism is indirect but

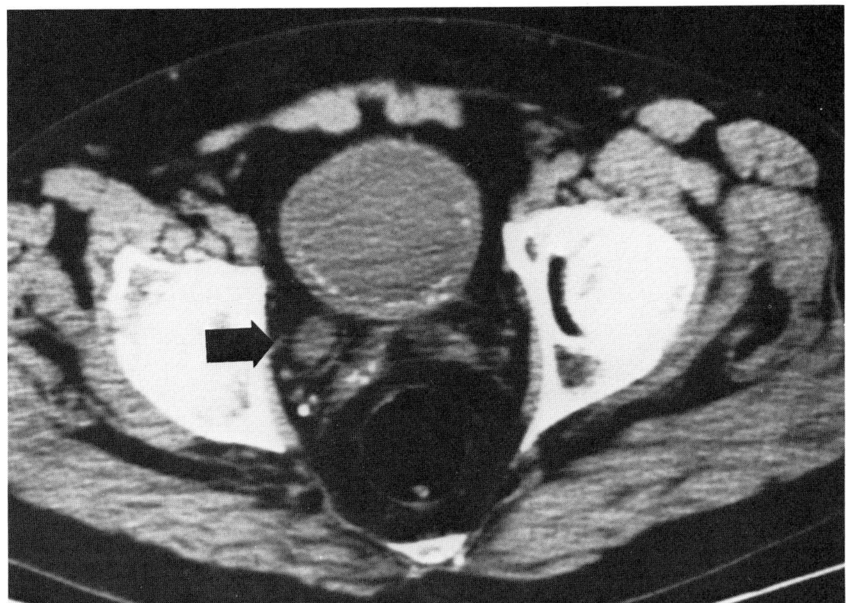

FIG. 10-6. Bladder wall thickening and calcification in TB cystitis. Note dilated right ureter (arrow). Seminal vesical calcifications are also present. The calcifications were not appreciated on the plain abdominal radiograph.

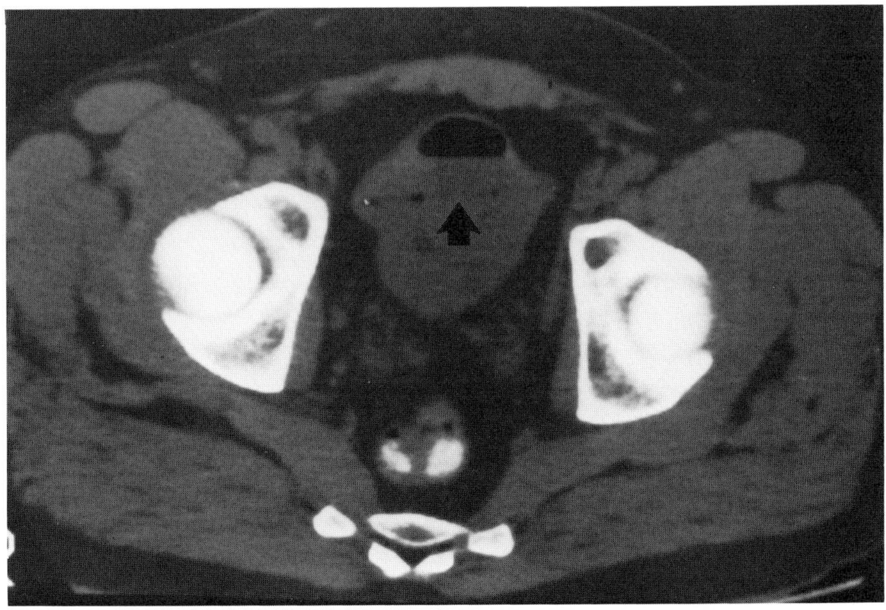

FIG. 10-7. A 41-year-old man with a suspected intravesical foreign body (Q-Tip). Plain radiographs, cystourethrography, and ultrasonography of the bladder were nondiagnostic. On noncontrast CT examination, the Q-Tip was readily evident, wedged transversely in the midportion of the bladder (arrow). Endoscopic removal was successfully accomplished. Note intravesical air from previous catheterization.

convincing evidence of communication with a hollow viscus, usually signifying an enterovesical fistula. Unlike plain radiography, CT detects even minute amounts of intravesical gas and can unequivocally determine whether the gas is in the bladder wall, in its lumen, or in adjacent bowel[30,31] (Figs. 10-7 and 10-8). In a series of 20 patients with enterovesical fistulas of various etiologies examined by CT, intravesical gas was documented in 90 percent of cases.[32] Other CT findings included focal bladder wall thickening (90 percent), thickening of adjacent bowel wall (85 percent), associated soft tissue mass often containing gas (75 percent), and passage of orally or rectally administered contrast medium into the bladder (20 percent). The fistulas secondary to colonic diverticulitia, rectosigmoid neoplasms, and uterine tumors usually involve the left and/or posterior aspects of the bladder. Those arising from Crohn's disease of the terminal ileum or from cecal and appendiceal lesions involve the right lateral or anterior aspects of the bladder.[32] Bladder involvement from adjacent inflammatory processes such as Crohn's disease or appendicitis, even in the prefistulous stage, can be detected with CT.[33,34] Early recognition of focal bladder wall thickening or contiguity of an inflamed loop of bowel to the bladder may result in prompt institution of appropriate therapy and perhaps prevent progression to frank fistula formation. The extent of associated soft tissue involvement is often predictive of whether a one-stage or two-stage operative repair is advisable.

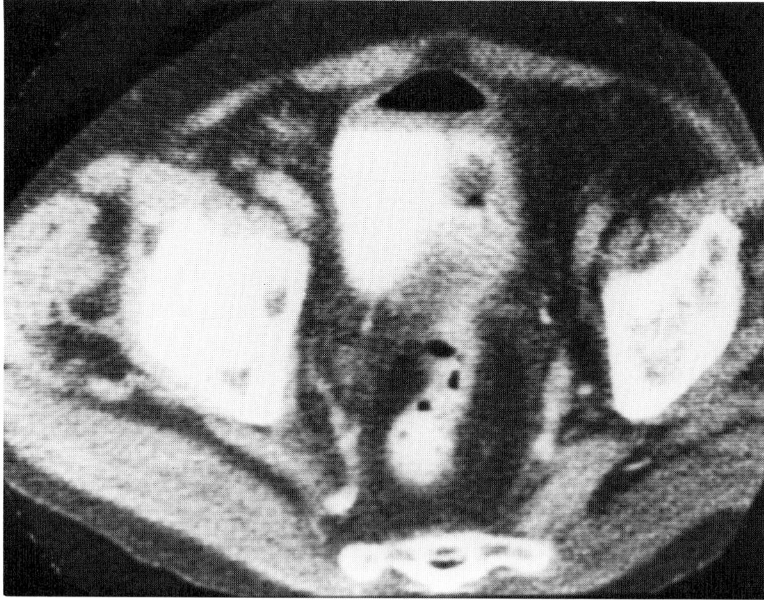

FIG. 10-8.   CT of colovesical fistula in a patient with sigmoid diverticulitis involving the left posterior aspect of the bladder. Note the continguous inflamed bowel and the CT depiction of intravesical gas.

Miscellaneous Conditions

Diffuse thickening of the bladder wall is a nonspecific finding that may be present in many conditions, usually benign, including acute and chronic infectious cystitis, edema, radiation fibrosis, endometriosis, extension from adjacent inflammatory processes, neuropathic bladder, and detrusor hypertrophy secondary to bladder outlet obstruction (Fig. 10-9). Benign and malignant tumors usually present with focal thickening of the bladder wall when demonstrated by CT. Nonepithelial tumors of the bladder constitute less than 5 percent of all primary bladder tumors.[35] Leiomyomas are the most common benign neoplasms in this subgroup and are three times more frequent in female than in male patients. In a few reported cases studied by CT, leiomyomas have appeared as lobulated, solid intraluminal masses arising from the region

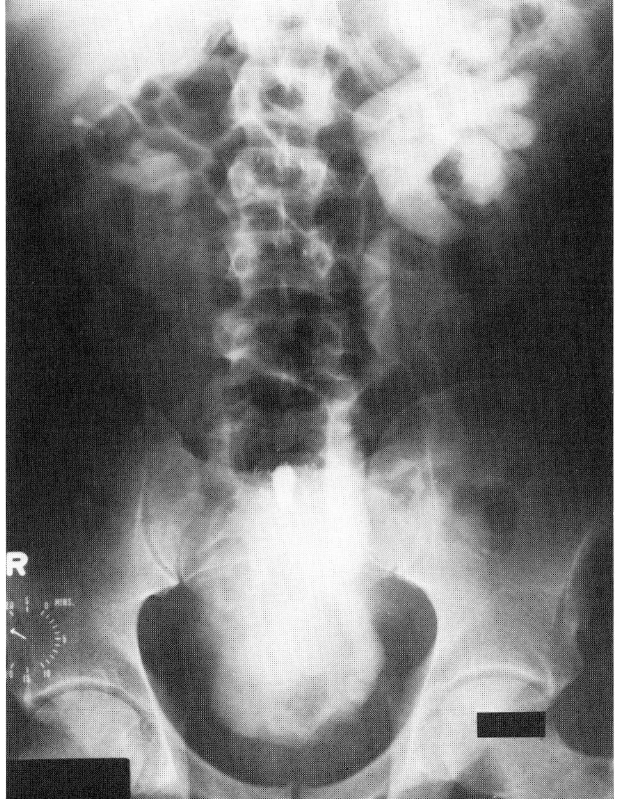

FIG. 10-9.   Marked diffuse thickening of the bladder wall representing detrusor hypertrophy in a patient with chronic bladder outlet obstruction. (A) Intravenous urogram (IVU) demonstrates elevation of the urinary bladder secondary to benign prostatic hyperplasia. The left ureter and renal collecting system are moderately dilated. Residual Pantopaque is seen in the lumbar subarachnoid space. (*Figure continues.*)

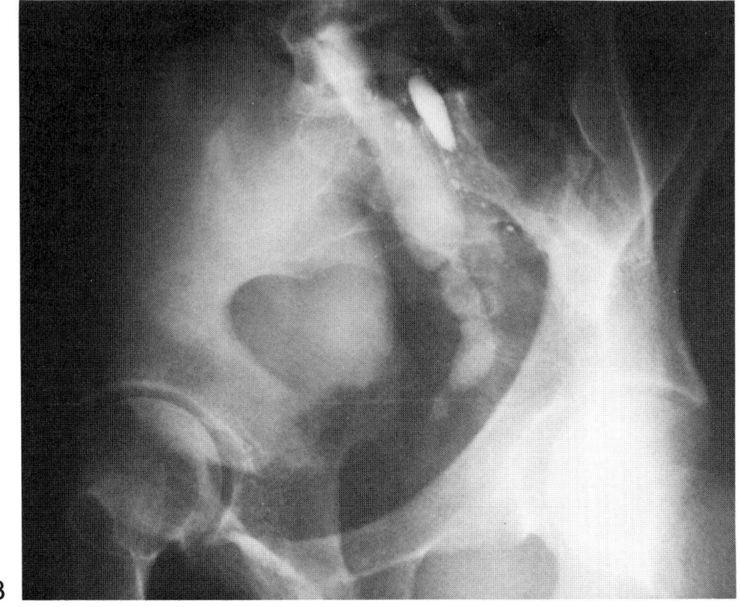

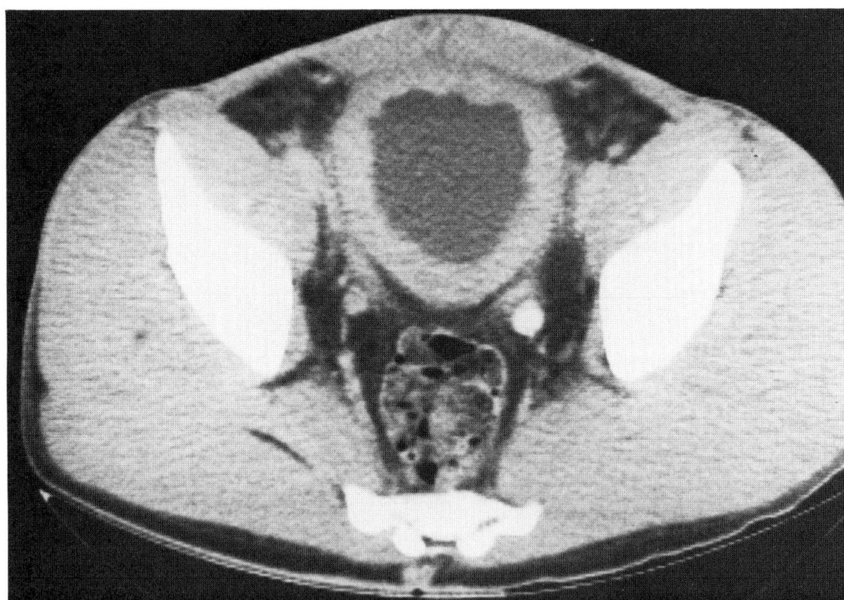

FIG. 10-9 (*Continued*). (B) Right posterior oblique view from IVU reveals the site of the left ureteral obstruction to be at the level of the bladder wall. (C) CT reveals diffuse mural thickening of the bladder. Trabeculation is evident, and there is retention of contrast medium in the dilated left ureter.

of the bladder base.[35–37] Their CT appearance is otherwise nonspecific. Other benign lesions of the bladder wall have also been demonstrated by CT, including cystitis cystica, cystitis glandularis, malakoplakia, and nephrogenic adenoma.[38–43] Differentiation of malignant lesions is not possible with CT, but determination of the extent of the lesion may be useful in preoperative planning.[44]

CT of Bladder Cancer

At CT, bladder carcinomas appear as sessile and/or polypoid intraluminal soft tissue masses, depending on whether their pattern of growth is primarily infiltrating or papillary. The CT attenuation values of bladder carcinomas range from 30 to 50 HU, similar to normal bladder wall density.[45] This, plus the fact that bladder tumors do not exhibit striking contrast enhancement, sharply limit the ability of CT to assess the depth of penetration of these neoplasms when they still lie completely within the bladder wall. Contrast differences among perivesical fat, bladder wall, and urine are sufficient to identify mural or mucosal bladder lesions, making complicated gas-filling techniques unnecessary. Intraluminal tumor extension of 1 to 1.5 cm in diameter can be identified against the background of low-density urine in a distended bladder. Rarely, surface calcification of the encrusting type is appreciable on CT.[46] Bladder carcinoma can merely appear as focal or diffuse thickening of the bladder wall. Focal mural thickening is a rather nonspecific finding that can be caused by many benign tumors and inflammatory conditions; the definitive diagnosis should be made on the basis of cystoscopy and biopsy. When neoplasms cause diffuse thickening of the bladder wall, the appearance can be confused with trabeculation and detrusor hypertrophy secondary to outflow obstruction or cystitis, although thickening is often more diffuse in the latter entities[47] (Fig. 10-9). Occasionally, it may be impossible to differentiate a primary bladder cancer invading the prostate from a prostatic carcinoma extending into the bladder. In lesions of the bladder base, prostatic carcinoma is actually a more likely lesion. However, the ultimate diagnosis awaits the results of biopsy. When other pelvic malignancies invade the bladder the extravesical origin of the primary (e.g., uterine cervix, colon) can be recognized because the main bulk of the tumor lies outside the bladder (Fig. 10-10). For these reasons and because cystoscopy is very sensitive in detecting small bladder neoplasms, this method remains the primary diagnostic procedure in patients with suspected bladder cancer. The main role of CT is in the evaluation of extent of tumor in patients with known bladder carcinoma to help determine the preferred treatment and prognosis, especially when radical surgery is contemplated. Whenever possible, CT should be performed prior to extensive or deep transurethral biopsy, lest postoperative reaction be mistaken for an advanced stage of malignancy.

The most important factors in the survival of the patient with bladder cancer are the histologic grade and the stage of the tumor at diagnosis.[48] Conventional

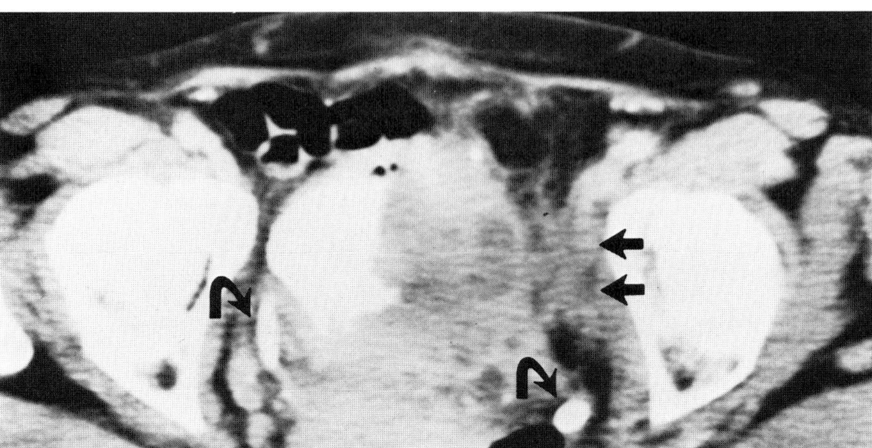

FIG. 10-10.   Advanced carcinoma of the cervix invading the urinary bladder. Note associated pelvic adenopathy (arrows) and bilateral ureteral obstruction (curved arrows). A small amount of intravesical air is present from recent cystoscopy.

clinical staging is carried out using bimanual examination under anesthesia and cystoscopy with biopsy, including sampling from the deepest extension of the tumor. Lower stages are often adequately classified by endoscopic methods; clinical staging becomes notoriously inadequate, however, in deeply invasive and advanced tumors when understaging and overstaging can occur in as many as 50 percent of patients.[49] (Understaging is the more common of these two inaccuracies.) Various radiographic techniques including excretory urography, arteriography, fractional double-contrast cystography, lymphangiography, and sonography have also been used but, except for the latter two techniques, all have been superseded by CT or MRI. Because it is more generally available and less expensive than MRI, CT is now the standard imaging modality for staging carcinoma of the bladder. Probably because of the limited view of the bladder available via the suprapubic approach, and the inconvenience of using the more informative transurethral approach, sonography has not gained as wide acceptance as CT for this purpose.

There are two staging systems for bladder cancer: the TNM classification (where T relates to the extent of the primary tumor, N to lymph node involvement, and M to distant metastases), originally proposed by the International Union Against Cancer (UICC), and the Jewett-Strong-Marshall system used primarily in the United States[50–52] (Tables 10-1 and 10-2). There are only minor differences between the two: the TNM system differentiates between

TABLE 10-1   Staging of bladder cancer: Jewett-Strong-Marshall system[a]

Stage	Tumor Description
O	Confined to mucosa
A	Infiltration of submucosa
B1	Infiltration of superficial muscle
B2	Infiltration of deep muscle
C	Perivesical infiltration
D1	Involvement of adjacent organs and pelvic lymph nodes
D2	Distant metastases or nodes above aortic bifurcation

[a] See Jewett and Strong[50] and Marshall.[51]

TABLE 10-2   TNM classification of bladder carcinoma (abbreviated)[a]

Stage	Tumor Description
Tis	Carcinoma in situ
Ta	Papillary, noninvasive carcinoma
T1	Lamina propria infiltration
T2	Extension to superficial muscle layer
T3A	Extension to deep muscle layer
T3B	Infiltration through bladder wall
T4A	Invasion of neighboring structures (prostate, uterus, or vagina)
T4B	Invasion of the pelvic or abdominal wall
N0	No regional lymph node metastases
N1	One homolateral solitary regional (internal or external iliac) lymph node metastases
N2	Contralateral or bilateral or multiple regional lymph node metastases
N3	Fixed regional lymph node metastases
N4	Juxtaregional (common iliac, inguinal, or aortic) lymph node metastases
M0	No (known) distant metastases
M1	Distant metastases present

[a] See American Joint Committee for Cancer Staging and End-Results Reporting.[52]

spread to the pelvic sidewall and visceral invasion, and between lymph node and distant metastases, while the Jewett classification does not. CT cannot reliably differentiate between lesions limited to the lamina propria (stage A or T1) from those that invade the superficial muscle (stage B1 or T2) or the deep muscle (stage B2 or T3A). For this reason, most reports group together the tumors staged B2 or T3A or lower in spite of the deficiencies of this practice, since muscle invasion to any degree significantly impacts on prognosis. The greatest value of CT in staging bladder carcinoma lies in its ability to differentiate between stages B2/T3A or lower (i.e., confined to the bladder) from higher-stage lesions with extravesical extension. When the carcinoma is confined to the bladder (stage B2 or T3A or less), CT shows an exophytic tumor or local thickening of the bladder wall with a smooth, well-defined outer border and preservation of the perivesical fat planes[53] (Fig. 10-11). The earliest sign of extravesical tumor spread on CT is poor definition of the outer aspect of the bladder wall in the region of the tumor with increased density in the adjacent perivesical fat.[54] Since streak artifacts from concentrated iodinated contrast can obscure subtle abnormalities in the perivesical fat, thin-section CT scans obtained prior to contrast administration are advisable.

Unresectable tumors can be demonstrated at CT when there is direct extension of the soft tissue mass into the pelvic sidewall with infiltration of the internal obturator muscle and/or pelvic bones, or into the anterior abdominal wall (stage D1/T4B). Early tumor invasion of adjacent viscera may be difficult to exclude with CT because normally no clear fat plane is present to demarcate the bladder wall from adjacent organs, such as rectum, prostate, uterus, and vagina. However, a structure or organ partially or completely surrounded by the tumor mass is considered to be involved[54] (Fig. 10-12). Obliteration of the normal fat plane between the posterior wall of the bladder and seminal vesicles (the "seminal vesicle angle sign") should be interpreted with caution in determining seminal vesicle invasion by tumor, since this sign can be simulated by a distended rectum and if CT scans are obtained in the prone position[53,55] (Fig. 10-13). Other important pitfalls in CT staging include the presence of edema and inflammatory changes from recent biopsies or perivesical fibrosis

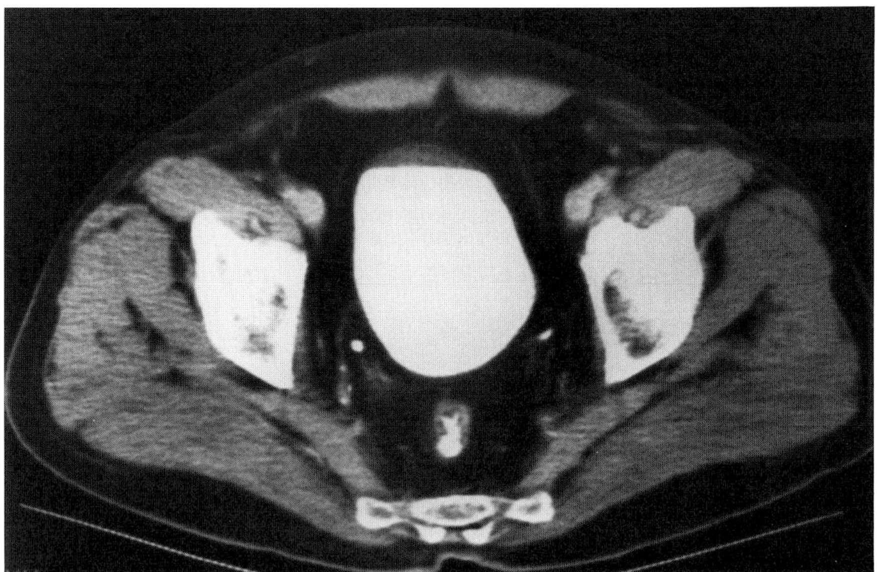

FIG. 10-11. Localized thickening of the bladder wall anteriorly. No extravesical extension. Pathologic examination of the radical cystectomy specimen showed bladder carcinoma with superficial muscle invasion (stage B1/T2).

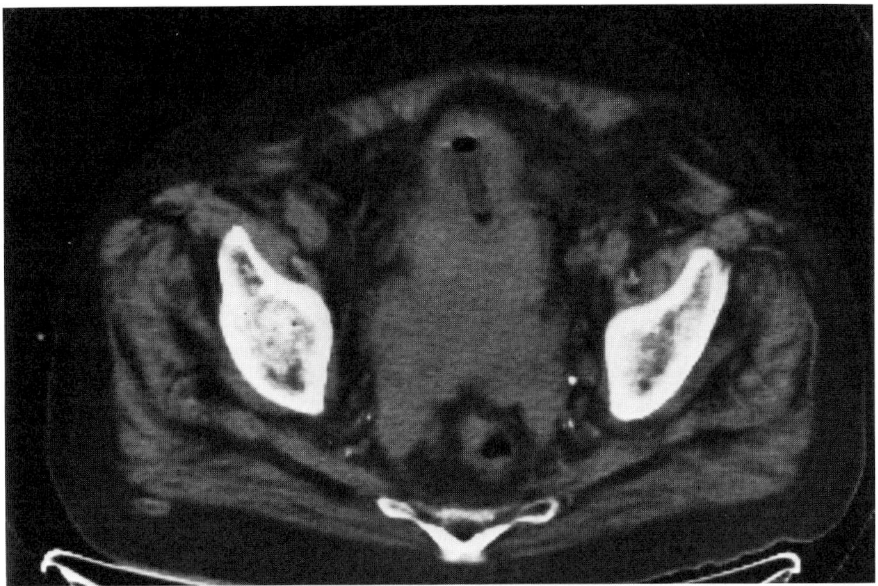

FIG. 10-12.   Extensive bladder carcinoma surrounding and infiltrating the seminal vesicles. There is a Foley catheter within the bladder.

caused by previous surgery or radiation therapy. These are a frequent source of overstaging of the lesions by CT. Although it has been suggested that local thickening and rigidity of the bladder wall signifies invasion of the deep muscle layer, this is not a reliable sign since previous diagnostic and therapeutic procedures, including radiotherapy, may produce similar changes. After pelvic irradiation or surgery, the bladder wall may become indistinct, resulting in overstaging.[56] Evaluation of recurrent tumor after radiation therapy may be difficult, since a small bladder capacity and a thickened wall are commonly present. Following deep mural transurethral resection or biopsy, the bladder may be thickened and the perivesical tissues edematous.

Because of its cross-sectional display, tumors at the bladder base and dome are difficult to see and stage confidently using CT. Multiplanar reconstruction with very fine sections (1.5 mm) have been used to overcome this problem but are not practical because of increased examination time and relatively high radiation dose. Errors resulting in understaging at CT emanate from the inability of CT to detect minimal or microscopic invasion of the perivesical fat, as well as small or microscopic foci of tumor in normal-size lymph nodes.[53,57] The overall accuracy of CT in staging (i.e., discriminating localized from extravesical tumor) invasive bladder carcinoma ranges from 64 to 92 percent.[53–60] Patients with invasion of sigmoid colon or uterus may or may not undergo cystectomy, depending on the clinical situation. The main value of CT, therefore, is in determining the presence of gross perivesical extension of tumor, including involvement of other pelvic organs, pelvic sidewall ex-

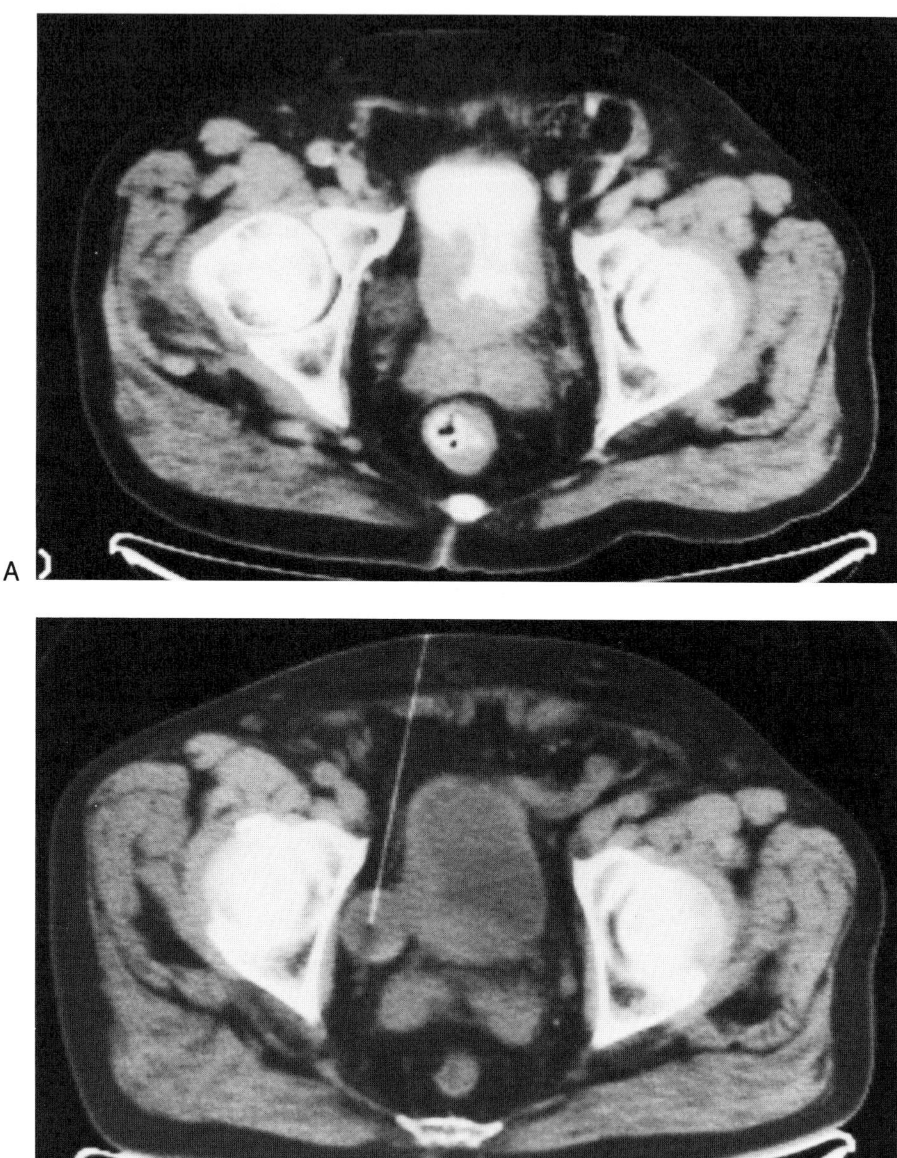

FIG. 10-13.   (A) Bladder carcinoma with false positive "seminal vesicle angle sign" on CT scan. (B) In another patient with tumor involving the posterior bladder wall, the fat plane separating it from the seminal vesicle is preserved. Note minimal rectal distention and enlarged obturator lymph node. CT-guided fine-needle biopsy of obturator adenopathy yielded positive results for metastatic tumor.

tension, and the presence of adenopathy, all indicators of advanced carcinoma and all having an important bearing on the prognosis and therapeutic management of those patients.

Lymph Node Metastases

The presence of regional lymph node metastases is a poor prognostic sign in patients with bladder cancer. The 5-year survival rates following radical cystectomy range from 7 to 17 percent when even limited nodal metastases are found.[61] This finding is consistent with the hypothesis that distant metastastic disease is probably present at the time of surgery but is not clinically detectable. The frequency of nodal involvement from transitional cell carcinoma relates directly to the depth of tumor infiltration of the primary bladder tumor. It is rare in superficial lesions, but the prevalence increases to 30 percent in tumors with deep muscle invasion (B2/T3A).[62] The obturator and external iliac nodes are the most frequently involved followed by the common iliac, hypogastric, and perivesical nodes[61] (Fig. 10-13). Further spread is to the para-aortic and inguinal nodes, but involvement above the aortic bifurcation in the absence of more distal node disease is virtually not seen. The obturator node is part of the medial chain of the external iliac nodes and is best seen on CT sections 1 to 3 cm superior to the acetabula, which depict the characteristic teardrop shape of the iliac bone.[63] The main external iliac nodes surround the external iliac artery and vein; asymmetry of the external iliac vascular bundle in one side of the pelvis is a useful sign of abnormality. Internal iliac adenopathy is seen more posteriorly adjacent to the gluteal vessels and anterior to the piriformis muscles.[54] Pelvic nodes 1.5 cm in diameter are considered abnormal at CT, and enlarged nodes of 2 cm or more on CT scans are important indicators of metastatic disease (Fig. 10-14). Minimal node enlargement is an important source of false-positive CT results, since benign conditions such as reactive hyperplasia and chronic lymphadenitis cannot be differentiated from metastases by CT scans. Other sources of error include lymph nodes with microscopic metastases and confusion between unopacified bowel loops or blood vessels and enlarged lymph nodes. The overall accuracy of CT in detecting lymph node metastasis has ranged from 70 to 92 percent in several published studies.[6] In problem cases or if histologic proof is deemed necessary, CT is a helpful tool to guide percutaneous fine-needle aspiration of suspicious nodal enlargement (Fig. 10-13).

CT Postradical Cystectomy

CT is the current imaging procedure of choice for the detection of tumor recurrence and of surgical complications in patients who have undergone radical cystectomy for bladder cancer.[64,65] The most common early surgical complications following radical cystectomy are abscess formation and urinomas from leakage of urine at anastomotic sites. An abscess cavity can be diagnosed unequivocally if an extra-alimentary tract mass containing gas is

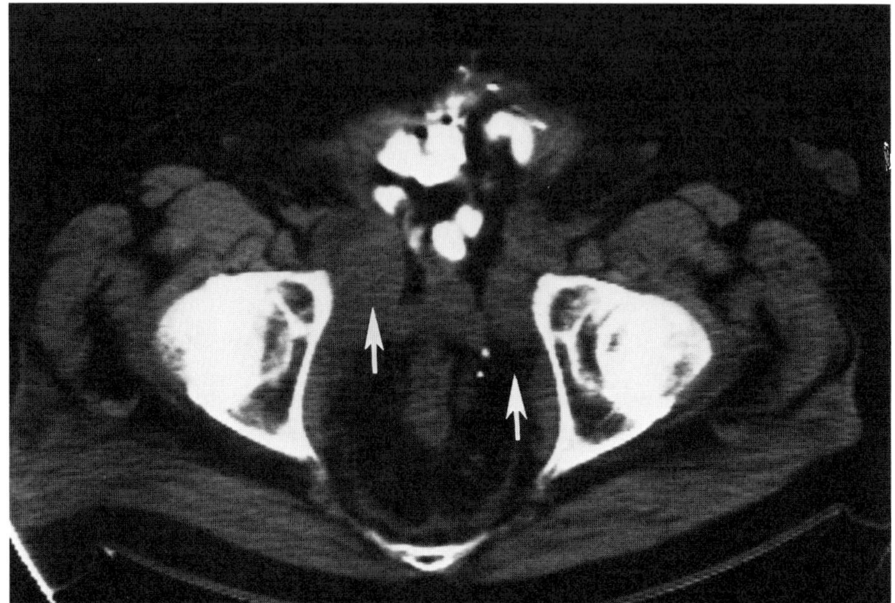

FIG. 10-14.   Bilateral pelvic adenopathy demonstrated at CT (arrows) signaling local recurrence in a patient one year status postradical cystectomy for bladder carcinoma.

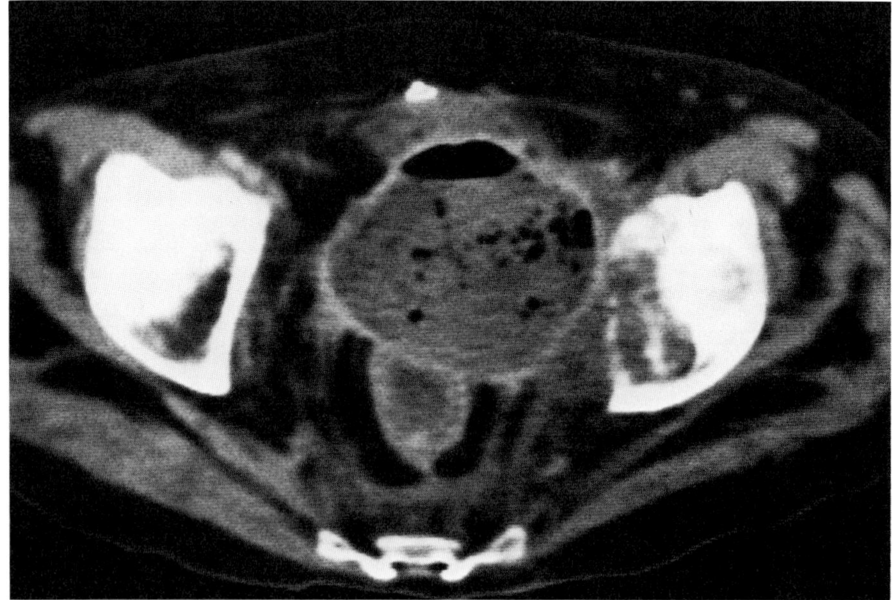

FIG. 10-15.   CT postradical cystectomy demonstrates a gas-forming pelvic abcess. Note also recurrent tumor causing lytic destruction of the adjacent bony pelvis.

shown on CT scans (Fig. 10-15). In the absence of gas, an abscess may be impossible to differentiate from other fluid collections (seroma, lymphocele, urinoma) or from necrotic tumor recurrence. The diagnosis may be expedited by analysis of aspirated material obtained by CT-guided needle aspiration. In men, after radical cystectomy, the bladder, prostate, and seminal vesicles are absent, and in women, the bladder, uterus, and fallopian tubes are removed. Small bowel loops and sigmoid colon fill the pelvic space previously occupied by those organs, and the bowel should be well opacified with oral and rectal contrast for optimal CT evaluation. The muscle groups lining the pelvic sidewall remain symmetric; any alteration of this symmetry may represent a clue to the presence of underlying pathology. On CT, a locally recurrent bladder carcinoma appears as a soft tissue density mass, separate from bowel, with or without central necrosis, or as recurrent pelvic or retroperitoneal adenopathy (Fig. 10-14). A potential problem with CT is the differentiation of a small recurrent tumor from postsurgical or postradiation fibrosis, especially when no immediate postoperative CT studies are available as a baseline. In these cases, a CT-guided needle biopsy may be necessary for definitive diagnosis of recurrent carcinoma.

MRI OF THE BLADDER

MRI Technique

For MRI of the bladder, no special preparation of the patient is needed, except for having a moderately distended bladder at the beginning of the examination. This is important for evaluation of the bladder wall and to facilitate identification of pelvic anatomy and pathology by displacing bowel loops out of the pelvis. However, an overdistended bladder is not advisable, since it may cause patient discomfort, resulting in body motion and even in interruption of the examination for voiding. Administration of 1 mg of glucagon given intramuscularly (IM) or IV immediately preceding the MRI study is a useful adjunct to improve image quality by decreasing bowel peristalsis.[66] In women, insertion of a vaginal tampon is helpful for localization. Insufflation of rectal air increases contrast between the rectum and adjacent pelvic structures. Scanning with the patient in the prone position may help alleviate claustrophobia and decrease respiratory motion artifact and at the same time help in retaining the insufflated air in the rectosigmoid colon.[67] Use of a flow-compensation algorithm is useful to eliminate artifacts from pulsatile blood vessels in the pelvis.

With the spin-echo technique, MRI scans obtained with short repetition time/echo-delay time (TR/TE) (i.e., TR 400 to 600 ms, TE 20 to 25 ms) are considered T_1 weighted. Long TR/TE spin-echo pulse sequences (i.e., TR 2,000 to 2,500 ms, TE 60 to 80 ms) are considered T_2 weighted. Our approach to imaging the bladder with MRI is to obtain both short and long TR/TE images in at least one plane (usually the axial plane) in order to assess the T_1 and T_2

relaxation times of the suspected abnormalities. This is complemented by images in other planes using T_2-weighted sequences in general. We usually start with a series of nine slices in the coronal plane, 10 mm in thickness, using a T_1-weighted sequence (TR/TE 600/15 ms), including both renal hila, obtained with a standard body coil. This is followed by a series of about 20 slices, 10 mm thick, in the axial plane from the pelvic brim to the pubic symphysis with a T_1-weighted sequence (i.e., TR/TE 600/20 ms), and also by a T_2-weighted sequence (TR 2,500 ms, TE 80 ms). Usually a series of scans in the sagittal plane are also obtained (TR 2,500 ms, TE 80 ms). A 128 matrix and two excitations are generally employed. Depending on the abnormality under study and its location in the bladder, additional views are obtained as needed. For example, the lateral walls of the bladder are better displayed on axial and coronal scans, while the regions of the bladder base and dome are better shown in the coronal and sagittal planes. The total time for the examination rarely exceeds 1 hour from beginning to end.

Normal MRI Appearance of the Bladder

In images obtained with short TR/TE (T_1 weighted), the urine-filled bladder appears as a structure of homogeneously low intensity in which it is difficult to identify the bladder wall (Fig. 10-16A). This is because both urine and the smooth muscle that predominantly forms the wall of the bladder have long T_1 relaxation times and have not achieved full recovery of magnetization between successive excitations. There is, however, a marked difference in T_1 values between bladder wall and perivesical fat, enabling a clear demonstration of extension of bladder lesions into the surrounding tissues. There is also a pronounced difference in T_2 values between bladder wall and urine; therefore, the contrast between bladder wall and urine improves when longer values of TE are used.[68] Since the T_1 value of urine is significantly longer than the T_1 value of muscle, intensity differences can also be shown using intermediate TR and TE sequences. With longer values of TR/TE (T_2 weighting), the bladder wall is visualized with low intensity because of its shorter T_2 relaxation time relative to urine, which now appears with high intensity (Fig. 10-16B).

When studying T_2-weighted images, it is important to recognize the low-intensity bladder wall from the low-intensity line created at one edge of the bladder by the so-called chemical shift artifact (Fig. 10-16B). This artifact is caused by the difference in precessional frequencies of the protons contained in water and in fat.[69,70] The chemical shift artifact occurs at the water-fat interface (bladder/perivesical fat) in the direction of the readout (frequency-encoded) gradient, which is different for different imaging planes. For transverse sections, the artifact will be seen in the lateral walls, while on coronal and sagittal images, it is usually located along the dome and base of the bladder. On transverse images obtained with most MRI units, the chemical shift artifact appears as a low-intensity dark band along the lateral wall on one side and a bright band along the lateral wall on the opposite side (Fig. 10-16B). This

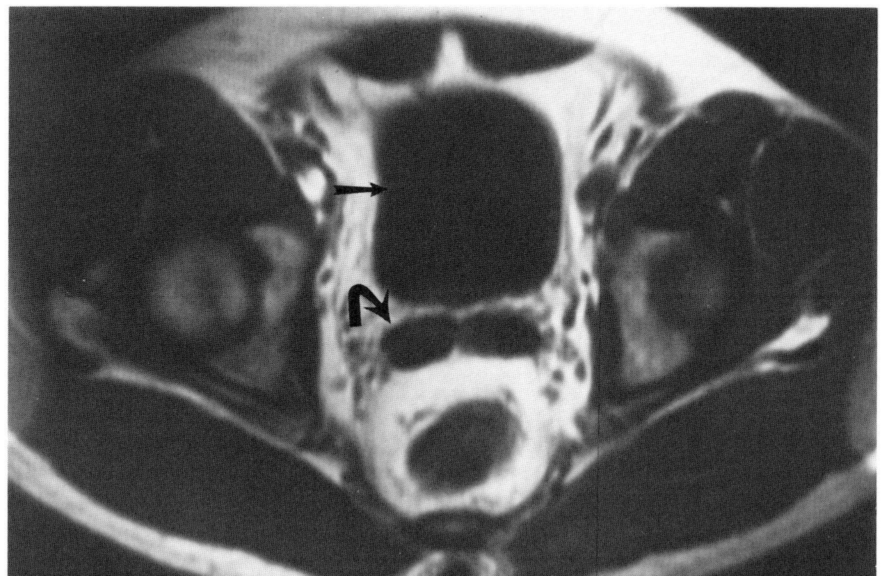

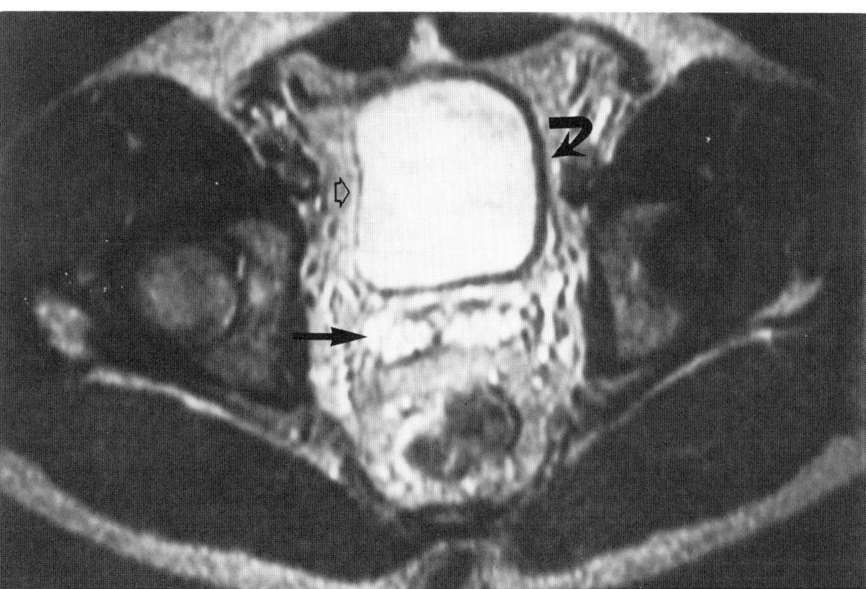

FIG. 10-16. (A) Normal urinary bladder. Axial T_1-weighted (TR/TE 600/20 ms) imaging through the lower pelvis. The urinary bladder has a homogeneously low signal intensity due to the long T_1 of urine (straight arrow) and the bladder wall cannot be discerned because of its relatively long T_1 value. The interface between the bladder wall and the perivesical fat is well demonstrated, however. The seminal vesicles also appear dark due to the presence of normal seminal fluid (curved arrow). (B) T_2-weighted (TR/TE 2,500/80 ms) scan at similar level. Both the bladder and seminal vesicle contents are now displayed with intense signal. Note multiseptated appearance of seminal vesicles (arrow). The bright line on the right side of the lateral bladder wall (open arrow) and the dark line on its left side (curved arrow) correspond to chemical shift artifacts (see text).

artifact is more pronounced in higher field-strength magnets and, in extreme cases, may simulate thickening of the bladder wall in one side and absence of the bladder wall on the opposite side.[71] Confusion between the chemical shift artifact and intrinsic bladder pathology can be dispelled, in the rare instances in which it becomes necessary, by reversing the phase-encoded and frequency-encoded gradients or by reversing the patient's position.

Benign Conditions

The signal intensity and relaxation times of thickened bladder wall secondary to vesical outlet obstruction are similar to those of normal bladder wall.[68,71] On T_1-weighted images, the hypertrophied bladder wall cannot always be distinguished from urine; however, it is well seen on T_2-weighted images. In patients with bladder outlet obstruction, mucosal congestion is sometimes seen within the region of the bladder base as one or more areas of high signal intensity on T_2-weighted images. This permits its separation from the lower signal intensity of the uninvolved bladder muscle.[68] Both inflammation and congestion cause prolongation of both T_1 and T_2 relaxation times of the bladder wall, although these values remain less than those of urine. Bladder congestion and inflammation are best demonstrated on images obtained with a long TR and long TE (i.e., T_2-weighted sequences). Congestion and inflammation cannot be distinguished from each other or from tumor on the basis of MRI signal-intensity differences.[72] Regarding chronic inflammation, in two patients with surgically proven radiation cystitis studied by Fisher et al.,[68] a variable appearance was found. In one patient, high signal intensity was seen in the mucosa of the bladder, while in the other no changes were evident. In patients with a pear-shaped bladder, MRI may clarify its etiology, confirming a suspected diagnosis of pelvic lipomatosis or one of its differential diagnostic possibilities as well as CT does. In addition, because of its multiplanar capability, MRI can nicely demonstrate the cephalad displacement of the bladder base and prostate and the elongation of the bladder neck and posterior urethra.[73] Currently, there is a paucity of information regarding the MRI appearance of benign bladder conditions, but in general it is not expected that specific diagnoses will be possible on the basis of MRI signal characteristics alone, except for pheochromocytomas, which should have characteristics similar to those in the adrenal.

MRI of Bladder Carcinoma

On MRI, bladder neoplasms are best demonstrated with a T_1-weighted image or with a balanced spin-echo or so-called proton-density image sequence (e.g., long TR, short TE: TR/TE 2,000/30 ms).[74] With these sequences, which are routinely obtained as the first echo of multiple echo spin-echo techniques, the tumors are of intermediate signal intensity, in contrast with the low-signal-intensity urine and high-signal-intensity perivesical fat. The signal intensity of bladder carcinoma is usually slightly lower than that of urine on T_2-weighted images, but the differences are not always pronounced, so the intraluminal component of the tumor may be significantly obscured in this sequence. However, the mural component of the tumor is best demonstrated in the T_2-weighted sequences, in which the infiltrating component of the tumor within the bladder wall is visualized with a slightly higher signal intensity than the wall itself. Visualization of the low-intensity line representing the uninvolved bladder wall between the tumor and the perivesical fat is an important determinant of MRI staging.[72] According to several investigators, disruption of this low-intensity line on the T_2-weighted images is indicative of deep muscle invasion (B2/T3A), whereas its preservation would imply a more localized lesion: superficial muscle invasion (B1/T2) or less.[72,74,75] Other workers have not been able to make that differentiation between superficial and deep bladder muscle invasion on their MRI studies.[76,77] The ability of MRI to differentiate tumors with deep muscle invasion from those without it may be potentially helpful in patient management to decide between performing a segmental cystectomy and a radical cystectomy and would be of significant prognostic value, since the incidence of associated pelvic node metastases is considerably greater in B2/T3A tumors than in B1/T2 lesions.[74]

For detecting tumor invasion of perivesical fat (stage C/T3B), the T_1-weighted images are the most sensitive, as they provide the greatest contrast between the lower-intensity tumor against the high-intensity signal from perivesical fat.[74] Perivesical fat invasion is occasionally confluent but more often has a wispy appearance seen as an area of diminished signal relative to pelvic fat[77] (Fig. 10-17). In the T_2-weighted images, a soft tissue mass with a signal intensity similar to the primary tumor is noted extending into the perivesical fat.

Criteria for MRI evidence of extension of the bladder tumor into adjacent pelvic organs include changes in the normal signal intensity or in the anatomic configuration of the affected organ on MRI scans. MRI provides an improved delineation of the seminal vesicles and prostate in comparison with CT. On T_1-weighted images, the seminal vesicles are of low signal intensity. However, on T_2-weighted sequences, they display an intense signal, owing to the fluid content in these structures, which allows for clear separation from adjacent bladder abnormalities (Fig. 10-18). Since on CT the seminal vesicles are generally of soft-tissue density, their involvement can be diagnosed at CT only by morphologic alteration and indirectly by obliteration of intervening fat planes. This has been shown to represent a major source of diagnostic error in CT and may help explain the low accuracy of CT in staging bladder carcinoma in some studies. For evaluation of seminal vesical extension, the axial plane is the preferred orientation with MRI as well as with CT; however, for assessment of tumor spread from the bladder to the prostate, rectum, and cervix, MRI scans in the sagittal and coronal planes are optimal (Fig. 10-19).

Pelvic adenopathy from bladder carcinoma is well demonstrated by MRI. Unfortunately, as with CT, the only criterion for abnormality is lymph node enlargement. At least two imaging sequences (T_1- and T_2-weighted) are needed for optimal demonstration of lymph nodes and discrimination from fat, blood

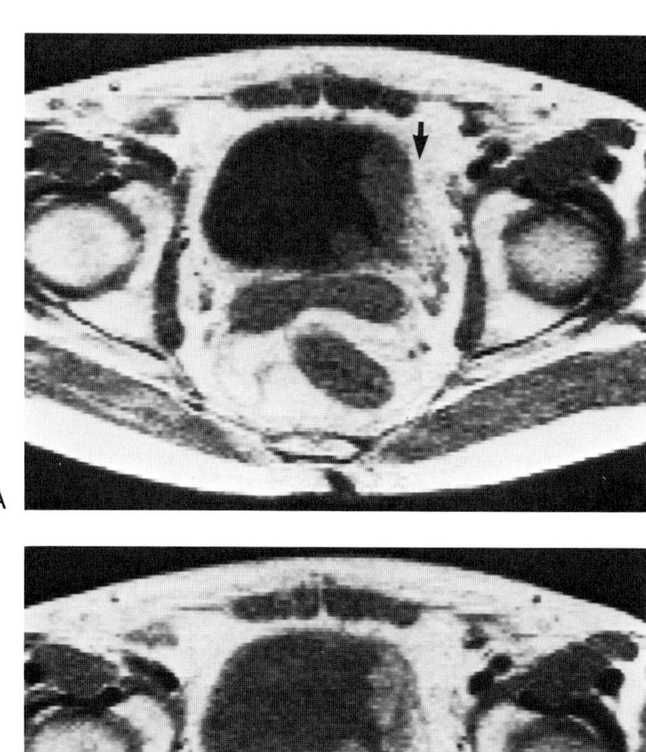

FIG. 10-17.   (A) Carcinoma of the bladder. Stage C/T3B. T_1-weighted MRI (TR/TE 500/28 ms). Irregular thickening of left lateral and posterior bladder wall with evidence of tumor extension into perivesical fat (arrow). No direct invasion of seminal vesicle is noted. (B) Corresponding MRI with proton-density spin-echo sequence (TR/TE 1,500/28 ms). Tumor infiltrating and breaching bladder wall with "wispy" extension into perivesical fat. Stage C/T3B confirmed at the time of radical cystectomy. (From Amendola et al.,[76] with permission.)

vessels, and muscle.[78,79] On the T_1-weighted sequence, lymph nodes have an intermediate signal intensity compared with the high intensity of pelvic fat and the signal void from adjacent pelvic vessels. On the T_2-weighted sequence, the lymph nodes will appear with a relatively high signal intensity compared with the low intensity of muscle. Lymphadenopathy is considered to be present

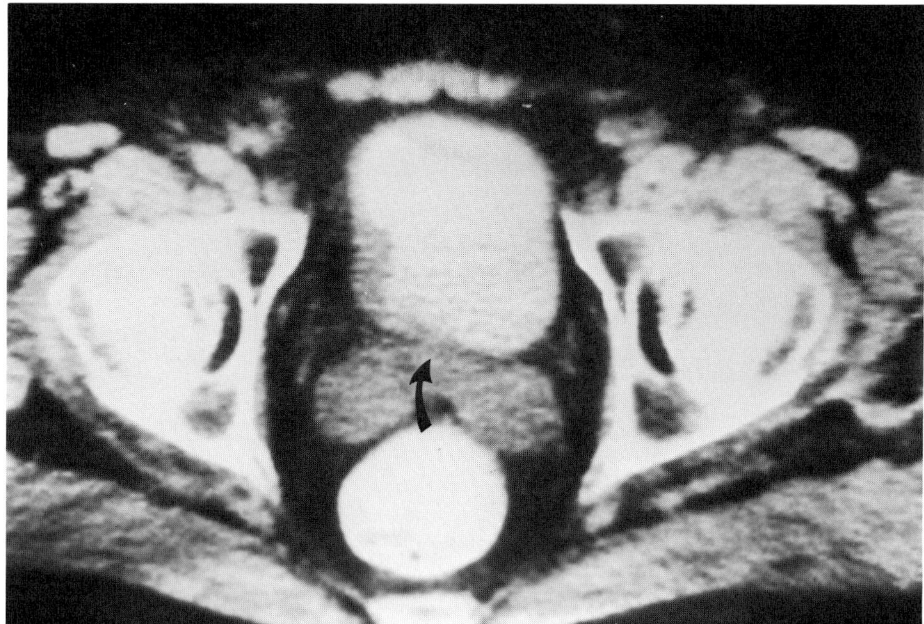

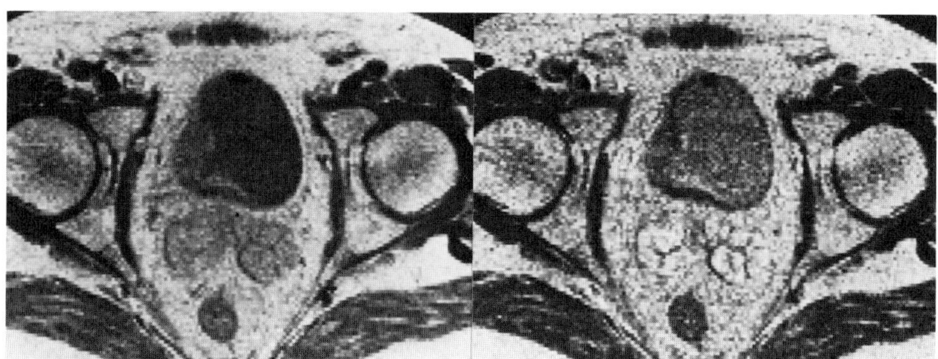

FIG. 10-18.   (A) Carcinoma of the bladder. Stage B/T3A. CT scans shows papillary and infiltrating tumor in the lateral and posterior wall of the bladder. The neoplasm appears to extend posteriorly into seminal vesicles near the midline with obliteration of intervening fat plane (arrow). (B) MRI (TR/TE 2,000/28 ms). The bladder tumor is well depicted by MRI. (C) MRI with relatively T_2-weighted sequence (TR/TE 2,000/56 ms). The tumor is confined to the bladder. Note the intact thin black line of the posterior bladder wall. Note also the bright signal from the uninvolved seminal vesicles. At surgery, the tumor stage was B2/T3A. (From Amendola et al.,[76] with permission.)

when the short axis is of a pelvic node in the transverse plane is 10 mm or more.[75]

An emerging body of work regarding MRI of bladder carcinoma suggests that MRI is at least as accurate as, if not superior to, CT for staging bladder

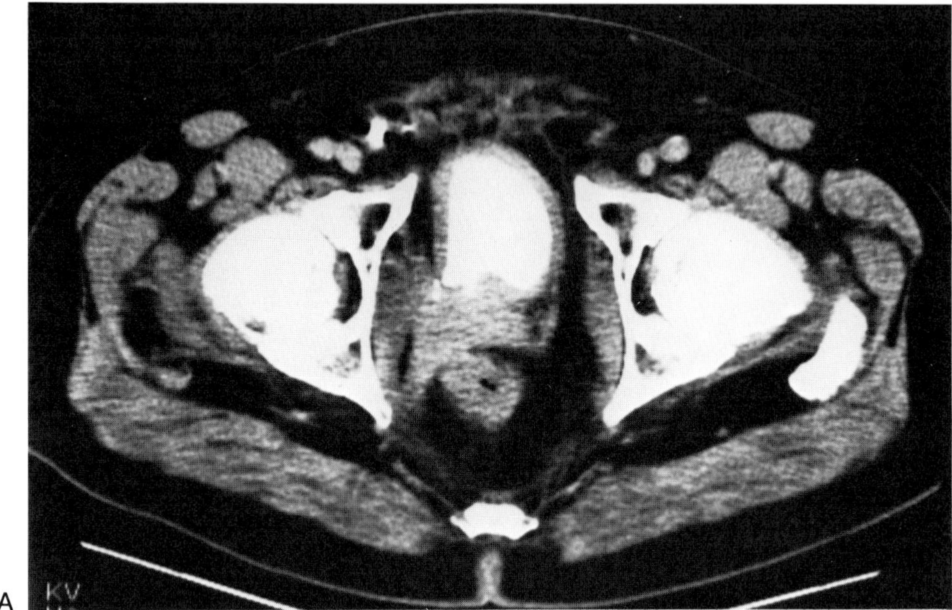

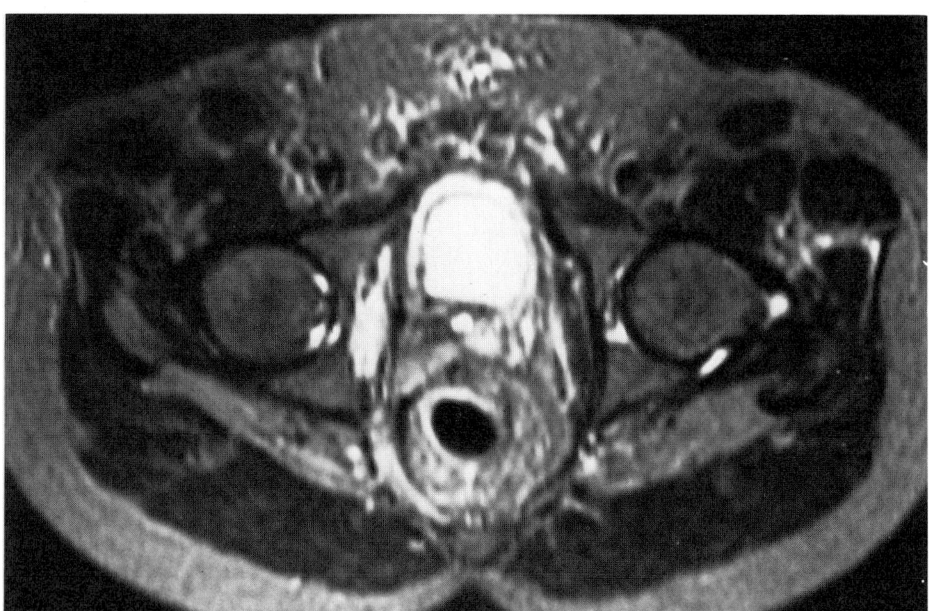

FIG. 10-19.   Bladder carcinoma extending into the right seminal vesicle, right internal obturator muscle, prostatic fossa, and central perineum inferiorly. (A) CT scan in the axial plane. (B) MRI at corresponding level (TR/TE 2,500/80 ms). (*Figure continues.*)

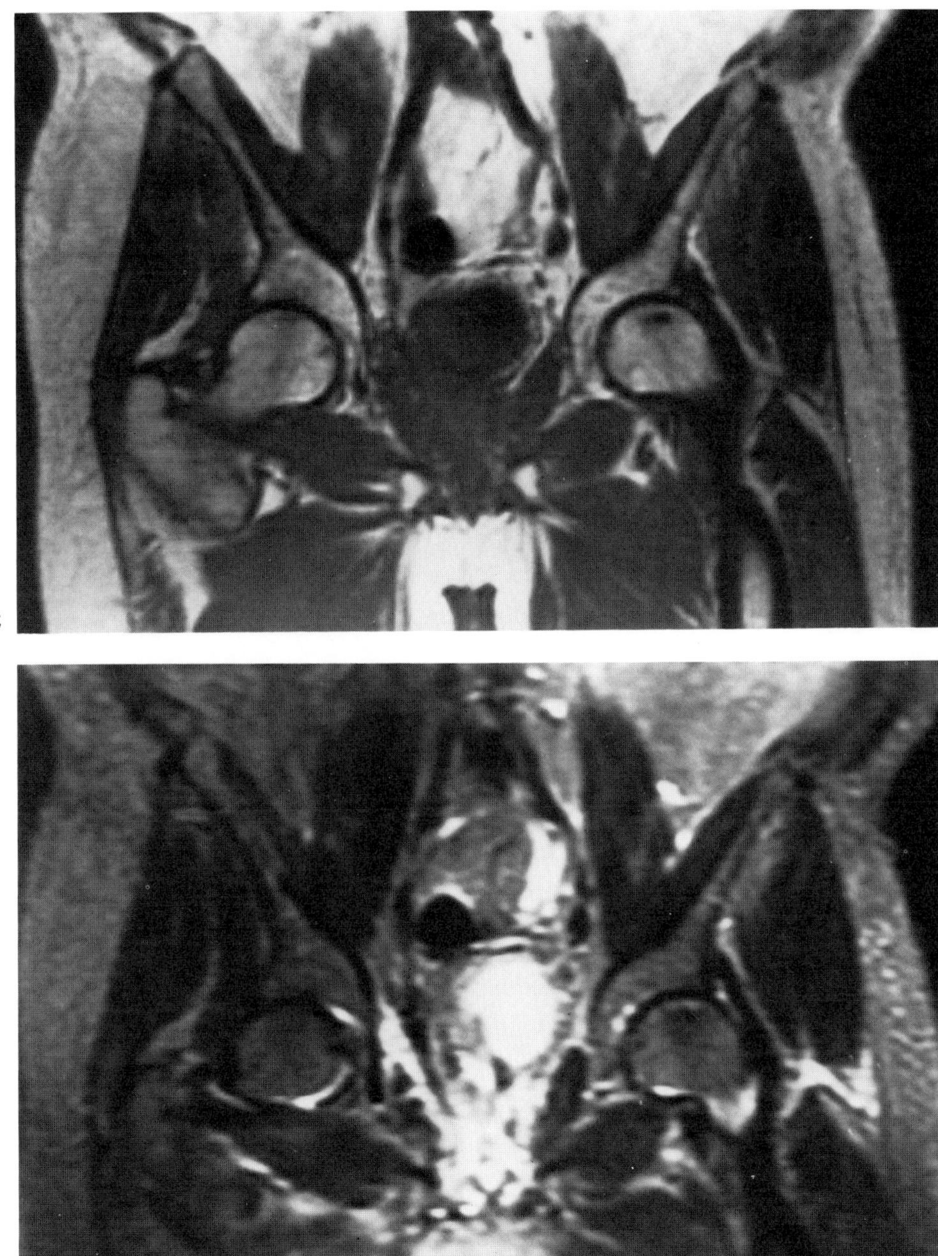

FIG. 10-19 (*Continued*).   (C) Coronal MRI with T_1-weighting (TR/TE 600/20 ms). (D) Coronal MRI with T_2-weighting (TR/TE 2,500/80 ms). Note the excellent depiction of the extensive lesion, which infiltrates laterally into the right pelvic sidewall and inferiorly into the perineum. (*Figure continues.*)

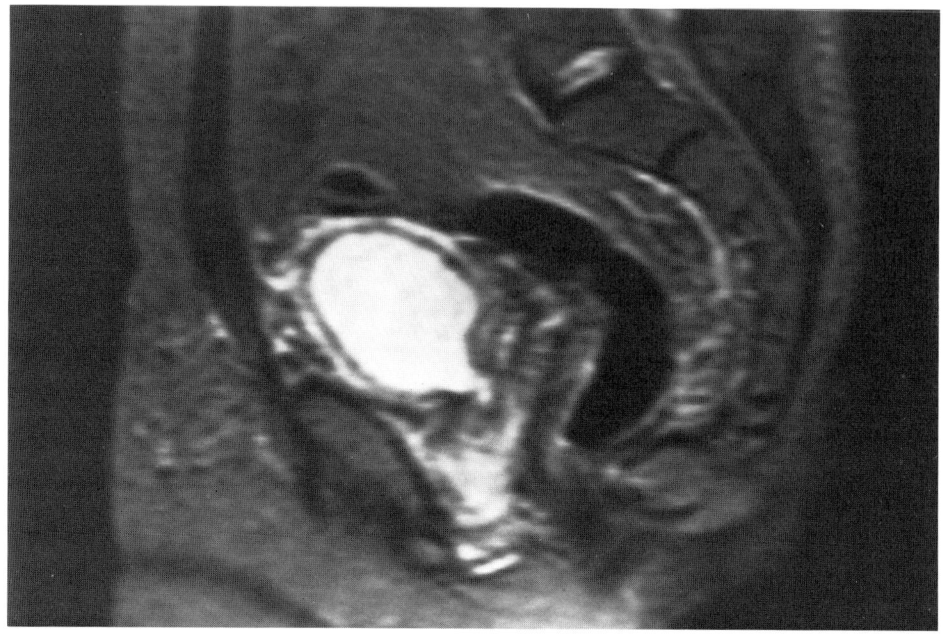

E

FIG. 10-19 (*Continued*).   (E) Sagittal MRI with T_2-weighting (TR/TE 2,500/80 ms) demonstrates similar findings.

carcinomas.[72,74–83] Using the detailed TNM staging classification, Fisher et al.[72] were able to stage correctly with MRI 12 of 14 patients (86 percent). In a larger series of 40 patients, all of whom underwent cystectomy and pelvic node dissection, Buy et al.[75] staged correctly with MRI 24 of 40 patients (60 percent). Employing the somewhat less detailed Jewett system, MRI staging accuracies for stages T3B or greater have ranged between 73 and 96 percent.[74,76] Pathways for future improvement in MRI of the bladder include (1) the use of surface and/or endocavitary coils to improve spatial resolution,[81] and (2) possible benefits from use of contrast enhancement with gadolinium-DTPA (Gd-DTPA) or other MRI contrast agents. Differentiation by MRI of postsurgical or postradiation changes versus recurrent tumor would be a highly significant contribution to the management of patients with bladder carcinoma. Although recent reports suggest the possible value of MRI in this area, further investigation is needed.[84]

REFERENCES

1. Jequier S, Rosseau O: Sonographic measurements of the normal bladder wall in children. AJR 149:563, 1987
2. Seidelmann FE, Cohen WN, Bryan PJ, et al: Accuracy of CT staging of bladder neoplasms using the gas-filled method: Report of 21 patients with surgical confirmation. AJR 130:735, 1978

3. Hildell JG, Nyman URO, Norlindh ST, et al: New intravesical contrast medium for CT: Preliminary studies with arachis (peanut) oil. AJR 137:777, 1981

4. Alhberg NE, Berlin T, Calissendorff B, et al: Intravesical fat emulsion at computed tomography of bladder tumors. Acta Radiol Diagn 22:645, 1982

5. Hamlin DJ, Crockett ATK: Computed tomography of bladder: Staging of bladder cancer using low density opacification technique. Urology 13:331, 1979

6. Weinerman PM, Arger PH, Coleman BE, et al: Pelvic adenopathy from bladder and prostate carcinoma: Detection by rapid sequence computed tomography. AJR 140:95, 1983

7. Morgan CL, Calkins RK, Cavalcanti EJ: Computed tomography in the evaluation, staging, and therapy of carcinoma of the bladder and prostate. Radiology 140:751, 1981

8. Hamlin DJ, Cockett ATK, Burgener FA: Computed tomography of the pelvis: Sagittal and coronal image reconstruction in the evaluation of infiltrative bladder carcinoma. J Comput Assist Tomogr 5:27, 1981

9. VanWaes PFGM, Feldberg MAM, Goldberg HI, et al: Direct coronal and direct sagittal CT of abdomen and pelvis: An approach to staging malignancies. Radiographics 6:213, 1986

10. Sandler CM, Hall JT, Rodriguez MB, Corriere JN Jr: Bladder injury in blunt pelvic trauma. Radiology 158:633, 1986

11. Carroll PR, McAninch JN: Major bladder trauma: The accuracy of cystography. J Urol 130:887, 1983

12. Mitty HA: CT for diagnosis and management or urinary extravasation. AJR 134:497, 1980

13. Sandler CM: Injuries of the bladder. p. 1505. In Pollack HM (ed): Clinical Urography. An Atlas and Textbook of Urological Imaging. WB Saunders, Philadelphia, 1989

14. Mee SL, McAninch JN, Federle MP: Computerized tomography in bladder rupture: Diagnostic limitations. J Urol 137:207, 1987

15. Pistoia F, Markowitz SK, Sussman SK. Contrast material in posterior vaginal fornix mimicking bladder rupture. J Comput Assist Tomogr 13:1533, 1989

16. Lebeskind AL, Elkin M, Goldman SM: Herniation of the bladder. Radiology 106:257, 1973

17. Curry NS, O'Connor KF, Tubbs CO: Scrotal cystocele diagnosed by computed tomography. Urol Radiol 9:247, 1988

18. Allen RP, Condon VR: Transitory extraperitoneal hernia of the bladder in infants (bladder ears). Radiology 77:979, 1961

19. Gerson ES, Gerzof SG, Robbins AH: CT confirmation of pelvic lipomatosis: Three cases. AJR 129:338, 1977

20. Wechsler RJ, Brennan RE: Teardrop bladder: Additional considerations. Radiology 144:281, 1982

21. Chang SF: Pear-shaped bladder caused by large ileopsoas muscles. Radiology 128:349, 1978

22. Pollack HM, Banner MP, Martinez LO, Hodson CJ: Diagnostic considerations of urinary bladder wall calcification. AJR 136:791, 1981

23. Jorulf H, Lindstedt E: Urogenital schistosomiasis: CT evaluation. Radiology 157:745, 1985

24. Lautin EM, Becker RD, Fromowitz FB, Bezahler GH: Computed tomography of the lower urinary tract in schistosomiasis. J Comput Assist Tomogr 7:164, 1983

25. Aisen AM, Gross BH, Glazer GM: Computed tomography of ureterovesical schistosomiasis. J Comput Assist Tomogr 7:161, 1983

26. Verguts V, Deconick K, Mortelmans LL: Alkaline encrusting cystitis. Urol Radiol 9:53, 1987

27. Patel PS, Wilbur AC: Nephrogenic adenoma presenting as a calcified mass. AJR 150:1071, 1988

28. Irwin GAL, Craig R, Novotny P: CT of calcified bladder masses. Comput Radiol 9:181, 1985

29. Pollack HM, Arger PH, Banner MP, et al: Computed tomographic of renal pelvic filling defects. Radiology 138:645, 1981

30. Goldman SM, Fishman EK, Gatewood OMB, et al: The CT demonstration of colovesical fistulae secondary to diverticulitis. J Comput Assist Tomogr 8:462, 1984

31. Ney C, Kumar M, Billah K, Doerr J: CT demonstration of cystitis emphysematosa. J Comput Assist Tomogr 11:552, 1987

32. Goldman SM, Fishman EK, Gatewood OMG, et al: CT in the diagnosis of enterovesical fistulae. AJR 144:1229, 1985

33. Merine D, Fishman EK, Kuhlman JE, et al: Bladder involvement in Crohn disease: Role of CT in detection and evaluation. J Comput Assist Tomogr 13:903, 1989

34. Wojtasek DA, Teixidor HS, Kazam E: Appendicitis with bladder involvement: CT appearance. Urol Radiol 9:237, 1988

35. Brant WE, Williams JL: Computed tomography of bladder leiomyoma. J Comput Assist Tomogr 8:562, 1984

36. Wenz W, Sommerkamp H, Dinkel E: Leiomyoma of the bladder. Urol Radiol 8:114, 1986

37. Illescas FF, Baker ME, Weinerth JL: Bladder leiomyoma: Advantages of sonography over computed tomography. Urol Radiol 8:216, 1986

38. Bidwell JK, Dunne MG: Computed tomography of the bladder malakoplakia. J Comput Assist Tomogr 11:909, 1987

39. Epstein BM, Patel V, Porteous PH: CT appearance of bladder malacoplakia. J Comput Assist Tomogr 7:541, 1983

40. Radin DR, Siskind SW, Weiner S, et al: Retroperitoneal malakoplakia. Urol Radiol 6:218, 1984

41. Zingas AP, Kling GA, Crotte E, et al: Computed tomography of nephrogenic adenoma of the bladder. J Comput Assist Tomogr 10:979, 1986

42. Kauzlaric D, Barmeir E, Campana A: Diagnosis of cystitis glandularis. Urol Radiol 9:50, 1987

43. Goff WB: Cystitis cystica and cystitis glandularis: Cause of bladder mass. J Comput Assist Tomogr 7:347, 1983

44. Binkovitz LA, Hattery RR, LeRoy AJ: Primary lymphoma of the bladder. Urol Radiol 9:231, 1988

45. Vock P, Haertel M, Fuchs WA, et al: Computed tomography in staging of carcinoma of the urinary bladder. Br J Urol 54:158, 1982

46. Lang EK: Neoplasms of the bladder, prostate and urethra. Semin Roentgenol 18:288, 1983

47. Lee JKT, Balfe DM: Pelvis. p. 393. In Lee JKT, Sagel SS, Stanley RJ (eds): Computed Body Tomography. Raven Press, New York, 1983

48. Schmidt JD, Weinstein SH: Pitfalls in clinical staging of bladder tumors. Urol Clin North Am 3:107, 1976

49. Olsson Ca, deVere White RW: Cancer of the bladder. p. 337. In Javadapour N (ed): Principles and Management of Urologic Cancer. Williams & Wilkins, Baltimore, 1979

50. Jewett HJ, Strong GH: Infiltrating carcinoma of the bladder. Relation of depth of penetration of the bladder wall to incidence of local extension and metastases. J Urol 55:366, 1946

51. Marshall VF: The relation of the preoperative estimate to the pathologic demonstration of the extent of vesical neoplasms. J Urol 68:714, 1952

52. American Joint Committee for Cancer Staging and End-Results Reporting: Manual for staging of cancer—1978. Whiting Press, Chicago, 1978

53. Koss JC, Arger PH, Coleman BG, et al: CT staging of bladder carcinoma. AJR 137:359, 1981

54. Husband JE: Staging of bladder and prostate cancer. p. 135. In Walsh JW (ed): Computed Tomography of the Pelvis. Churchill Livingstone, New York, 1985

55. Seidelman FE, Cohen WN, Bryan PJ: Computed tomographic staging of bladder neoplasms. Radiol Clin North Am 15:419, 1977

56. Salo Jo, Kivisaari L, Lethonen T: CT in determining the depth of infiltration of bladder tumors. Urol Radiol 7:88, 1985

57. Jeffrey RB, Palubinskas AJ, Federle MP: CT evaluation of invasive lesions of the bladder. J Comput Assist Tomogr 5:22, 1981

58. Kellet MJ, Oliver RTD, Husband JE, Kelsey-Fry I: Computed tomography as an adjunct to bimanual examination for staging bladder tumors. Br J Urol 52:101, 1980

59. Ahlberg NE, Calissendorff B, Wikjstrom H: Computed tomography in staging of bladder carcinoma. Acta Radiol Diagn 23:47, 1982

60. Sager EM, Talle K, Fossa S, et al: The role of CT in demonstrating perivesical tumor growth in the preoperative staging of carcinoma of the urinary bladder. Radiology 146:443, 1983

61. Smith JA, Whitmore WF Jr: Regional lymph node metastases from bladder cancer. J Urol 126:591, 1981

62. Lieskovsky G, Skinner DG: Role of lymphadenectomy in the treatment of bladder cancer. Urol Clin North Am 11:709, 1984

63. Walsh JW, Amendola MA, Konerding KF, et al: Computed tomographic detection of pelvic and inguinal lymph node metastases from primary and recurrent pelvic malignant disease. Radiology 137:157, 1980

64. Lee JKT, McClennan BL, Stanley RJ, et al: Use of CT in evaluation of postcystectomy patients. AJR 136:483, 1981

65. Oliva L, Cariati M, Reggiani L, et al: CT evaluation of cavity after cystectomy. J Comput Assist Tomogr 8:734, 1984

66. Winkler ML, Hricak H: Pelvis imaging with MR: Technique for improvement. Radiology 158:148, 1986

67. Spritzer CE, Kressler HY, Mitchell D: Magnetic resonance imaging of the female pelvis. p. 203. In Kressel HY (ed): Magnetic Resonance Annual 1987. Raven Press, New York, 1987

68. Fisher MR, Hricak H, Crooks LE: Urinary bladder: MR imaging. I. Normal and benign conditions. Radiology 157:467, 1985

69. Lee JKT, Rholl KS: MRI of the bladder and prostate. AJR 147:732, 1986

70. Babcock EE, Brateman L, Weinreb JC, et al: Edge artifacts in MR images: Chemical shift effect. J Comput Assist Tomogr 9:252, 1985

71. Heiken JP, Lee JKT: MR imaging of the pelvis. Radiology 166:11, 1988

72. Fisher MR, Hricak H, Crooks LE: Urinary bladder: MR imaging. II. Neoplasm. Radiology 157:471, 1985

73. Demas BE, Avallone A, Hricak H: Pelvic lipomatosis: Diagnosis and characterization by magnetic resonance imaging. Urol Radiol 10:198, 1988

74. Rholl KS, Lee JKT, Heiken JP, et al: Primary bladder carcinoma: Evaluation with MR imaging. Radiology 163:117, 1987

75. Buy JN, Moss AA, Guinet C, et al: MR staging of bladder carcinoma: Correlation with pathologic findings. Radiology 169:695, 1988

76. Amendola MA, Glazer GM, Grossman HB, et al: Staging of bladder carcinoma: MRI-CT surgical correlation. AJR 146:1179, 1987

77. Bryan PJ, Butler HE, Lipuma JP, et al: CT and MR imaging in staging bladder neoplasms. J Comput Assist Tomogr 11:96, 1987

78. Dooms GC, Hricak H, Crooks LE, et al: Magnetic resonance imaging of lymph nodes: Comparison with CT. Radiology 153:719, 1984

79. Lee JKT, Heiken JP, Ling D, et al: Magnetic resonance imaging of abdominal and pelvic lymphadenopathy. Radiology 153:181, 1984

80. Koelbel G, Schmiedl U, Griebel J, et al: MR imaging of bladder neoplasms. J Comput Assist Tomogr 12:98, 1988

81. Barentz JO, Lemmens JAM, Ruijs SHJ, et al: Carcinoma of the urinary bladder: MR imaging with a double surface coil. AJR 151:107, 1988

82. Salo JO, Kivisaari L, Lethonen T: Comparison of magnetic resonance imaging with computed tomography and intravesical ultrasound in staging bladder cancer. Urol Radiol 10:167, 1988

83. Smith FW, Sarkar TK, Hewitt BR: Monitoring of bladder uroplasia by low field magnetic resonance imaging. Br J Radiol 61:166, 1988

84. Ebner F, Kressel HY, Mintz MC, et al: Tumor recurrence versus fibrosis in the female pelvis: Differentiation with MR imaging at 1.5T. Radiology 166:333, 1988

85. Amendola MA: Conventional radiographic contrast procedures. p. 96. In Fisher MR, Kricum ME (eds): Imaging of the Pelvis. Aspen, Rockville, MD, 1989

11 CT and MRI of Urachal Carcinoma

STEVEN H. BRICK
ARNOLD C. FRIEDMAN
HOWARD M. POLLACK
PAUL D. RADECKI

The urachus is a vestigial remnant of the fetal genitourinary tract. Benign urachal anomalies are rare and usually present in early childhood. These include patent urachus, which is most common, urachal cyst, umbilicourachal sinus, and vesicourachal diverticulum. The least common, but most serious, complication of persistent urachal remnants is the development of carcinoma.

ANATOMY AND EMBRYOLOGY

The urachus is a midline tubular structure that extends cephalad from the anterior dome of the bladder. It is extraperitoneal in location, lying within the space of Retzius, which is bordered anteriorly by the transversalis fascia and posteriorly by the peritoneum. The urachus is a remnant of at least two embryonic structures: (1) the cloaca, which is derived from the terminal portion of the hindgut and is the cephalad extension of the urogenital sinus (the precursor of the fetal urinary bladder), and (2) the allantois, a derivative of the yolk sac.[1–5]

In the adult, the urachus can range in length from less than 2 cm up to 15 cm and can have a variety of appearances. The urachus can extend from the bladder apex to the umbilicus, independent of the obliterated umbilical arteries. It can merge in the midline with both obliterated umbilical arteries and continue to the umbilicus as a common ligament, or it can deviate from the midline to merge with one obliterated umbilical artery. It can also be very short (< 2 cm) and end freely or in a fine fibrous plexus.[6]

HISTOLOGY AND PATHOLOGY

Histologic evaluation of the urachus reveals a multilayered structure. An inner layer of transitional cell epithelium lines a real or potential lumen, although one-third of dissected specimens reveal columnar metaplasia. The mucosa is covered by a connective tissue layer of blood and lymph vessels, and an outer layer of smooth muscle. A serosal coat of peritoneum is seen only on the posterior surface and is absent along its intramural course in the bladder wall.[2,7,8]

Even though the urachal mucosa consists of transitional epithelium, 85 to 95 percent of all urachal cancers are adenocarcinomas. This is most likely a result of metaplasia of the urachal mucosa into columnar epithelium and subsequent malignant transformation. Seventy-five percent of urachal adenocarcinomas are mucin-producing. Other types of urachal neoplasms, which are considerably less common, include sarcomas, transitional cell carcinomas, and squamous cell carcinomas.[1,8]

CLINICAL FINDINGS

Urachal carcinoma is extremely rare, representing only 0.01 percent of all adult cancers, 0.17 to 0.34 percent of all bladder cancers, and 20 to 39 percent of all primary bladder adenocarcinomas.[1] Most patients with urachal carcinoma are 40 to 70 years of age, although it has been reported at all ages. Sixty-five to 75 percent of patients are male. The signs and symptoms of urachal carcinoma are nonspecific and include hematuria (found in 71 percent of patients), suprapubic mass, abdominal pain, irritative voiding symptoms, and discharge of blood, pus, or mucus from the umbilicus. The discovery of gross or microscopic mucus in the urine is highly suspicious for adenocarcinoma, but is found in only 25 percent of cases and can occur with either bladder or urachal tumors.[1,8]

Urachal carcinoma has a considerably worse prognosis than does primary bladder transitional cell carcinoma. Local invasion has frequently occurred prior to diagnosis, most often to the space of Retzius, peritoneum, regional lymph nodes, abdominal wall, and/or bladder. This local invasion is certainly facilitated by the lack of a serosal covering of peritoneum on the anterior surface of the urachus and along its intramural course in the bladder wall. Local recurrence following surgery is not uncommon, although distant metastasis is usually a late event.[1,8]

CT AND MRI APPEARANCE

The CT appearance of urachal carcinoma has been described in several case reports[9–17] and in two larger studies.[18,19] The most frequent appearance by far is that of a predominantly supravesical mass (Fig. 11-1). Although considerably less common, the tumor can predominantly involve the intramural portion of the urachus[18] (Fig. 11-2). The location of the tumor in relation to the anterior

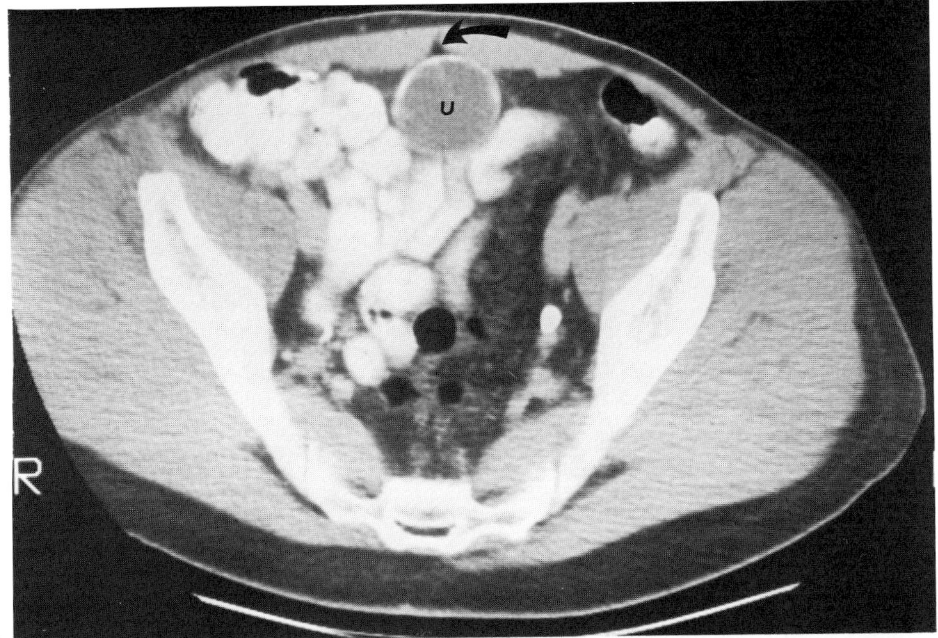

A

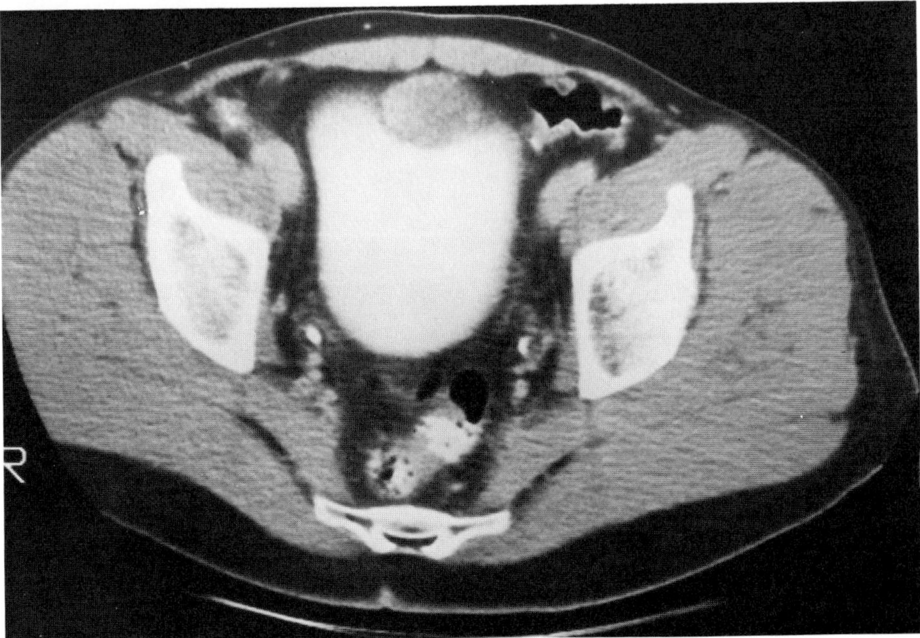

B

FIG. 11-1.   Cystic urachal carcinoma. (A) Image at level of iliac crests shows a supravesical low attenuation mass (u) with a thin peripheral rim of calcification directly posterior to the linea alba (curved arrow). (B) Scan obtained 1 cm lower shows the intramural component of the tumor. (From Brick et al.,[18] with permission.)

abdominal wall is also characteristic. The midline position of the urachus within the space of Retzius places it just posterior to the linea alba, the fibrous sheath between the two rectus abdominus muscles. Most urachal carcinomas therefore lie directly posterior to the linea alba, an easily recognized landmark on CT (Figs. 11-1 and 11-3). The few cases in which the tumor is minimally deviated

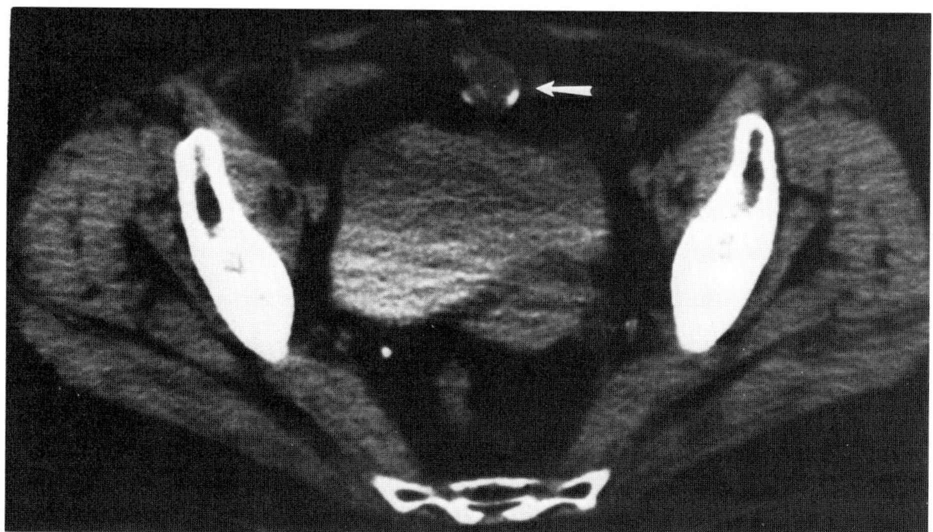

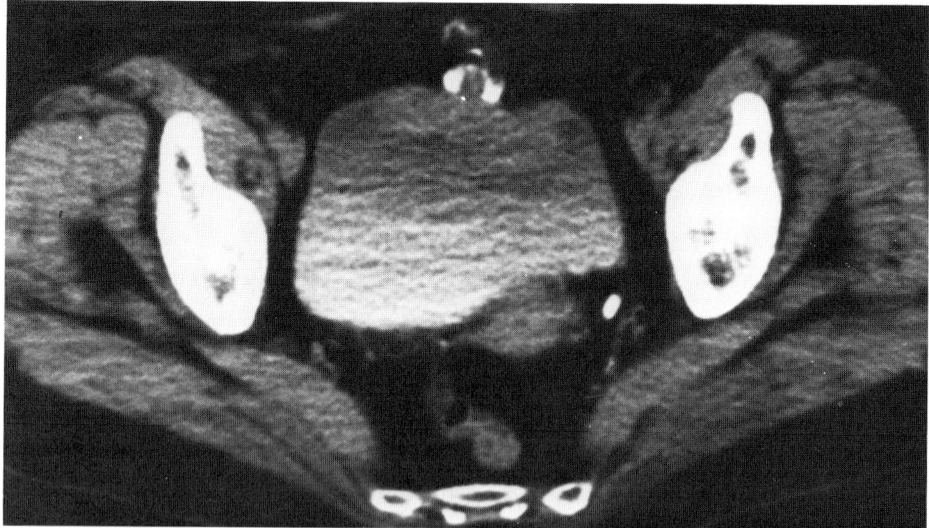

FIG. 11-2.   Urachal carcinoma with large intravesical component. (A) Image at level of iliac crests shows calcified supravesical mass (long arrow) in expected location of urachus. (B) Image 1 cm lower shows junction of mass with bladder wall. (*Figure continues.*)

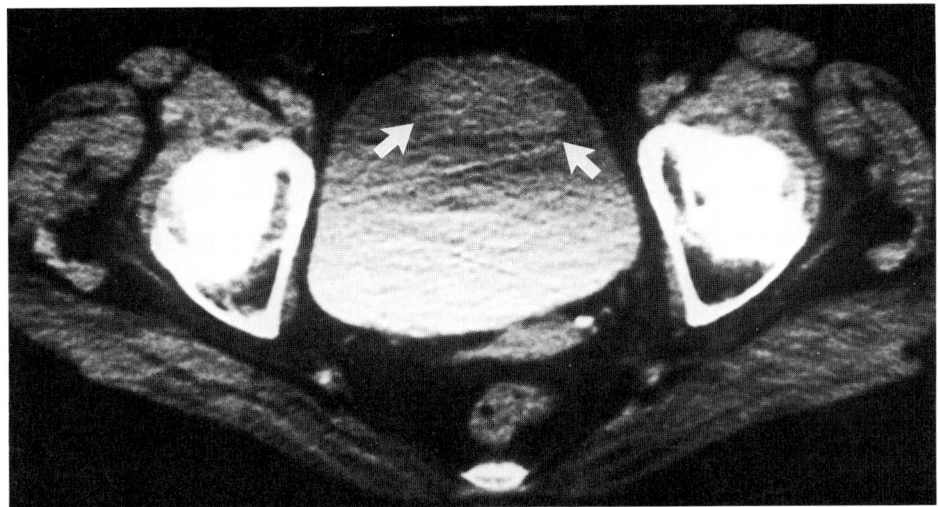

C

FIG. 11-2 (*Continued*).   (C) Image 1 cm lower shows large intravesical component of tumor (short arrows). (Courtesy of Elliott K. Fishman, M.D., Johns Hopkins Hospital, Baltimore, Md.)

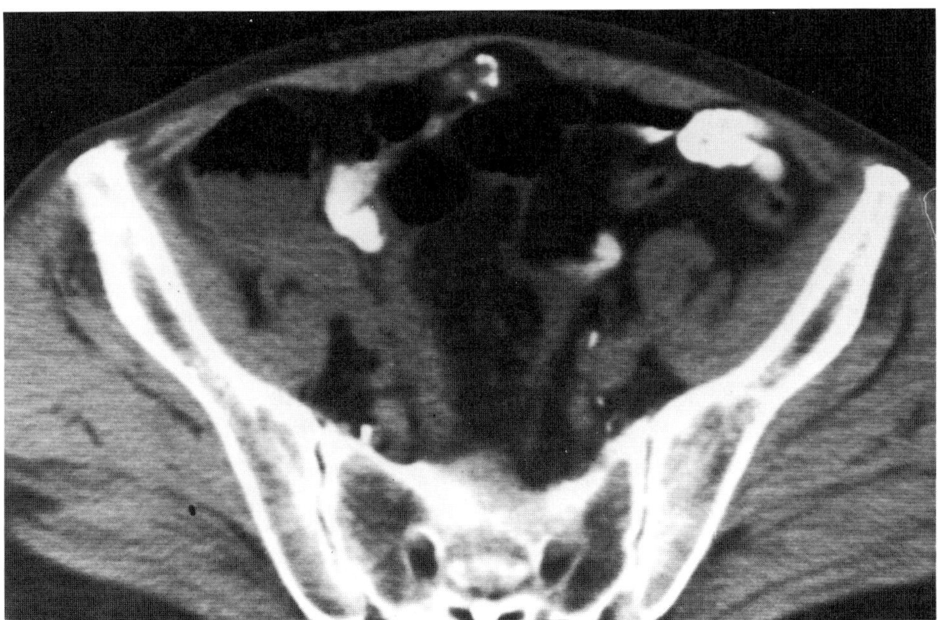

A

FIG. 11-3.   Solid urachal carcinoma following the course of the urachus. A solid mass containing multiple thick flakes of calcification is seen arising several centimeters below the umbilicus (A). (*Figure continues.*)

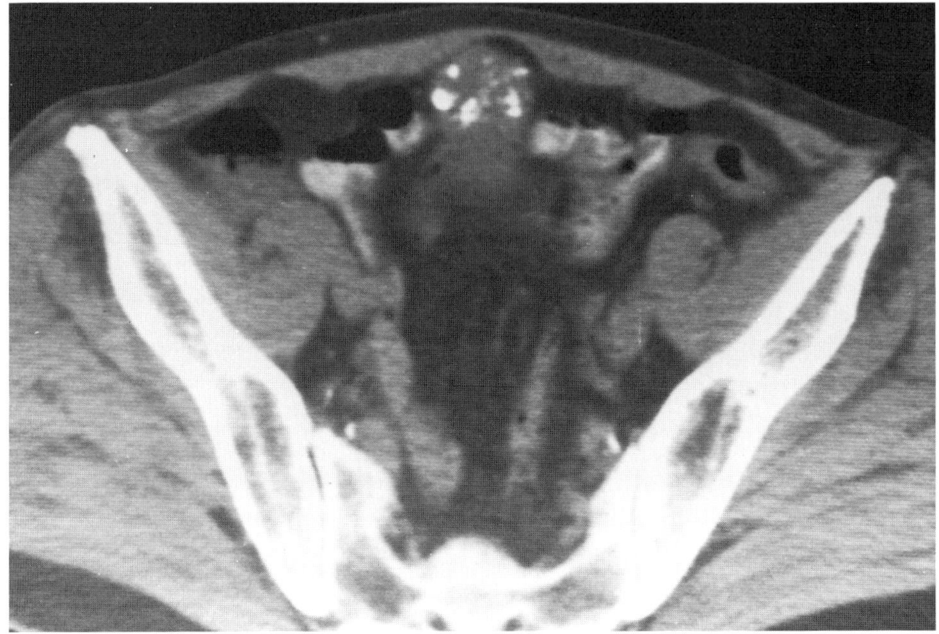

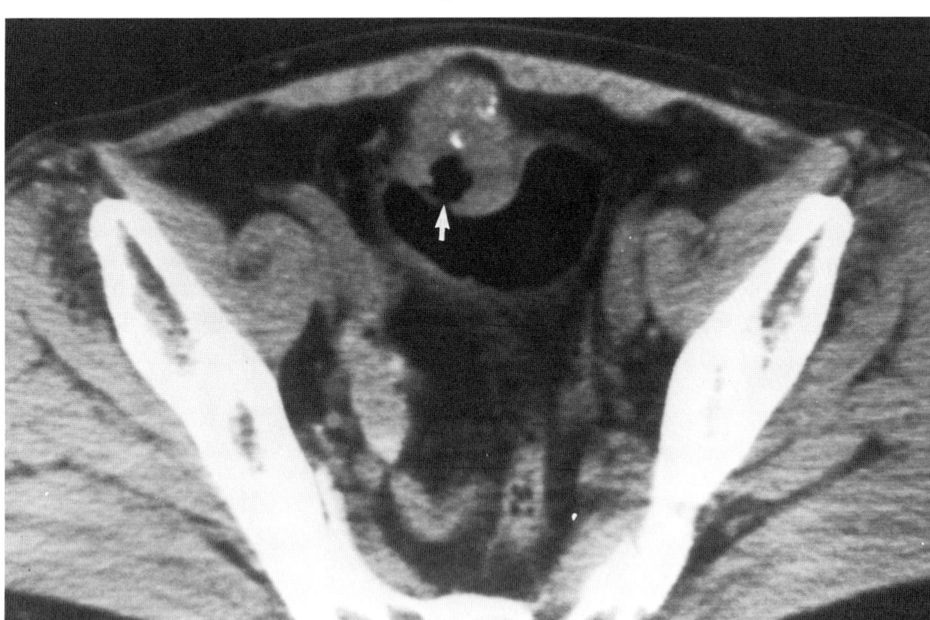

FIG. 11-3 (*Continued*). The mass follows the expected position of the urachus (B & C) down into the bladder dome (D). (*Figure continues.*)

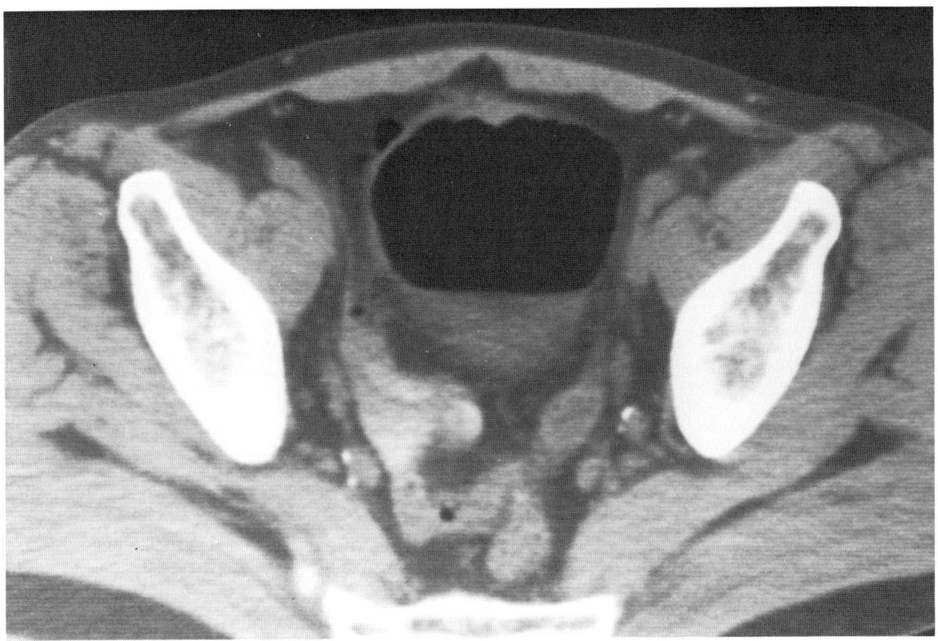

D

FIG. 11-3 (*Continued*).   The bladder was filled with air prior to this study. The ulceration in the posterior aspect of this mass (Fig. C, arrow) was at the site of a previous biopsy. (From Brick et al.,[18] with permission.)

toward one side can be explained embryologically, since the urachus occasionally moves slightly off midline to merge with one of the obliterated umbilical arteries.[18]

Urachal carcinomas can appear cystic or solid on CT. Up to 60 percent of cases have been described as being partially or predominantly low attenuation, most likely due to the large pools of mucin seen pathologically. Calcification is not uncommon in mucinous tumors and has been described in 50 to 70 percent of cases. Types of calcification include central or peripheral, punctate or curvilinear[18,19] (Figs. 11-1 to 11-4).

CT plays an important role in some aspects of preoperative staging of urachal carcinoma. CT is excellent for evaluating the gross intravesical and extravesical extent of tumor and its effect on surrounding structures. Since the main bulk of the tumor is frequently outside of the bladder, tumor size can be considerably underestimated by intravenous (IV) urography, cystography, or cystoscopy. CT can also determine whether gross invasion of the abdominal wall is present. However, CT has been shown to be limited in its ability to diagnose spread of tumor into the periurachal fat or bladder mucosa.[18] The integrity of the bladder mucosa is best evaluated by cystoscopy and biopsy.

The MRI appearance of urachal carcinoma (Fig. 11-5) has only been reported in two papers.[18,20] The anatomic location and appearance is similar to that

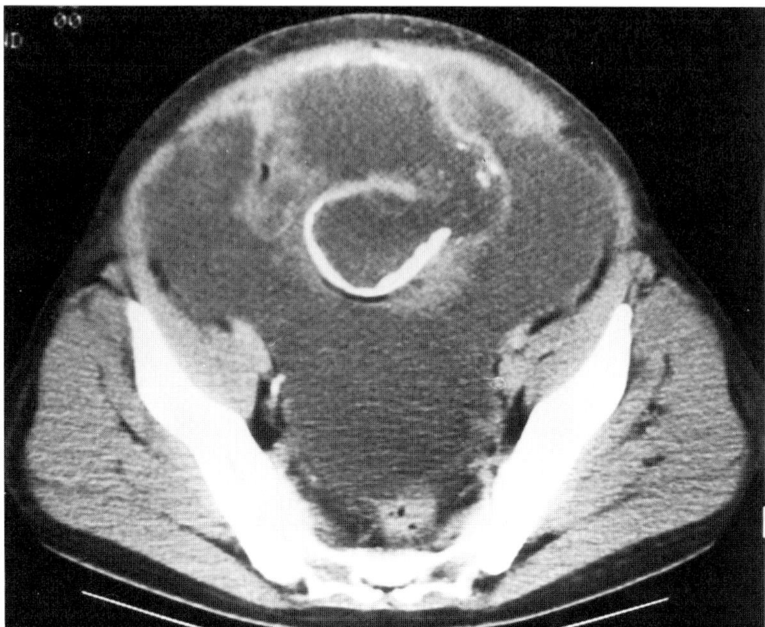

FIG. 11-4.   Cystic urachal carcinoma with peritoneal metastases. A large calcified cystic mass is seen in the anterior upper pelvis. The large amount of ascites is due to peritoneal metastases, which were seen on other images. (Courtesy of Donald G. Mitchell, M.D., Philadelphia, Pa.)

described by CT. The signal characteristics are similar to those of other tumors with low signal on T_1-weighted images and increased signal on T_2-weighted images. Heavily T_2-weighted images may show markedly increased signal from the tumor, possibly due to the large amount of mucoid material often found. MRI offers the added advantage over CT of multiple scan planes, which may permit improved preoperative staging. However, the detection of calcifications, whose presence is essential when formulating a differential diagnosis, is very difficult with MRI.

DIFFERENTIAL DIAGNOSIS

Nonurachal Bladder Tumors

A predominantly supravesical midline tumor most likely represents a urachal carcinoma, since it is very unusual for a primary bladder tumor to extend above the bladder dome along the course of the urachus.[19] Although less common, urachal carcinoma can be limited to the intramural portion of the urachus, and differentiation from a primary bladder dome tumor can be difficult. A tumor located off the midline most likely has originated in the bladder,

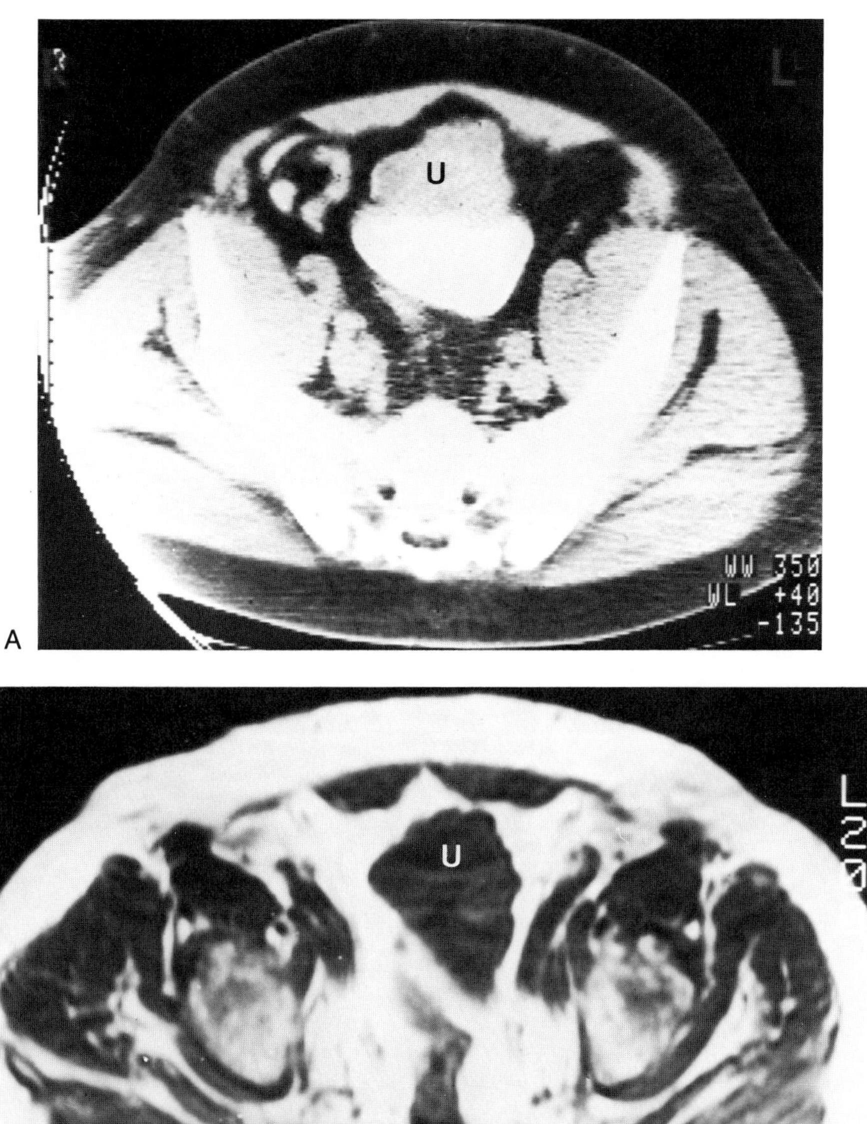

FIG. 11-5.   Lobulated cystic tumor with pools of mucin best seen with MRI. (A) CT
scan shows multiple low attenuation regions within the tumor and minimal peripheral
calcification. The characteristic location posterior to the linear alba is again seen. (B)
T_1-weighted (SE 600/20) axial image shows a mass with low signal intensity similar to
muscle but slightly less than urine. (*Figure continues.*)

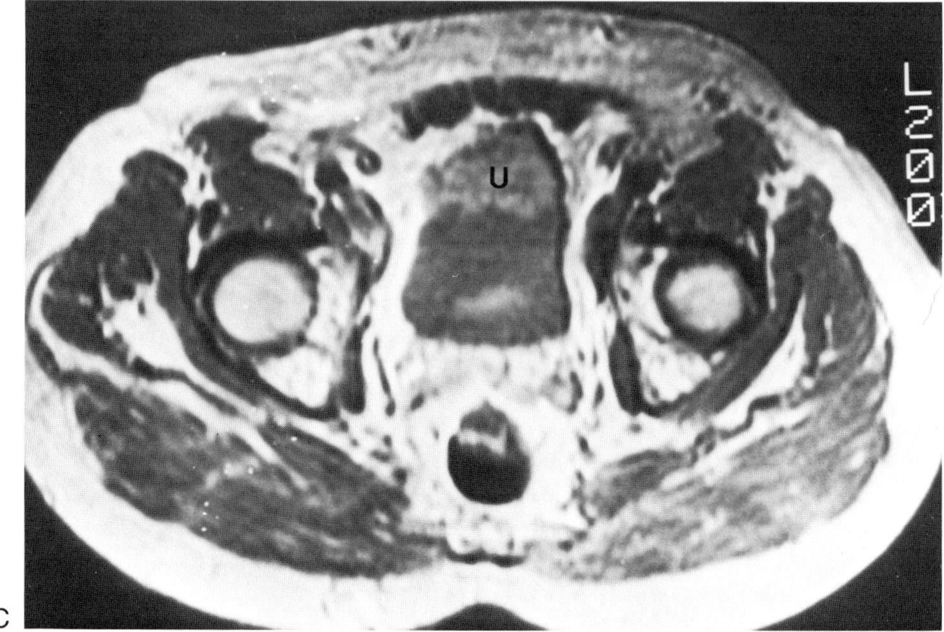

C

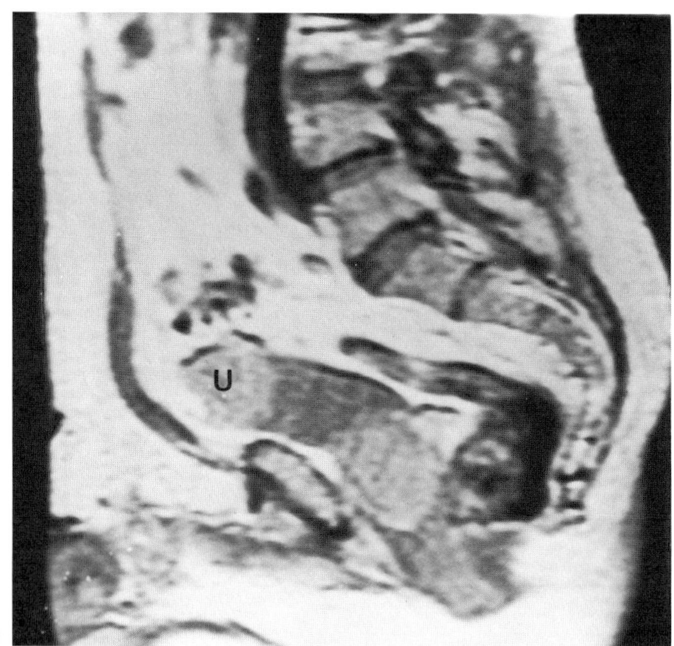

D

FIG. 11-5 (*Continued*). On proton density (SE 2,500/20) axial (C) and sagittal (D) images, the signal intensity increases to slightly greater than muscle and urine. (*Figure continues.*)

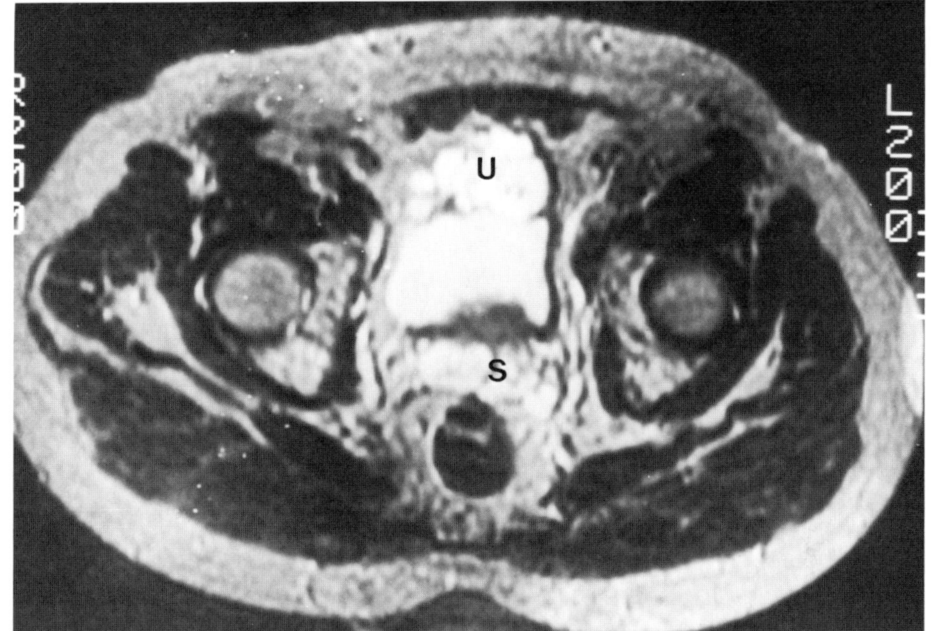

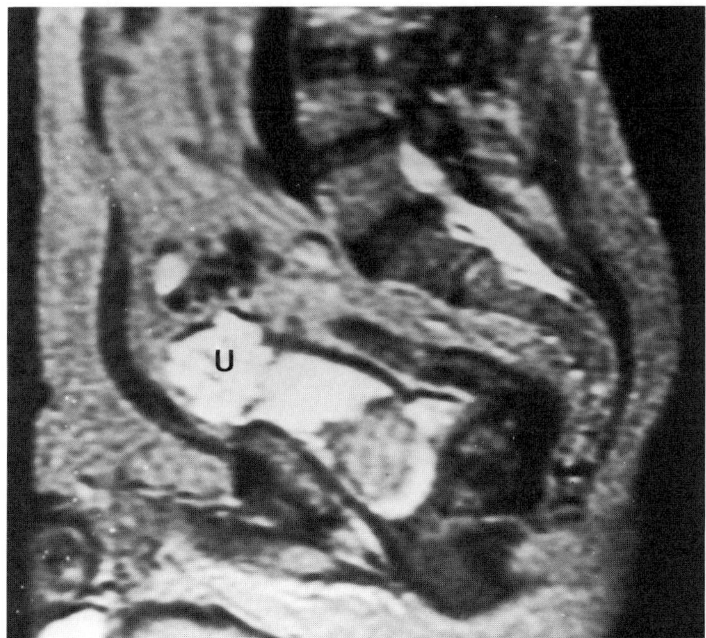

FIG. 11-5 (*Continued*).   T$_2$-weighted (SE 2,500/80) axial (E) and sagittal (F) images show the high signal produced by the mucinous fluid in the tumor, which is similar to urine and the seminal vesicles. U, urachal carcinoma; S, seminal vesicle. (From Brick et al.,[18] with permission.)

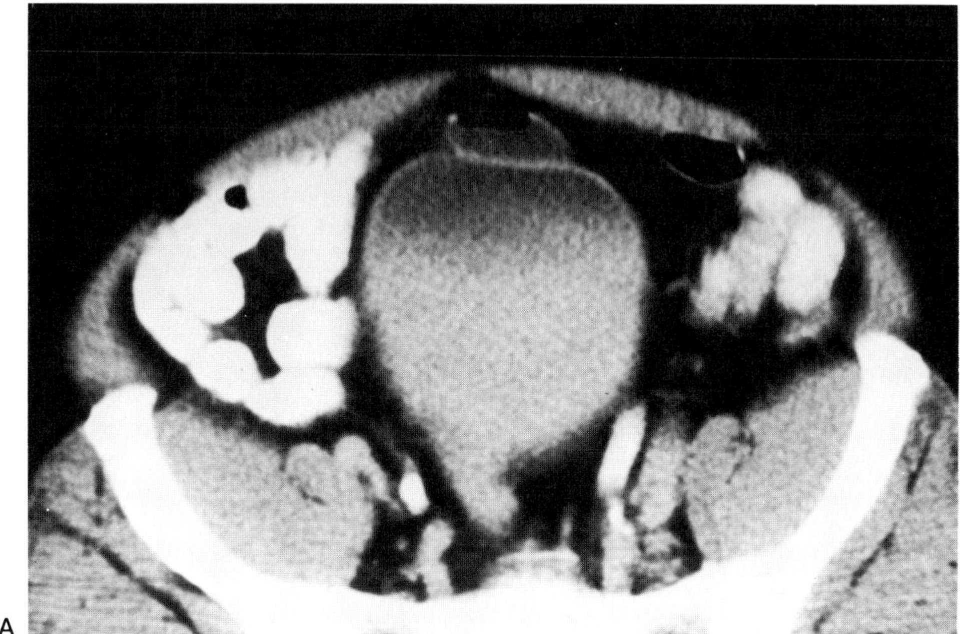
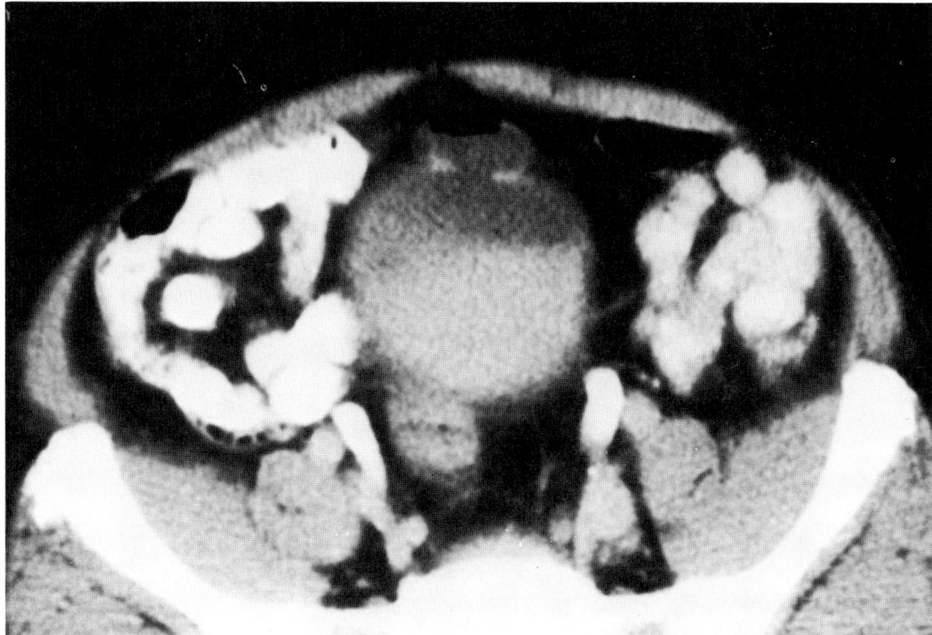

FIG. 11-6. Incidental vesicourachal diverticulum discovered on CT in a 69-year-old man being staged for carcinoma of the prostate. (A) A small cystic structure containing an air-fluid level is seen anterior to the bladder. (B) The communication between the cyst and the bladder is shown 10 mm cephalad to the cyst in Fig. A. The location and the communication are diagnostic of vesicourachal diverticulum. The air is residual from the cystoscopy done 1 day prior to the CT.

although urachal tumors can occasionally be deviated slightly to one side. If calcifications are seen by CT, urachal adenocarcinoma is considerably more likely than transitional cell bladder carcinoma, and the diagnosis can be easily confirmed by biopsy. However, adenocarcinoma of the bladder can also calcify and differentiation between adenocarcinomas of urachal and bladder origin can be difficult even with pathologic evaluation. If the tumor is completely supravesical, or if it is located within the bladder dome wall beneath a normal layer of urothelium, urachal origin is obvious. However, since an intramural urachal carcinoma has frequently invaded the mucosa by the time of diagnosis, and since 15 percent of adenocarcinomas of the bladder are confined to the dome, determining the site of origin can become problematic.[8,18]

Other Urachal Abnormalities

Urachal cysts result from segmental persistence of the urachus with closure at both ends. Uncomplicated urachal cysts can be uniloculated or septated, and calcification of the wall can be seen. When complicated by infection, the walls can be thickened and irregular, and the CT attenuation of the cyst can increase.[9] Although the number of reported cases is relatively small, there appears to be overlap in the CT appearance of urachal cysts and carcinoma, and a cystic urachal mass should not be considered benign on the basis of the CT appearance alone. A vesicourachal diverticulum (Fig. 11-6) results from obliteration of the cephalic portion of the urachus only. This diagnosis is confirmed when CT demonstrates filling of the diverticulum with intravenously administered contrast or gas introduced by a bladder catheter.[21]

REFERENCES

1. Sheldon CA, Clayman RV, Gonzalez R, et al: Malignant urachal lesions. J Urol 131:1, 1984

2. Bauer SB, Retik AB. Urachal anomalies and related umbilical disorders. Urol Clin North Am 5:195, 1978

3. Moore KL: The urogenital system. p. 220. In Moore KL (ed): The Developing Human. 2nd Ed. WB Saunders, Philadelphia, 1977

4. Begg RC: The urachus: Its anatomy, histology, and development. J Anat 64:170, 1930

5. Begg RC: The colloid adenocarcinomata of the bladder vault arising from the epithelium of the urachal canal: With a critical survey of the tumours of the urachus. Br J Surg 18:422, 1931

6. Blichert-Toft M, Koch F, Nielson OV: Anatomic variants of the urachus related to clinical appearance and surgical treatment of urachal lesions. Surg Gynecol Obstet 137:51, 1973

7. Nadjmi B, Whitehead ED, McKiel CF Jr, et al: Carcinoma of the urachus: Report of two cases and a review of the literature. J Urol 100:738, 1968

8. Peterson RO: Urachus. p. 288. In Peterson R, Stein B (eds): Urologic Pathology. JB Lippincott, Philadelphia, 1986

9. Spataro RF, Davis RS, McLachlan MSF, et al: Urachal abnormalities in the adult. Radiology 149:659, 1983

10. Thomas AJ, Pollack MS, Libshitz HI: Urachal carcinoma: Evaluation with computed tomography. Urol Radiol 8:194, 1986

11. Mekras GD, Block NL, Carrion HM, Ishikoff M: Urachal carcinoma: Diagnosis by computerized axial tomography. J Urol 123:275, 1980

12. Sarno RC, Klauber G, Carter BL: Computer assisted tomography of urachal abnormalities. J Comput Assist Tomogr 7:674, 1983

13. Kwok-Liu JP, Zikman JM, Cockshott WP: Carcinoma of the urachus: The role of computed tomography. Radiology 137:731, 1980

14. Ghazizadeh M, Yamamoto S, Kurokawa K: CT scan in the diagnosis of urachal carcinoma. Urol Int 37:358, 1982

15. Zagoria RJ, Higgins WJ, King GT, Williams CD: Elderly man with hematuria and a pelvic mass. Invest Radiol 22:424, 1987

16. Rao BK, Scanlon KA, Hinke ML: Abdominal case of the day. AJR 146:1074, 1986

17. Baumgartner BR, Frederick HM, Austin HM: Adenocarcinoma of the urachus with vesicoenteric fistula. Urol Radiol 6:55, 1984

18. Brick SH, Friedman AC, Pollack HM, et al: Urachal carcinoma: CT findings. Radiology 169:377, 1988

19. Narumi Y, Sato T, Kuriyama K, et al: Vesical dome tumors: Significance of extravesical extension on CT. Radiology 169:383, 1988

20. Rosen L, Hoddick WK, Hricak H, Lue TF: Urachal carcinoma. Urol Radiol 7:174, 1985

21. Schnyder P, Candardjis G: Vesicourachal diverticulum: CT diagnosis in two adults. AJR 137:1063, 1981

12 MRI of the Male Genitalia: Testes, Seminal Vesicles, and Urethra

ROBERT MATTREY

High-resolution sonography is the primary imaging modality for the assessment of the testes and scrotum.[1-5] The success of sonography is based on its depiction of scrotal anatomy and disease in any plane, its low cost and accessibility, and its lack of ionizing radiation. MRI provides multiplanar images with sufficient contrast and spatial resolution to evaluate the scrotum[6-10] and, like sonography, is non-ionizing. Since our first reports,[6,7] our experience and that of others has increased,[8-10] with more than 120 cases with a variety of scrotal diseases having been studied at our institution alone. The ability of MRI to characterize scrotal disease, as had been described,[7] has been substantiated with our added experience and that of others.[8,9] While many disease processes have had characteristic appearances, the exact specificity of MRI is not yet clear. In a report in which 14 tumors were imaged by both sonography and MRI, sonography missed four, whereas MRI failed to miss a single lesion.[10] The ability of MRI to display normal intrascrotal anatomy with specificity, to include on the same image the right and left hemiscrotum and the inguinal region, and to do so with high contrast makes the interpretation of MRI studies less subjective than sonograms. MRI has changed the sonographic diagnosis of testicular disease from normal to cancer in 4 of 23 (17 percent) subjects,[10] and from cancer to benign disease in nearly 6 percent of our cases (data not yet published). The proven efficacy of sonography built over several years of experience has slowed the advance of this new application to truly assess its impact on patient care. The key to the success of MRI is to reduce cost, which could be achieved by shorter examination time, and to improve accessibility. At our institution, we have been able to decrease examination time to less than 30 minutes in most patients without compromising diagnostic quality, and have reduced the charge to $500, which is 1.8 times that of scrotal sonography. It seems inevitable, given its sensitivity and convincing display of disease to the referring physician that MRI will become the imaging modality of choice.

MRI is both sensitive and specific in the assessment of seminal vesicle invasion by prostate cancer. In that setting, MRI can not only assess all the parameters depicted by CT, but can also assess signal behavior. Furthermore, the multiplanar capability of MRI adds to its ability to evaluate this anatomically complex region.

This chapter is intended to describe the imaging techniques found to be most optimal, present the normal appearance of these structures on MRI, and demonstrate some common pathologic conditions.

TESTES

Imaging Technique

Patient Positioning and Preparation

The patient is positioned supine on the scanning table, feet first, and the scrotum elevated by placing a wedge between the thighs. The penis is angled to the side and the whole region draped. A 12.5-cm standard equipment circular surface coil is centered over the scrotum and placed horizontally on a 1-cm standoff. The entire area is then wrapped with a 14-inch strap that is attached to the table to minimize patient motion. In infants, the standard 9-cm circular coil is used in lieu of the 12.5-cm coil.

Pulsing Sequence

Imaging is done in the sagittal and coronal planes. The sagittal series is T_1-weighted (TR 600, TE 20 ms). It is acquired with a 256 × 128 matrix, 20-cm field of view, and two excitations requiring 2.5 minutes to acquire. It provides T_1 contrast for tissue characterization and serves as a localizer to plan the longer and most important T_2-weighted coronal sequence.[6,7] The coronal series covers from the posterior aspect of the scrotum to the anterior aspect of the external inguinal ring. It is obtained with a field of view of 16 cm and slice thickness of 3 mm, with 1.5-mm interslice gap to ensure proper T_2 weighting. Thinner interslice gaps produce cross-talk, increasing T_1 contrast, which is undesirable. This sequence is acquired with a TR of 2,000 and a TE of 20 and 70 ms. The data-acquisition matrix of 256 × 256 obtained with two excitations results in an imaging time of 17.5 minutes. To shorten examination time, we have found that a 256 × 192 matrix, which was recently added to our system, provides sufficient resolution and decreases imaging time to 12.8 minutes. The sagittal T_1-weighted and coronal T_2-weighted series are sufficient for better than 80 percent of cases. Axial T_2-weighted series are reserved for patients with complex findings or those with a suspected mass whose coronal series was normal.

Normal Anatomy

The normal testis on MRI is sharply demarcated and has homogeneous signal intensity slightly brighter than water and darker than fat on T_1-weighted images, becoming equal to or slightly brighter than water, but darker than fat on hydrogen density-weighted images (Fig. 12-1). Testes become equal to or slightly darker than water but brighter than fat on T_2-weighted images (Fig. 12-1). The intensity of the testis on T_2-weighted images is contrasted with the fluid frequently present between the layers of the tunica vaginalis, allowing the assessment of its signal behavior.

The testis is completely surrounded by the tunica albuginea, a layer of dense fibrous tissue that is thin and of low signal intensity (Fig. 12-1). The tunica albugenia can adopt a slightly brighter signal due to partial volume when the slice plane is oblique to the testicular surface. The tunica vaginalis, an extension of peritoneum, is fused to the tunica albuginea except along the "bare area" of the testis, which becomes highlighted by hydrocele (Fig. 12-2). Along the bare area, the tunica albuginea invaginates the testis to produce the mediastinum testis, which is of lower signal than testis and is 2 to 3 cm in length (Fig. 12-2). Intrinsic testicular signal, although homogeneous, in some patients displays internal texture outlining lobules and rete testes (Fig. 12-2). Intratesticular vessels are infrequently seen in normal testes.

On proton density-weighted images, the epididymis is inhomogeneous with intermediate intensity less than or equal to the signal of normal testicular tissue. On T_2-weighted images, the normal epididymis is moderately less intense than normal testis (Figs. 12-1 and 12-2). The head, body, and tail of the normal epididymis can be recognized but are best delineated when highlighted by fluid.

The outer parietal and inner visceral layers of the tunica vaginalis are frequently separated by a small amount of fluid (Fig. 12-1). On T_2-weighted images and in the presence of hydrocele, the fluid completely surrounds the testes, except along the bare area (Fig. 12-2). The scrotal sac structures, such as fat and dartos muscle, can at times be seen (Fig. 12-1); however, most commonly the scrotal sac assumes a black signal on T_2-weighting (Fig. 12-2).

The spermatic cord is seen in all cases. Tortuous tubular structures of low signal intensity located at the posterior-superior aspect of the scrotal sac represent the pampiniform plexus (see Figs. 12-13 and 12-20). Serpiginous high signal intensity areas within the cord on hydrogen density and T_2-weighted images represent phase shift from slow blood flow in the cord vessels as well as chemical shift artifact (Fig. 12-1). Because of the cremasteric reflex, mild tortuosity of the cord is acceptable (Fig. 12-1). The deferent duct can be seen in some patients. When seen it is a smooth undulating tubular structure similar in signal intensity to that of testis (Fig. 12-3). It is not clear whether only ectatic ducts are seen, since the deferent duct is not visualized in most patients. It is also possible that this tubular structure represents a dilated vein with stagnant blood. Further experience and clinical correlation are required to resolve these questions.

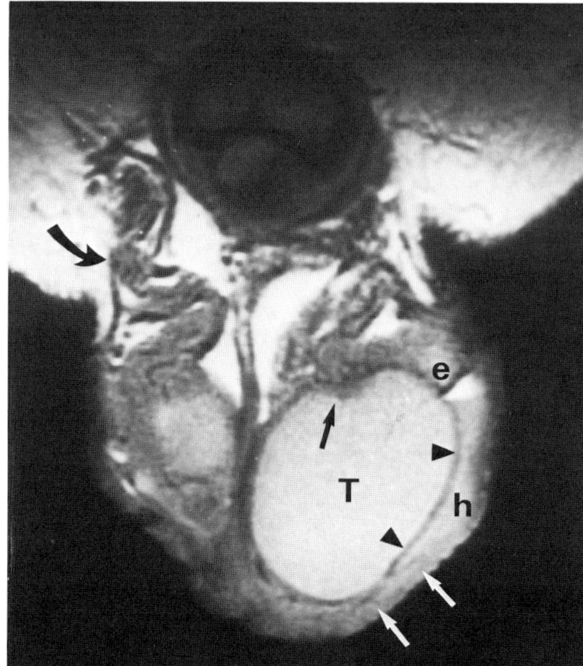

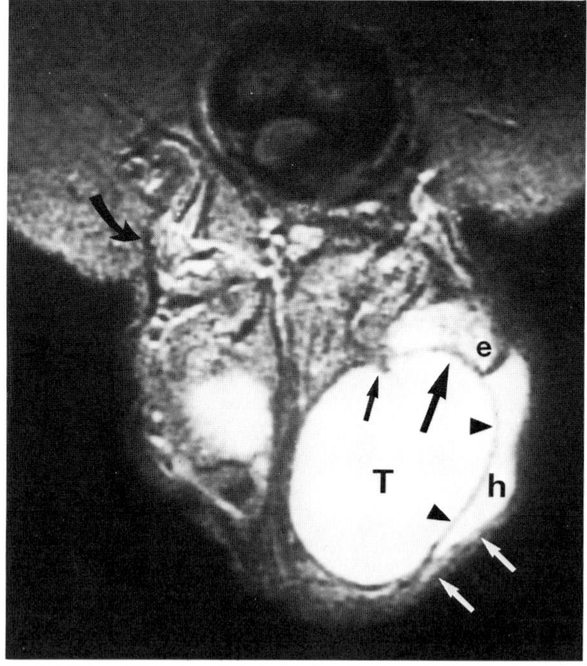

FIG. 12-1. Normal testis (T), epididymis (e), tunica albuginea (arrowheads), and mediastinum testis (black arrow), shown in the coronal plane on (A) hydrogen density-weighted and (B) T_2-weighted images. A small amount of fluid between the tunical layers (hydrocele, h), shown best on the T_2-weighted image, outlines the epididymal head (e). Note the accordion-shaped spermatic cord (curved arrow) entering the base of the right hemiscrotum. Also note the dark signal of the dartos muscle, seen as a black line in the scrotal wall with T_2 weighting (white arrows). (From Baker et al.,[6] with permission.)

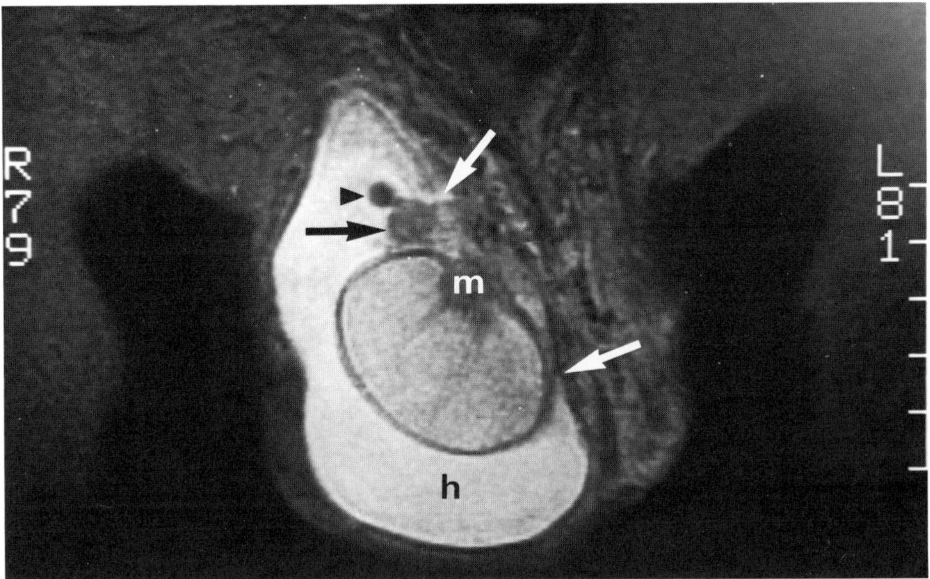

FIG. 12-2.   Acute simple hydrocele (h) is shown on a T_2-weighted image. Note that the signal of hydrocele is consistent with that of water, intermediate on hydrogen density (not shown), and bright on T_2 weighting. This sympathetic hydrocele is thought to be due to torsion of the epididymal appendix (arrowhead), shown to be attached to the normal epididymis (black arrow) and to be hemorrhagic. It was bright on T_1 weighting (not shown) and is dark on T_2 weighting. In this example, the lobular septa can be seen emanating from the mediastinum testes (m). Note the presence of a sizable hydrocele, and the demonstration of the bare area of the testis, the edges of which are marked by white arrows. (From Baker et al.,[7] with permission.)

Pathology

The homogeneous high signal intensity of the normal testes on T_2-weighted images provides an excellent background for visualizing intratesticular pathology. Except for old hematoma, all intratesticular pathology has been less intense than normal testicular tissue on T_2-weighted images.

Neoplasms

General Comments.   In our studies, all tumors were of inhomogeneous signal intensity consistently equal to or lower than that of normal testis on hydrogen-density images and moderately lower on T_2-weighted images. Extension of mass into extratesticular locations such as epididymis or cord was clearly shown.[7] While MRI was shown to stage incorrectly 4 of 11 cases and sonography 6 of 11,[10] this seeming handicap is not important preoperatively, since testicular cancer, regardless of the stage of disease, requires orchiectomy for

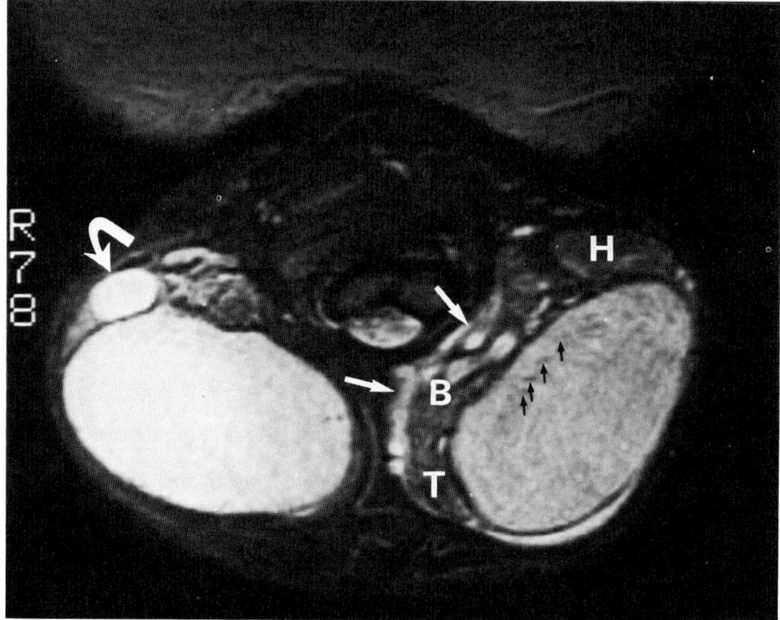

FIG. 12-3.   Coronal T$_2$-weighted image shows a prominent serpentine structure in the body of the epididymis (white arrows). Its signal was similar to testis on all sequences (not shown). This is presumed to represent the vas deferens as it courses towards the lower pole of the testis. It could, however, also represent a dilated vein with stagnant blood. Note that the entire epididymis can be seen: head (H), body (B), and tail (T). Also note the clear delineation of testis from epididymis by the dark tunica albuginea. Small linear dark signals (small arrows) within the testis are interlobular septa converging toward the mediastinum, seen on the following slice (not shown). Also note the presence of an epididymal cyst (curved arrow) on the right. Since it was dark on hydrogen density (not shown), its signal behaved like that of water. (From Mattrey and Trambert,[63] with permission.)

pathologic staging. The only local extension of concern preoperatively is to the scrotal wall. This degree of invasion is rare and by its nature may be easily assessed clinically and by imaging.

Cancer has typically left a rim of normal testicular tissue, even when large.[11] Of the more than 25 cancers reported in the literature,[7–10] and an additional 13 at our institution,[11] primary cancers totally replaced normal testicular tissue in only one patient with Leydig cell tumor.[10] It is possible in infiltrative disorders (lymphoma/leukemia) for the testis to become totally replaced.[10] In such instances, the signal of the affected testis can be compared with the contralateral testis or surrounding structures and hydrocele. While MRI has not missed any lesion seen sonographically and detected all 14 cancers, including the four missed by sonography,[10] it is not clear what would be its ultimate sensitivity and specificity and the minimum consistently detectable lesion size. Because of the lengthy imaging time and the continuous contraction of the dartos muscle, causing testicular motion, partial volume may obscure small lesions. The smallest lesion detected by MRI prospectively and proven surgically was a 3-mm germ cell tumor (Fig. 12-4). Any study compromised by motion that was aimed at detecting testicular neoplasm should be repeated if no lesions are found. On the other hand, when clear depiction of intratesticular morphology is achieved, it should be regarded as evidence of sufficient quality to negate the presence of disease (Fig. 12-2).

Testicular neoplasms can be primary or metastatic and frequently afflict males under 10 years of age, between 20 and 40 years, and then over 60. They have peak incidence and are the most common solid tumors between the ages of 20 and 34. Primary neoplasms are grouped into germ cell and stromal tumors, accounting for 95 percent of all testicular lesions. Germ cell tumors are in turn grouped into seminomatous and nonseminomatous lesions, accounting for 40 percent and 50 percent, respectively.[12] Seminomatous and nonseminomatous elements can infrequently be mixed. When mixed, the lesion is regarded and treated as a nonseminomatous tumor. Germ cell tumors of yolk sac origin are the predominant lesions of infancy.[12] Testicular lymphoma is the most common testicular neoplasm affecting the testis of men over 50 years of age.[12] Testicular tumors are bilateral, either at diagnosis or on follow-up evaluation, in 1 to 3 percent of cases.[13] Therefore, careful examination of the contralateral testis at the time of diagnosis and close follow-up management is mandatory.

The differentiation of seminomatous from nonseminomatous lesions is critical in that patients with pure seminomatous lesions are often radiated and those with nonseminomatous lesions undergo retroperitoneal dissection and chemotherapy. While these modes of therapy remain controversial,[12] they are standard practice in many institutions. Since seminomatous lesions may harbor small islands of nonseminomatous histology in 10 to 15 percent of cases,[12] treatment is planned following detailed histologic analysis of the resected testis. This is particularly true when there is elevation of β-HCG or α-fetoprotein, findings suggesting the presence of nonseminomatous elements. While treatment cannot be determined preoperatively, preoperative differentiation and staging may help in planning patient management.[14] From our data[11] and that presented in the literature to date,[8-10] it appears that MRI may offer such differentiation.

Germ Cell Tumors.   Seminomatous lesions are sheets of cells intermixed with fibrous strands presenting a homogeneous histologic pattern. The MRI appearance of this tumor type, like its histology, has been consistent. Their signal is mildly inhomogeneous. Their intensity is lower than normal testicular tissue or hydrocele fluid on T_2-weighted images (Fig. 12-5). At times they contain well-defined regions of low signal thought to be due to increased fibrosis.[11] While atypical, some seminomatous lesions may bleed internally, resulting in a focus of different signal dependent on the age of the bleed. This was seen in one of six seminomas.[11] A single focus of higher signal should be suspected as being hemorrhage or necrosis rather than a focus of nonseminomatous

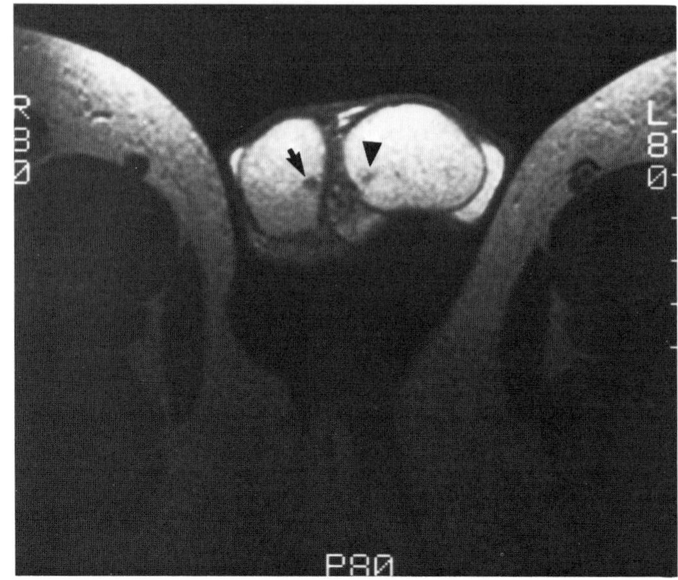

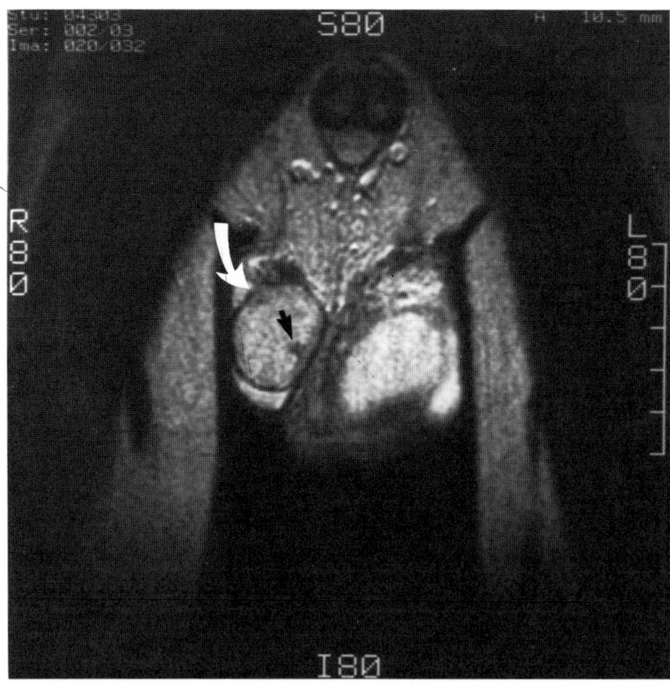

FIG. 12-4.   (A) Transaxial and (B) coronal T_2-weighted images show a small 3-mm focus (black arrow) in the right testis. This lesion was an embryonal cell tumor with hemorrhage at pathology. The left (arrowhead, Fig. A) and right (curved arrow, Fig. B) mediastinum testis can also be seen. This lesion was too small to allow for proper characterization.

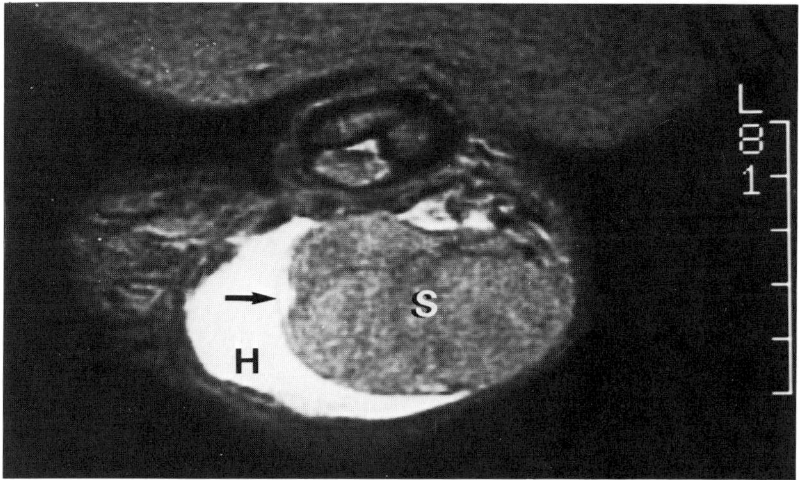

FIG. 12-5.   Left testicular seminoma (S) is mildly inhomogeneous on a T_2-weighted image and of markedly lower signal than the remaining normal testicular tissue (arrow) and hydrocele (H).

elements, since the latter, when mixed with seminomatous tissue, presents as multiple microscopic foci. A small rim of normal testicular tissue was always visible and was clearly demarcated from lesion providing contrast[11] (Fig. 12-5).

Lumped in the category of nonseminomatous lesions and listed in order of occurrence are teratocarcinomas, embryonal cell, teratomas, and choriocarciomas. Nearly 40 percent of nonseminomatous lesions are a mixture of two or three elements. They all carry similar prognosis and are treated in a similar fashion. Therefore, preoperative distinction of the cell type is not necessary. These lesions present heterogeneous histology owing to their mixed cellularity, their attempt at tubular formation, the mixed elements that may be contained in teratomatous lesions, and their high propensity to invade vessels causing internal hemorrhage and necrosis. These tumors are markedly heterogeneous on MRI, which represents their most distinctive feature when compared with seminomatous lesions.[11] Over a background that is isointense or slightly brighter than normal testis on T_2-weighted images, multiple areas of high and low signal intensities on both hydrogen density and T_2-weighted images are seen. These areas represent hemorrhage of various ages within the mass so characteristic of these lesions (Fig. 12-6). In studies at our institution, the degree of heterogeneity and the overall signal intensity were much greater than was seen with seminoma. A band of low signal intensity was visible circumscribing the mass in most cases. This was shown histologically to represent the fibrous tumor capsule, also typical for these lesions. Remaining normal testicular tissue was easily differentiated from tumor by its homogeneous and characteristic intensity, even when the lesion was very large.[11]

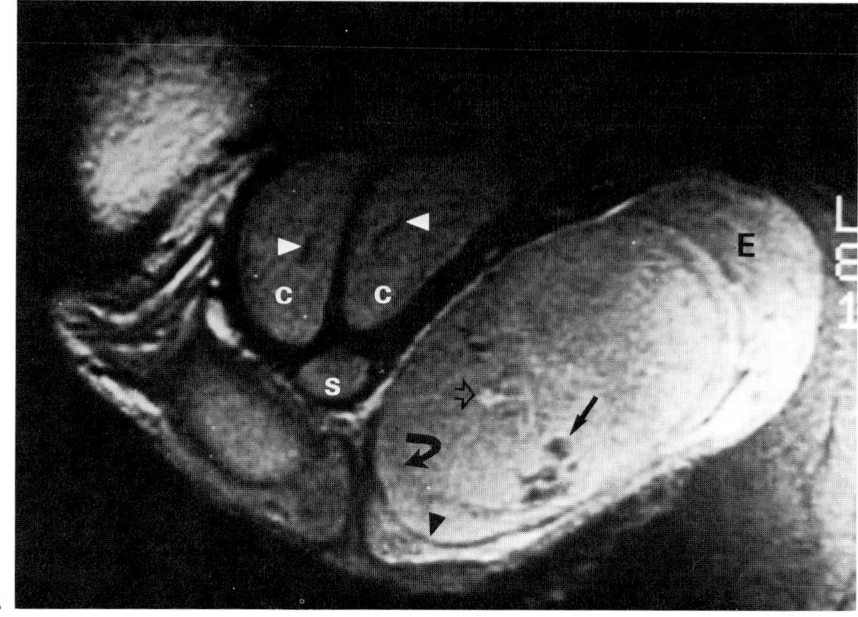

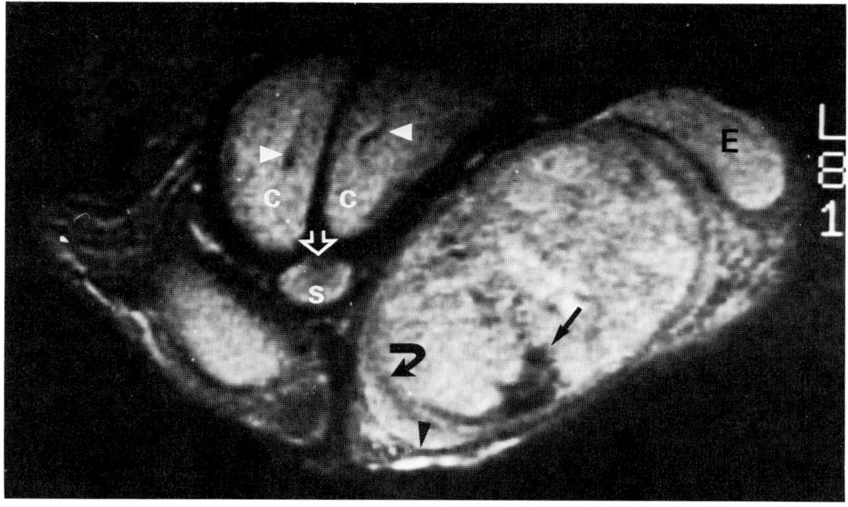

FIG. 12-6. Coronal views of mixed nonseminomatous tumor-embryonal cell and cho-riocarcinoma. Note the presence of normal testicular tissue between the tunica albugenia (black arrowhead) and pseudocapsule of tumor (curved arrow), shown on (A) hydrogen density-weighted and (B) T_2-weighted images, proven pathologically. Note region of high signal (Fig. A, small open arrow) and another region of dark signal on hydrogen density weighting (Fig. A, arrow). The dark region becomes darker with T_2-weighting (Fig. B, arrow). These are areas of hemorrhage of different ages characteristic of this tumor type. Also note incidental finding of a spermatocele in the head of the left epididymis (E). Normal penile anatomy is well seen in this patient in oblique section. The penis is composed of two corpora cavernosa (c) and one corpora spongiosa (s), through which courses the urethra, better seen on T_2-weighting (Fig. B, large open arrow). The corpora cavernosa is surrounded by a thick dark band, the tunica albuginea of the penis. Well seen in this patient are the cavernosal arteries (white arrowheads) with shift artifact from flow seen best as a white companion line to the left of the left cavernosal artery on T_2-weighting. (From Baker et al.,[6] with permission.)

Stromal Tumors.   Stromal tumors account for nearly 5 percent of all primary testicular tumors, with peak incidence between 20 and 60 years of age. They are well circumscribed and rarely exhibit hemorrhage or necrosis. Since these lesions generally produce hormones, prepubertal boys can present with precocious puberty and adults with gynecomastia. The cell types include Leydig and Sertoli cells. These lesions are malignant in 10 percent of cases. Malignancy is suspected histologically when lesions are large, necrotic, infiltrative, or invading blood vessels and is clearly established when there are metastases. One could hypothesize that given their homogeneous histology and lack of hemorrhage and necrosis their appearance on MRI would mimic that of seminomatous lesions.[7,10] However, when malignant, the hemorrhage and necrosis would change their appearance to mimic nonseminomatous lesions.

Two published proven cases of Leydig cell tumor show the mass on T_2-weighted images to be of moderately darker signal intensity than normal testis.[7,10] One was small and well defined[7] (Fig. 12-7), and the other totally infiltrated the testis in a prepubertal boy.[10] It is not yet clear whether MRI will be able to distinguish stromal tumors from germ cell lesions.

Other Tumors.   Lymphomatous or leukemic infiltration of the testis is common. Lymphoma accounts for nearly 5 percent of all testicular neoplasms and

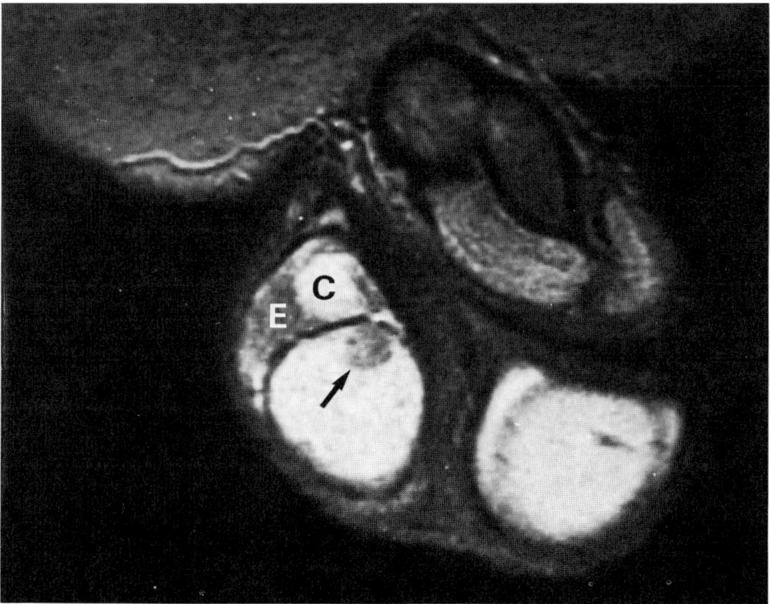

FIG. 12-7.   Mildly inhomogeneous well-marginated testicular tumor (arrow), which proved histologically to be a Leydig cell tumor, that was better seen on the T_2-weighted image. Epididymal cyst (C) within the normal epididymal head (E) has MRI characteristics similar to water. It was dark on hydrogen density (not shown). (From Baker et al.,[7] with permission.)

is the most common testicular lesion in men over 50 years of age.[12] It may be primary in the testis, or the manifestation of occult disease seated elsewhere, or a late manifestation of disseminated disease. The majority are infiltrative and may extend into or originate in the epididymis. The major cell type is histiocytic lymphoma.

The testis, like the central nervous system (CNS), may be the site of relapse of leukemia in children. A blood-testis barrier exists that prevents chemotherapeutics from eradicating its disease. While ultrasound can detect leukemic infiltration,[15] it has poor sensitivity.[10] While the sensitivity of MRI in detecting leukemic infiltration is not yet clearly defined, four cases have been detected by MRI that were missed by sonography.[10] Leukemia in these cases affected the entire testis diffusely and decreased its signal.[10]

Inflammation

Epididymitis. Epididymitis is the most common intrascrotal infection. It may be diffuse or focal and is frequently secondary to prostatitis. Most cases of epididymitis are treated conservatively. Surgery is reserved for complications such as abscess formation. Therefore, diagnostic follow-up in patients with poor response to therapy may be warranted. Testicular infarction secondary to epididymitis has also been reported.[16]

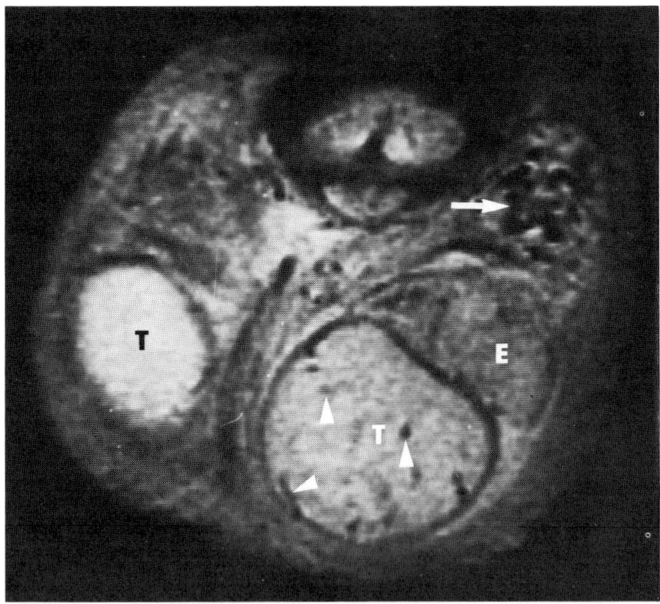

FIG. 12-8. Patient with acute epididymitis shown on a T_2-weighted image in the coronal plane. Testis (T) is of slightly lower signal than the contralateral side and is hypervascular (arrowheads). The epididymis (E) is enlarged and assumes a higher signal on T_2-weighting than is normally observed. Note the hypervascularity in the cord typical of this condition (arrow). (From Trambert et al.,[22] with permission.)

Patients with clinical evidence of epididymitis at our institution consistently showed epididymal enlargement (Figs. 12-8 to 12-11). The epididymis, which is normally of lower signal intensity than testis on T_2-weighted images, maintained a higher signal in patients with acute epididymitis, nearly equal to that of testis (Fig. 12-8). Acute epididymitis, particularly when severe, may be associated with hemorrhage within the epididymis (Fig. 12-9) and hypervascularity (Figs. 12-8 and 12-10), thickening, and swelling of the spermatic cord (Fig. 12-10). While the degree of hypervascularity has been variable, it has been consistently present in all patients. Hypervascularity is seen as multiple serpiginous vessels with signal void due to high flow (Figs. 12-8 and 12-10). This is in contradistinction to normal vessels, which are usually thinner and lack the very dark signal because of their slower flow (Fig. 12-1). Hypervascularity of the testis associated with epididymitis has also been observed in some patients (Fig. 12-8). Sympathetic hydrocele was present in most patients and manifested signals identical with those of water. When sufficiently large, it demonstrated the bare area (Fig. 12-10), excluding testicular torsion, the most common differential diagnostic question. Inguinal adenopathy is frequent (Fig. 12-10) but is nonspecific.

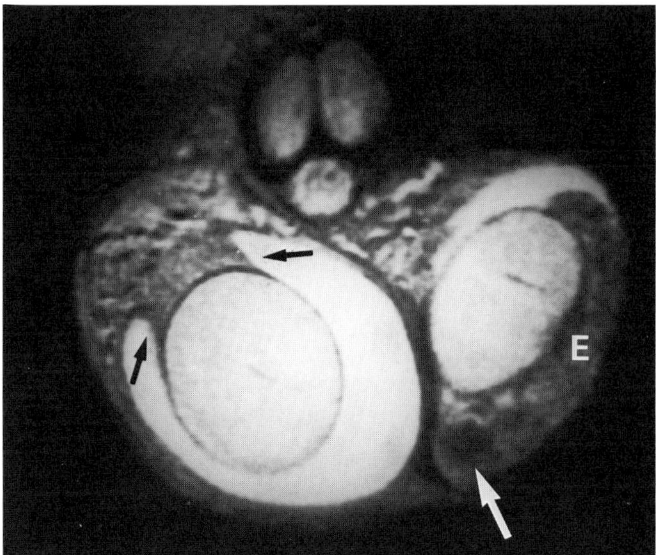

FIG. 12-9.   Diffuse chronic epididymitis involving the entire epididymis on the left and shown in the coronal plane on a T_2-weighted image. Note diffuse enlargement of the entire epididymis (E) with possible hemorrhage in the tail (white arrow). The epididymal tail was intermediate in signal on hydrogen density (not shown). Mild ipsilateral and moderate contralateral hydroceles are present. The right hydrocele outlines the bare area in its transverse direction, which covers nearly 25 percent of the testicular circumference in this patient. Also note prominent epididymal body on the right (black arrows) presumed to be from chronic epididymitis. (From Mattrey and Trambert,[63] with permission.)

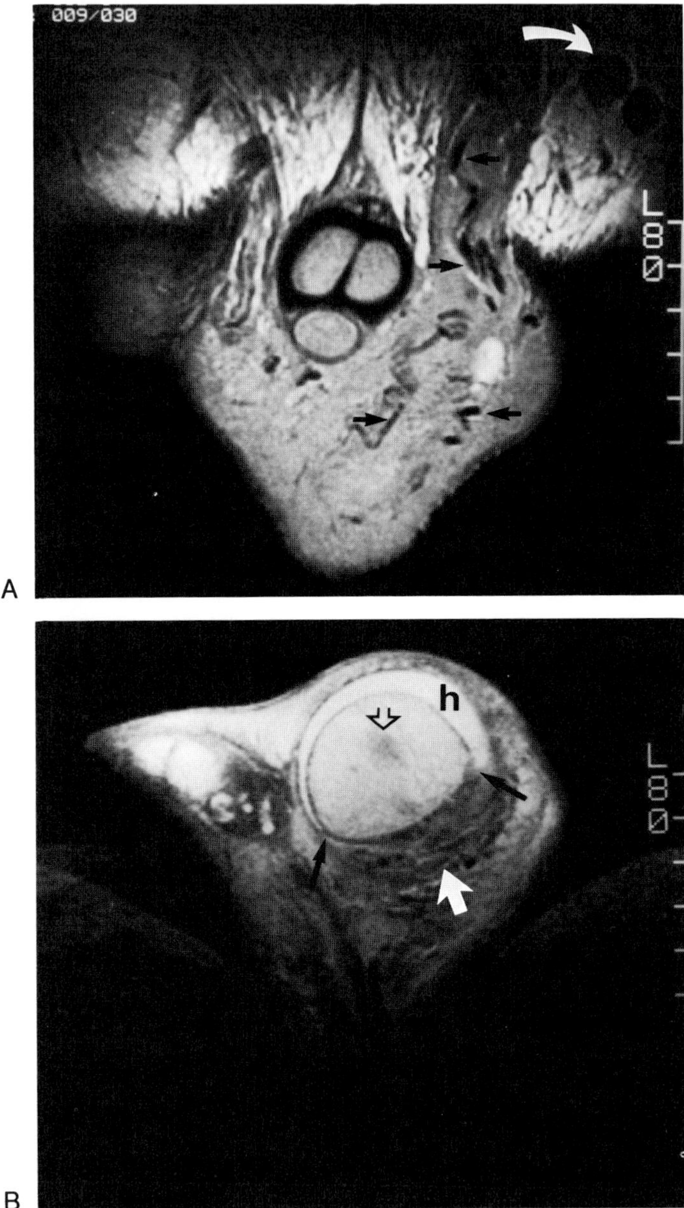

FIG. 12-10.   Acute scrotal pain due to epididymitis with associated orchitis. (A) Coronal hydrogen density-weighted image shows hypervascular (arrows) and thickened extra- and intrascrotal spermatic cord. It also shows inguinal adenopathy (curved arrow). (B) T_2-weighted image shows prominence of the epididymal body (white arrow) and a mild hydrocele (h) that outlines the bare area of the testis, the edges of which are marked by black arrows, excluding torsion. Note the small poorly defined focus of low signal in the testis (open arrow) compatible with infection. (From Trambert et al.,[22] with permission.)

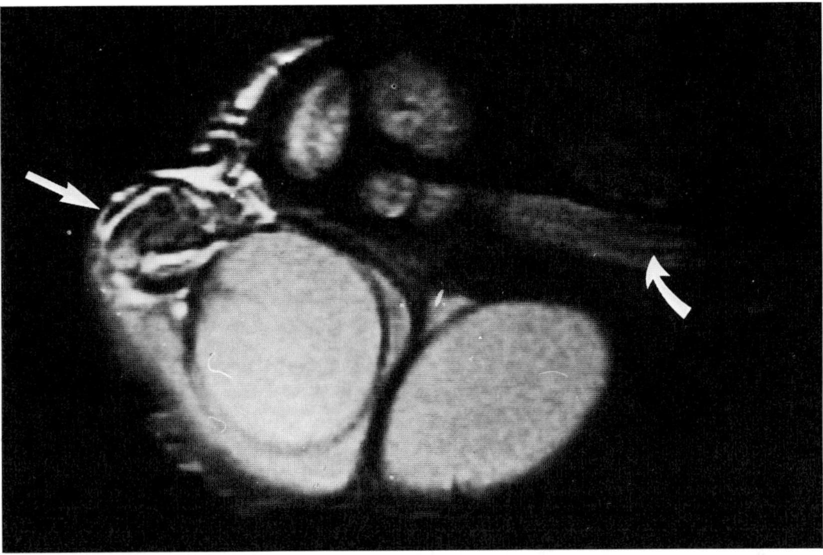

FIG. 12-11.   Focal chronic epididymitis involving the head of the right epididymis shown on a T_2-weighted image. Note the enlarged dark epididymis (arrow). Patient known to have chronic epididymitis now presents with acute exacerbation. There is mild reactive ipsilateral hydrocele. Oblique view of the penis shows urethra (curved arrow) traveling through corpora spongiosa. (From Baker et al.,[6] with permission.)

In chronic epididymitis, the epididymis was enlarged in a focal (Fig. 12-11) or diffuse manner (Fig. 12-9) and became darker than normal on T_2-weighted images. In the setting of chronic epididymitis, acute exacerbation may not affect the signal (Fig. 12-9).

Orchitis.   Orchitis is frequently the sequel of epididymitis. Pure orchitis without epididymitis suggests a viral etiology. When orchitis accompanies epididymitis, treatment is extended over a longer period of time due to the blood-testis barrier. Since orchitis, even when appropriately treated, can develop into an abscess (Fig. 12-12), follow-up evaluation is necessary in cases with poor response to therapy. The focus of infection within the testis is of lower signal than testis (Fig. 12-10), is less sharply demarcated than tumor, and is at times heterogeneous in signal.[7]

Tuberculous orchitis is also associated with tuberculous epididymitis. We have imaged three such patients with proven tuberculous scrotal infection. All had epididymal and testicular involvement. Testicular changes were patchy, poorly marginated areas of slightly lower signal than testis. Epididymal changes were less severe than bacterial epididymitis, and the degree of hypervascularity was less prominent. In one patient with surgically proven diffuse chronic tuberculous orchitis missed on sonography, the testis was dif-

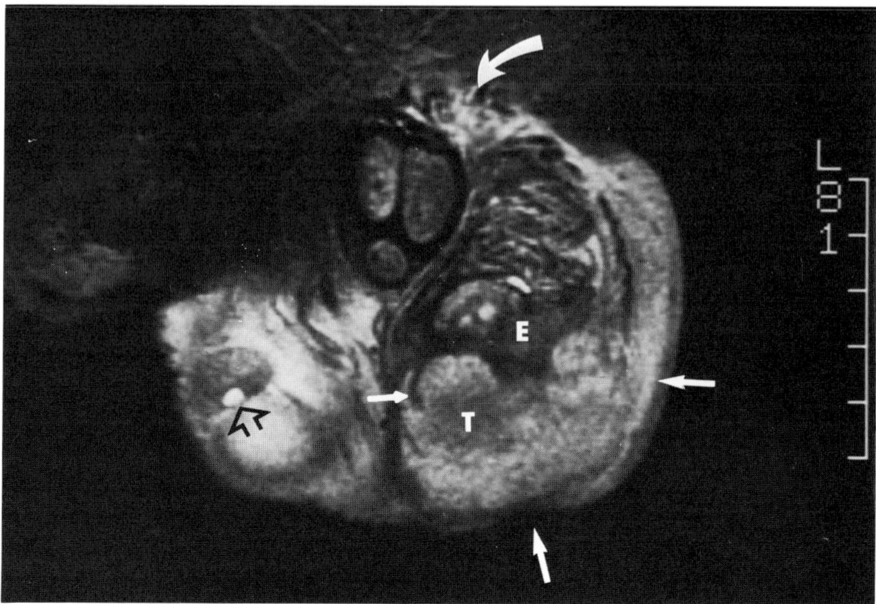

FIG. 12-12. T_2-weighted image shows complete destruction of the testis (T) and loss of intrascrotal anatomic detail (arrows) in a patient with scrotal abscess secondary to epididymo-orchitis (E, epididymis). Note the cephalic extension of scrotal wall involvement and the spread of edema to the base of the penis (curved arrow). Also note a small presumed hemorrhagic cyst (open arrow) in the right epididymis; this cyst was bright on hydrogen density (not shown). (From Mattrey and Trambert,[63] with permission.)

fusely inhomogeneous with low signal intensity on T_2-weighted images but without mass effect (Fig. 12-13).

Trauma

Surgical intervention in scrotal trauma is reserved for patients with testicular rupture or when the intratesticular hematoma is extensive. MRI is well suited to assess both the integrity of the tunica albuginea and the degree of intratesticular hematoma. In this setting, multiple imaging planes may be required to ensure that all surfaces are optimally imaged without partial volume.

Overall, for our patients the traumatized testes were highly inhomogeneous with high and low signal intensity regions compared with normal testicular tissue on both hydrogen density and T_2-weighted images secondary to hemorrhage of different degrees of organization (Fig. 12-14). Hematocele frequently accompanies trauma and assumes signals commensurate with the age of hemorrhage (Fig. 12-14). Intratesticular trauma has caused more linear than spherical changes, decreasing its confusion with mass lesions. Furthermore, associated clinical and scrotal changes with trauma differ from those of tumors.

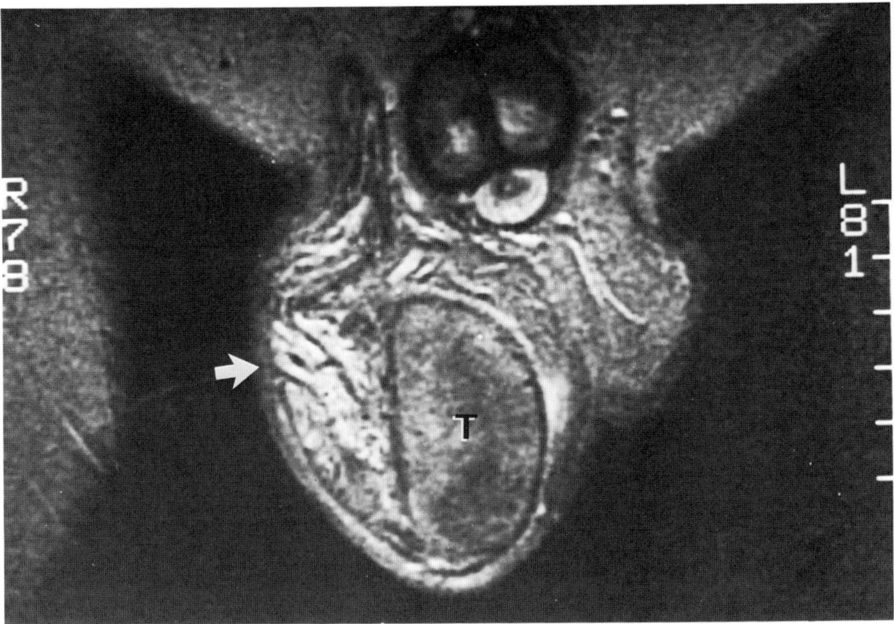

FIG. 12-13.   Chronic tuberculous orchitis shown in the coronal plane on a T_2-weighted image displays a diffuse poorly defined process involving the entire testis (T). Note the prominent cord and pampiniform plexus at the base of the scrotum (arrow) compatible with the palpable varicocele. The left testis had been removed because of a tuberculous infection. (From Baker et al.,[7] with permission.)

Torsion

Intravaginal Spermatic Cord Torsion.   The testis, like other abdominal organs, is retroperitoneal and is covered by the tunica vaginalis, except for the bare area. The bare area extends from the upper to lower pole (Fig. 12-2) and has a variable width nearly one-third that of the testicular circumference (Fig. 12-10). This bare area serves as a passage for support structures and as an anchor attaching the testis to the scrotal wall, preventing the testis from twisting. The tunica vaginalis can, however, undermine the support structures and epididymis to a variable degree and to a point that the bare area could be reduced to a thin stalk. This anomalous condition, called the "bell-clapper" deformity, which could be bilateral in 40 percent of cases,[17] predisposes the testis to twist and strangulate. When the testis makes one or more turns on its stalk, the veins become occluded and the testis swells. When intratesticular pressure exceeds arterial pressure, blood flow ceases, and the testis undergoes hemorrhagic necrosis.

Torsion typically occurs in the teens and 20s, affecting 1 in 4,000 men.[18] If torsion is suspected, immediate surgery is required, since salvage of testicular funciton decreases with time. While nearly all testes can be salvaged if ischemic

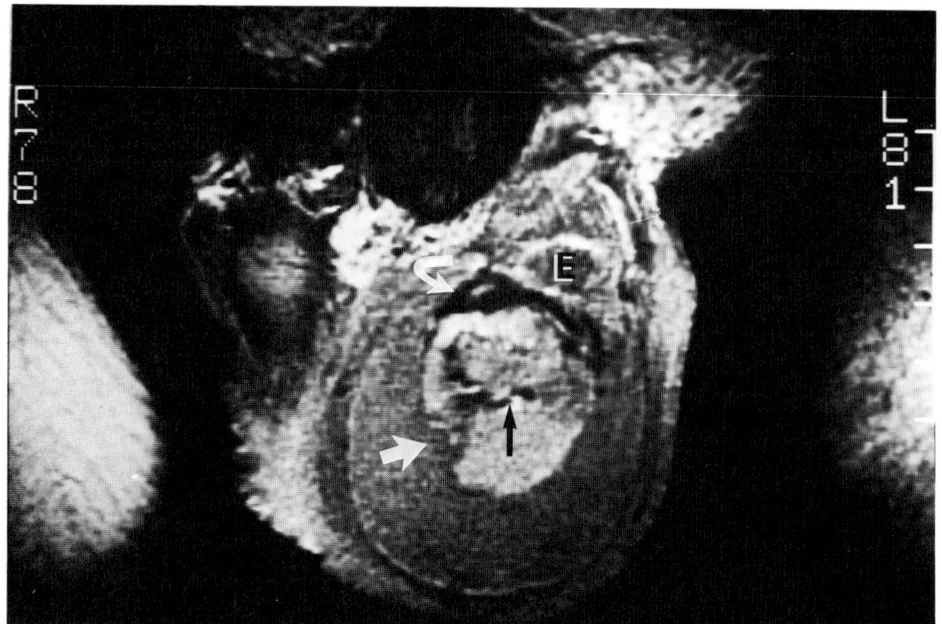

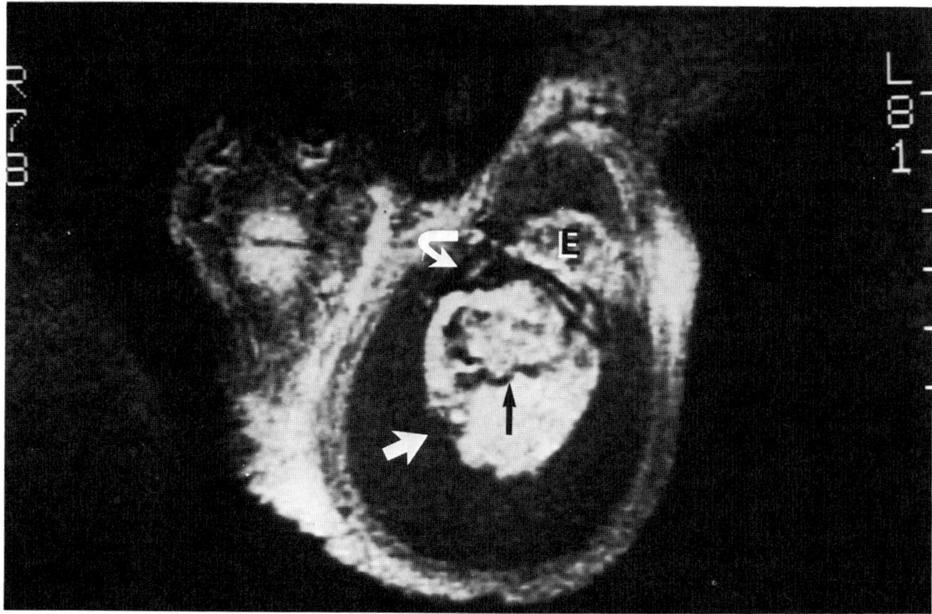

FIG. 12-14. Three-day-old scrotal trauma is shown in the coronal plane on (A) hydrogen density-weighted and (B) T₂-weighted images. Note that the hematoma outlining the tunica along the upper pole of the testis is very dark (curved arrow) and the intratesticular hematoma, although darker than testis, is brighter than upper pole collection (black arrow). The reason for the discrepancy of signals is not clear. The central hemorrhage is incompletely surrounded by a dark band. Given the age of these hematomas (3 days), these cannot represent hemosiderin-filled macrophages. Note that the tunica is interrupted along the medial lower pole (thick white arrow). A hematocele is also present with signals consistent with subacute hemorrhage (intermediate on hydrogen density weighting [Fig. A] and dark on T₂-weighting [Fig. B]). Also note that the epididymis (E) is also enlarged, swollen, and inhomogeneous. (From Baker et al.,[7] with permission.)

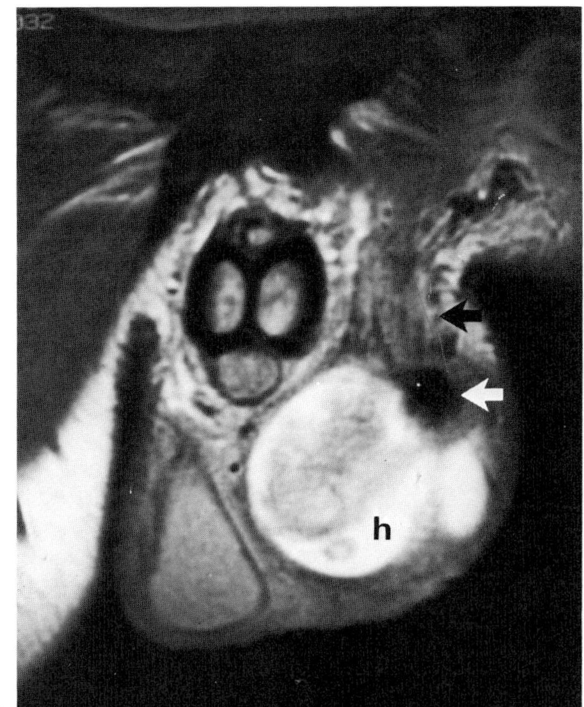

FIG. 12-15.   Five-day old torsion. (A & B) Hydrogen density-weighted coronal images and (C) a T_1-weighted axial image. This case demonstrates the following: (1) torsion knot (Fig. A, thick white arrow), a dark region that represents the point of twist, it is thought to be due to the wringing out of water from the cord at the point of twist; (2) whirlpool pattern (Fig. B, small arrows), representing the twisted facial planes of the cord emanating from the point of twist seen just anterior to Fig. A; (3) the swollen hypovascular cord (Figs. A & B, thick black arrows);

(Figure continues.)

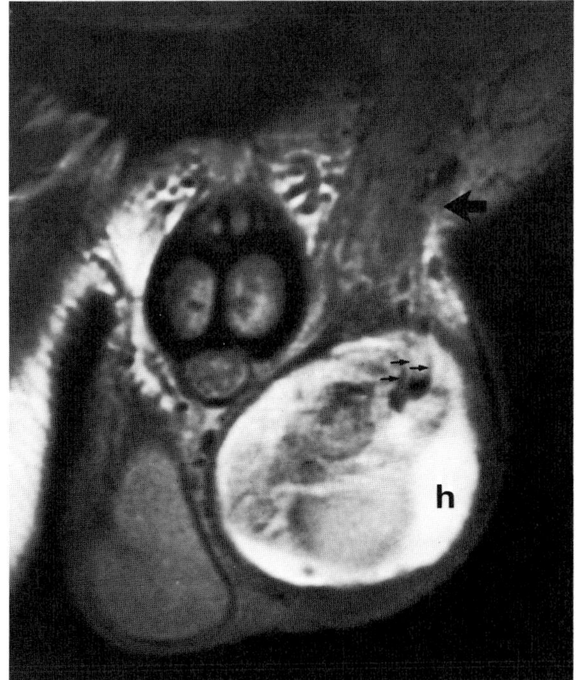

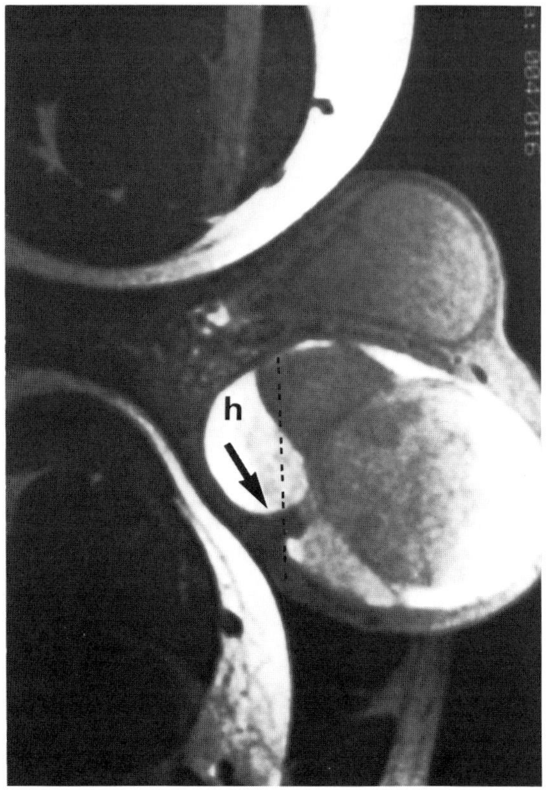

(FIG. 12-15 (*Continued*). (4) the bell-clapper deformity, seen because the hematocele (h) in Fig. C highlights the stalk (arrow), proven surgically, perpendicular to which the images in Figs. A and B were obtained (dashed line is level of image in Fig. A); (5) the hematocele (h), seen as bright fluid on T_1-weighting (Fig. C) and hydrogen density and T_2-weighting (Figs. A & B). (From Trambert et al.,[22] with permission.)

for 5 hours or less, the salvage rate decreases to 20 percent if surgery is done at or beyond 12 hours.[19–21] When patients present in the subacute phase (beyond 24 hours), surgery is still required to remove the torsed testis, stop the pain, and fix the contralateral testis to the scrotum. Epididymitis is the only significant differential problem clinically and with imaging, particularly in the subacute setting when the hyperemic response may hide the avascular testis on nuclear scans. In a recent series, six patients with subacute torsion 5 to 30 days following their event were accurately distinguished from seven patients with epididymitis.[22] Torsion presented with characteristic findings, three of which were specific for torsion.[22]

The first is the appearance of the point of twist itself. The twisted stalk becomes very dark at the point of twist. This is presumably because of the water being squeezed out of the tissues, similar to the wringing of a wet towel (Fig. 12-15). From this dark point emanate several curvilinear dark lines, presumably representing the spiraling facial planes resembling a whirlpool. To best demonstrate the "whirlpool" pattern, the stalk must be imaged perpendicular to its axis. This pattern was clearly seen in five of the six cases. In a rat study, the whirlpool pattern was the most consistent finding that allowed the recognition of all the torsed testis from their sham controls[23] (Fig. 12-16).

The second finding is the appearance of the testis and epididymis. In all

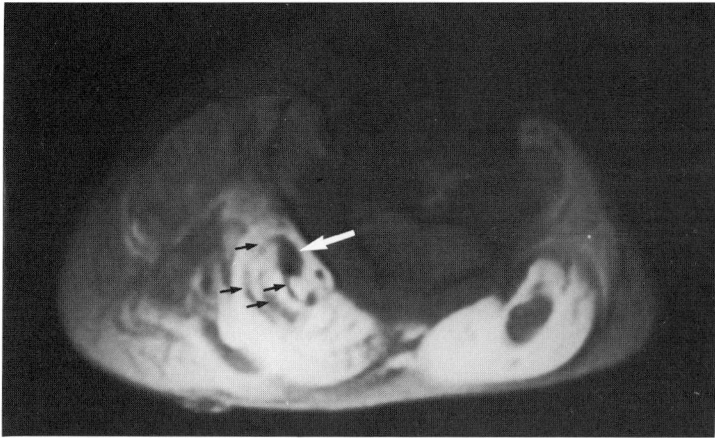

FIG. 12-16.   Torsion knot (white arrow) and whirlpool pattern (small arrows) shown in a rat with surgically induced spermatic cord torsion. Note the similarity with the case shown in Figure 12-15. These two findings allowed the recognition of all torsed testes in the rat study from the normal contralateral side and from sham controls.

cases, the epididymis was markedly thickened with areas of swelling and subacute hemorrhage (Fig. 12-17). The testis in the subacute phase (more than 5 days) was smaller than the contralateral testis. Its signal on T_2-weighted images was diminished and inhomogeneous. The inhomogeneity was due to linear bands of slightly diminished signals separated by thin lines of increased signal emanating from the mediastinum testis possibly representing the affected lobules (Fig. 12-17). In some cases, there was thickening of the tunica albuginea, which became striking 3 weeks from the episode (Fig. 12-18). When the episode was remote in time the testis became small and exceedingly dark both diffusely and homogeneously on T_2-weighted images, probably as a result of the significant accumulation of hemosiderin and fibrosis. The combination of tunical thickening, loss of testicular volume, and darkening of the entire testis is characteristic of old torsion (Fig. 12-18).

The third finding is the appearance of the proximal cord, which was thickened in all cases. All cords had absent or diminished vascularity (Figs. 12-15 and 12-18). This is in contradistinction to the hypervascular cord associated with epididymitis (Figs. 12-8 and 12-10).

Other associated findings that are helpful include a hematocele, which may be seen in torsion (Fig. 12-17) in lieu of a hydrocele, which may be present with epididymitis (Fig. 12-10). When these fluid collections are large, they could demonstrate the bell-clapper deformity (Fig. 12-15) or the testicular bare area (Fig. 12-10), ruling in or out testicular torsion. P-31 MR spectroscopy is currently being studied to identify ischemia after testicular torsion, and may someday, along with MRI, replace the more commonly used ultrasonography and scintigraphy as it becomes more readily available.[23–26]

Extravaginal Torsion.   Extravaginal torsion is a spontaneous event that occurs

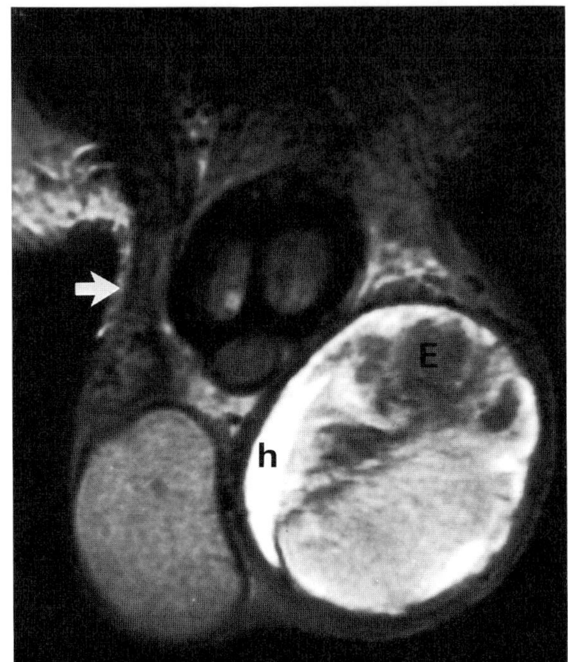

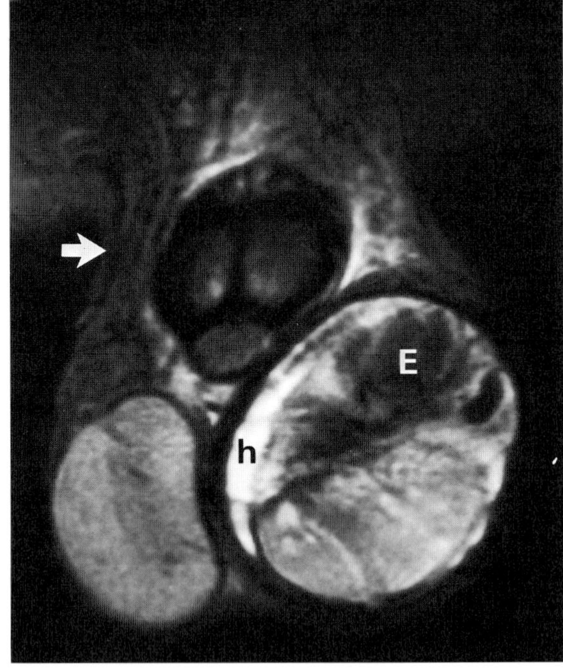

FIG. 12-17. (A) Hydrogen density-weighted and (B) T_2-weighted images of the patient in Figure 12-15 show the epididymal and testicular changes characteristic of torsion. Compare the normal cord (arrow) with the swollen cord seen in Figure 12-15. The enlarged hemorrhagic and swollen epididymis (E) can be seen. The superior and transverse position of the epididymis can be also appreciated. This finding, however, is not specific. Note that intratesticular changes, seen as linear stripes of high and low signal, are oriented in the direction of the interlobular septa emanating from the region of the mediastinum. Also note the hematocele (h). (From Mattrey and Trambert,[63] with permission.)

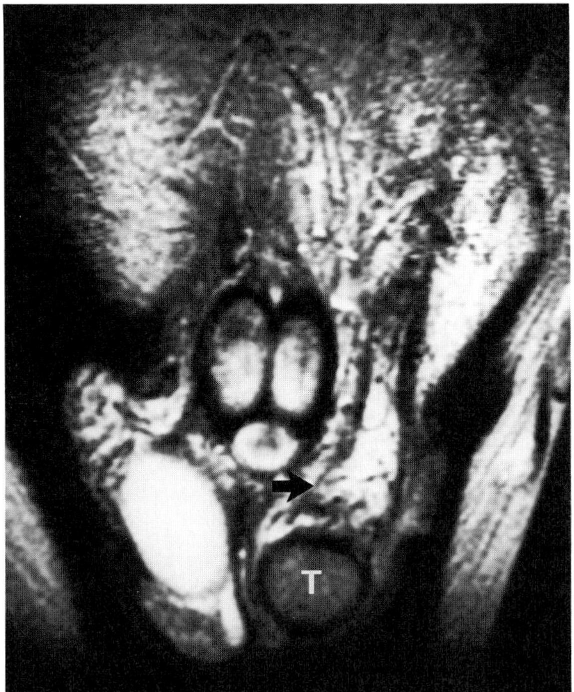

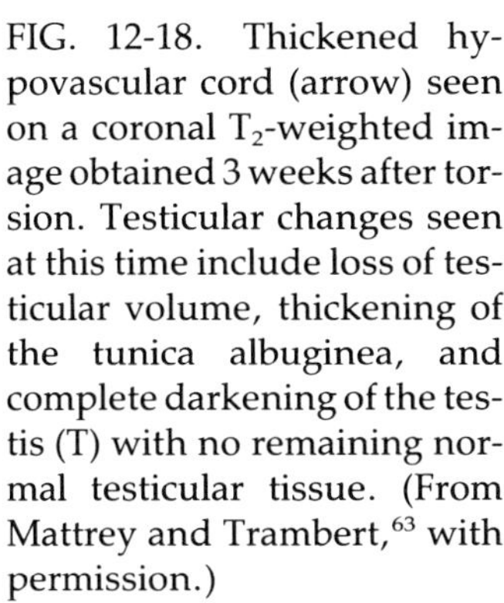

FIG. 12-18. Thickened hypovascular cord (arrow) seen on a coronal T_2-weighted image obtained 3 weeks after torsion. Testicular changes seen at this time include loss of testicular volume, thickening of the tunica albuginea, and complete darkening of the testis (T) with no remaining normal testicular tissue. (From Mattrey and Trambert,[63] with permission.)

perinatally during testicular descent and involves the testis, its support structures, and the vaginal process.[17] The torsed vaginal process in the inguinal or spermatic canal can mimic strangulated intestinal hernia. While the clinical presentation is clear in many cases, at times imaging is required to confirm the diagnosis. This condition is generally not treated surgically, since it is discovered too late to preserve testicular function, and is not associated with developmental anomaly such as the bell-clapper deformity to warrant contralateral orchiopexy.[17]

We have imaged three infants with this condition, all of whom were late in their course. All testes were small, dark, and associated with thickened tunica albuginea, similar to changes seen in chronic torsion in adults (Fig. 12-19). As in the adult, the entire testis was dark without any spared areas. These testes, with time, become a streak of fibrous tissue.

Extratesticular Lesions

Spermatocele. On MRI, patients with spermatoceles studied at our institution were easily identified within the epididymis, with the most frequent site of involvement being the globus major (head). These round, well-circumscribed structures display signal intensity similar to that of water (Figs. 12-3, 12-6, and 12-7). In a minority of cases, they were brighter than water on hydrogen density-weighted images and remained bright on T_2-weighted images (Fig.

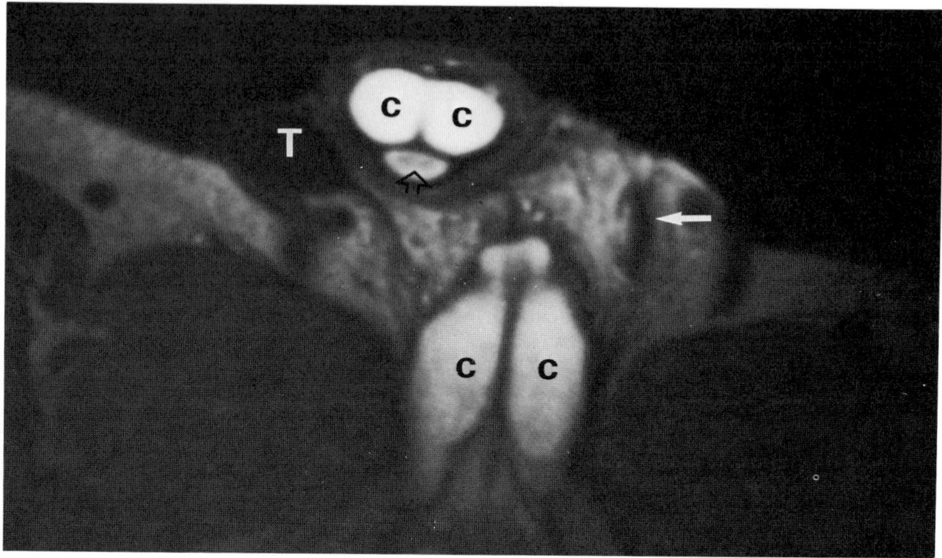

FIG. 12-19.　Axial T_2-weighted image obtained in a 6-month-old infant with neonatal extravaginal torsion at the level of the affected testis (T). Note the loss of testicular volume, the thickened tunica albuginea, and the complete darkening of the testis with no remaining normal testicular tissue, similar to the testis seen in Figure 12-18. Also note that the testis is located in the spermatic canal at the level of the normal contralateral cord (arrow). Also well seen is the penile anatomy. Corpora cavernosa (c) and spongiosa are bright and the urethra (open arrow) is seen within the corpora spongiosa. The lesser signal of the corpora at the base of the penis is due to increased distance from the surface coil. (From Mattrey and Trambert,[63] with permission.)

12-12). We are uncertain as to whether the contents were old blood or high proteinaceous fluid.

Hydrocele.　Simple hydrocele has typical fluid characteristics on MRI that are intermediate on hydrogen density and high on T_2-weighted images relative to fat (Fig. 12-2). While fluid is normally present within the layers of the tunica vaginalis (Fig. 12-1), the assessment of increased volume is subjective. Complicated hydroceles will demonstrate septae and signals characteristic of their content.

Varicocele.　MRI clearly shows the entire spermatic cord from the inguinal ring to the mediastinum testis. Our patients with varicocele had widening of the spermatic canal and prominence of the intrascrotal spermatic cord and/ or pampiniform plexus. The spermatic cord was more heterogeneous, with a greater number of serpiginous structures with increased signal, due to a phase-shift artifact from slow blood flow in these vessels. This was observed on both hydrogen density and T_2-weighted images. An insufficient number of patients have been studied with this condition to ascertain the role of MRI in this

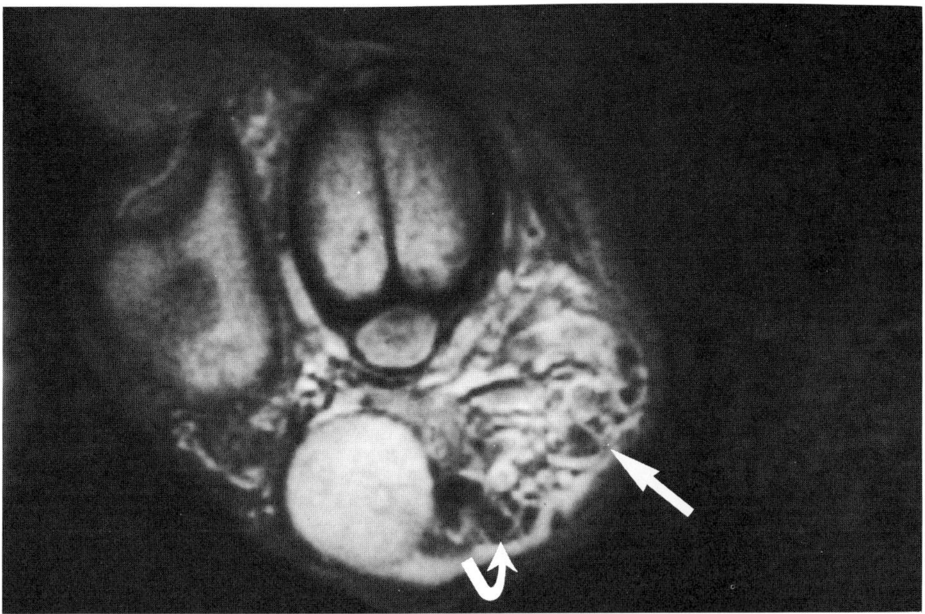

FIG. 12-20.   Left varicocele is seen on a coronal T_2-weighted image (arrow) as a prominent cord and pampiniform plexus at the base of the scrotum. Note mild hypervascularity in the intrascrotal cord (curved arrow) in this patient. (From Mattrey and Trambert,[63] with permission.)

setting. In a prepubertal boy with varicocele, vessels with flow void in the cord as well as prominence of the pampiniform plexus at the base of the scrotum were evident (Fig. 12-20). In a recent study, abdominal compression, similar to that applied during intravenous urography, exaggerated the appearance of vessels in the cord in patients with varicoceles.[27] While clinically palpable varicoceles were easily depicted on MRI, it is not clear whether MRI will be able to diagnose subclinical varicoceles with sufficient accuracy.

Undescended Testis

Cryptorchidism occurs in 2.7 to 6 percent of full-term males, with 0.8 percent prevalence at 1 year of age. Spontaneous descent is unlikely after the first year.[28–30] Because of a significantly increased risk of malignancy[31,32] and impaired spermatogenic function in the contralateral descended testis,[33] many techniques have been developed to aid in the diagnosis and treatment of the cryptorchid testis so as to monitor the testis for neoplasia and diminish the incidence of infertility. An undescended testis may be either intra-abdominal, intracanalicular, ectopic, atrophic, or congenitally absent. Undescended testes may be located anywhere from the renal hilum to the superior scrotum. They may also be found in an ectopic location such as a superficial abdominal wall or perineum. Testes located proximal to the external inguinal ring are usually impalpable, as there may be small or atrophic testes located distal to the external inguinal ring. Neonatal extravaginal torsion results in complete replacement of testicular tissue with scar. If neonatal extravaginal torsion is missed at birth, the patient may present later in life with a nonpalpable undescended testis, but possibly a palpable cord. Such a patient would require surgery for diagnosis. If the diagnosis of testicular atrophy could be reliably made preoperatively, surgery could be avoided or limited to those wanting prosthetic replacement.

The adequate preoperative assessment and localization of the undescended testis is useful since it may obviate surgery, may make a more limited operative procedure possible, or may allow for preoperative planning, particularly with the increased popularity of autotransplantation. Various diagnostic modalities, such as ultrasound,[34,35] CT,[35–37] spermatic venography, and arteriography,[37–39] have been used to localize the cryptorchid testis. These modalities have been accompanied by such disadvantages as invasiveness, technical difficulties, poor sensitivity and/or specificity, and exposure to ionizing radiation. Laparoscopy has been introduced to evaluate the nonpalpable testis prior to exploration.[40] If testicular vessels and vas deferens end blindly in the abdomen, no exploration is required. If tissue is present at the end of the vas deferens, exploration follows. While laparoscopy is 100 percent accurate in localizing the potential location of the testis, and may obviate surgery in some patients, it is not useful if the cord enters the internal inguinal ring.[40]

From a recently completed study at our institution with 35 patients,[41] and those published by others,[42–44] MRI seems to be the most accurate noninvasive examination.

Imaging Techniques

Patients between 6 months and 6 years of age require sedation. They are placed directly in the head coil if they are small enough to fit. A standard 5-inch circular surface coil is centered approximately over the symphysis pubis to ensure that the base of the scrotum and lower pelvis are included in the field of view. A 16-cm field of view (FOV), a 256 × 256 acquisition matrix, and a 3-mm-slice thickness are used. In small infants, the 3-inch surface coil is used and the FOV is reduced to 12 cm.

Two series are sufficient in most cases, requiring a total examination time of 30 minutes. Keeping imaging time short is important, since most cases require sedation. The first is a transaxial T_1-weighted series (TR 600, TE 20 ms) obtained from the base of the scrotum to midbladder. It is used to assess the entire spermatic cord to the level of the internal inguinal ring and to graphically prescribe the coronal series, which covers the region from the posterior aspect of the scrotum to the anterior abdominal wall. The coronal series (TR 2,000, TE 20/70 ms) is obtained with a slice thickness of 3 mm and an interslice gap of 50 percent to ensure proper T_2 weighting. The 256 × 256 matrix obtained with two excitations requires a 17.5-minute acquisition time.

It allows further assessment of the cord within the spermatic canal and provides testicular tissue characterization. These two series are sufficient if the testes and cord are atrophic and are in the spermatic canal, or if the testis is located intracanalicular or more distal. This was true in 23 of the 35 cases (66 percent) in our series. However, if the testes are not seen or are intra-abdominal, a third series is required.

If testes are seen and are intra-abdominal in location near the internal inguinal ring, the third series is obtained in the transaxial plane with similar technique as the coronal plane, except TR is increased to 3,000 ms and the number of excitations reduced to 1. It serves to characterize testicular tissue further and locate more precisely the position of the testis relative to the inguinal canal. If, on the other hand, neither the cryptorchid testis nor its cord structures could be seen on the coronal series, the third series is obtained from the symphysis pubis to the upper pole of both kidneys using either the head or body coil, dependent upon patient size. The pulsing sequence for this series is TR 2,000 ms and TE 20 and 70 ms, four excitations, 20 to 34 cm FOV, with either 10-mm slice thickness every 15 mm or 5 mm every 7.5 mm to ensure full coverage of the region of interest and proper T_2 weighting.

Role of MRI in Cryptorchidism

High-resolution MRI with surface coils clearly delineates the spermatic cord, inguinal canal, inguinal ring, pubic tubercle, testes, and regional lymph nodes.[6–10,41–44] At our institution, undescended testes were best seen and recognized on coronal images.[41,42] The 32 undescended testes in our series with surgical or clinical proof were either intra-abdominal or not visualized in 19 percent, intracanalicular in 37 percent, or atrophic in 44 percent. Except for the group with atrophic testes, these relationships were nearly similar to the experience of others.[43,44] Four of the six intra-abdominal testes were correctly located. Errors made by others were also related to testes in intra-abdominal locations.[43,44] We believe that those errors should be avoidable with added experience. The overall accuracy of MRI in our prospective series was 93.8 percent (30 of 32 testes),[41] which is comparable to previously published reports of 94 percent (15 of 16)[43] and 93 percent (retrospective data) (13 of 14).[44] Accuracy was lowest for intra-abdominal testes in all three series.

The task of locating intra-abdominal testes when proximal to the internal inguinal ring is the most difficult on MRI. Confusion with lymph nodes and bowel in the abdomen becomes possible. With the advent of MRI oral contrast and with added experience, this problem could be partially overcome. However, when testes are near the internal inguinal ring, which is the most common intra-abdominal location, they are well depicted and distinguished with higher confidence from lymph nodes. While it is important to visualize high intra-abdominal testes,[45] I believe that there will always be a certain degree of uncertainty such that laparoscopy should precede surgical exploration. Therefore, the inability to visualize the high intra-abdominal testis is less critical for patient management, since patients with absent cord and testis will have to undergo laparoscopy and surgical exploration. When the testis and/or cord are well evaluated, laparoscopy is not necessary. MRI in our series could have potentially decreased laparoscopy from 100 percent to 13 percent.[41]

In our experience, assessment of the spermatic cord and testis together seems essential for proper diagnosis. An empty spermatic canal is visible on MRI. It appears as a thin line extending from the inguinal canal to the base of the scrotum (Fig. 12-21) most likely representing the gubernaculum, a thin fibrous strand. This should not be mistaken for an atrophic cord. The latter has significant width but is thinner than the normal contralateral cord (Fig. 12-22). While an empty canal and an absent cord suggested the possibility of an intra-abdominal testis, the presence of cord structures in the canal does not exclude this possibility. Cord structures may precede the testis, or the testis if attached to a long mesentery may flip-flop between an intracanalicular and an intra-abdominal location. Since most intra-abdominal testes will be found near the internal inguinal ring, where MRI should be reasonably accurate, the goal of the imaging schemes should be to maximize assessment

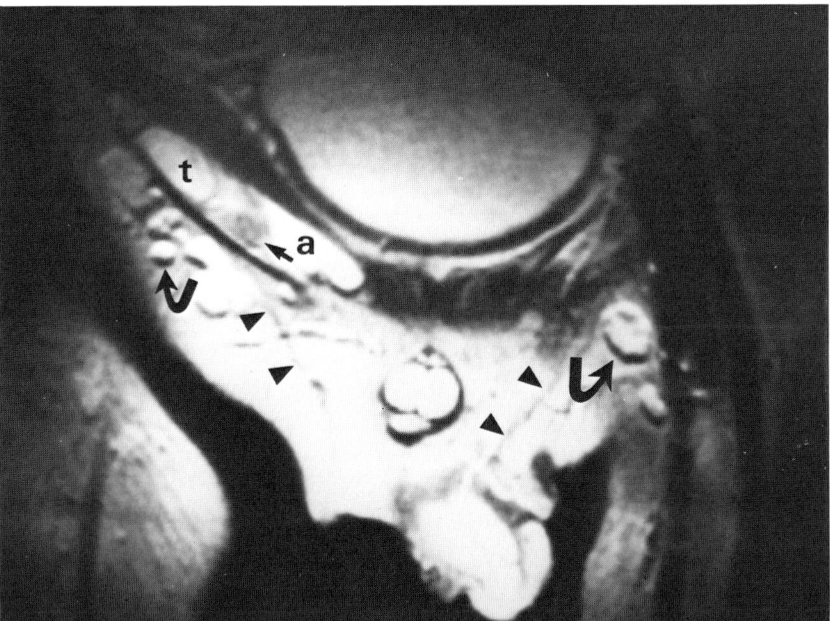

Fig. 12-21. Undescended nonpalpable right testis in a typical intracanalicular location. Note that the testis (t) has normal signal behavior when seen on a T_2-weighted image and has an associated normal epididymis (arrow) and ascites (a). In this location, fluid is technically ascitic since the vaginal process is patent. The other testis was intra-abdominal (not shown here). Note the gubernaculum bilaterally extending from the external inguinal ring to the base of the scrotum (arrowheads). Note the presence of inguinal adenopathy lateral to the right and left canals (curved arrows). (From Gylys-Morin et al.,[44] with permission.)

FIG. 12-22. Atrophic left testis (arrow) seen on (A) hydrogen density-weighted and (B) T_2-weighted images. Note the presence of an atrophic cord that is thinner than the normal contralateral cord (arrowhead) and thicker than the gubernaculum seen in Figure 12-21. Also note that the atrophic cord reaches the base of the scrotum. Note the presence of inguinal adenopathy lateral to the right cord (curved arrow). Heterogeneous signal seen below the scrotum is urine in a diaper. (From Gylys-Morin et al.,[44] with permission.)

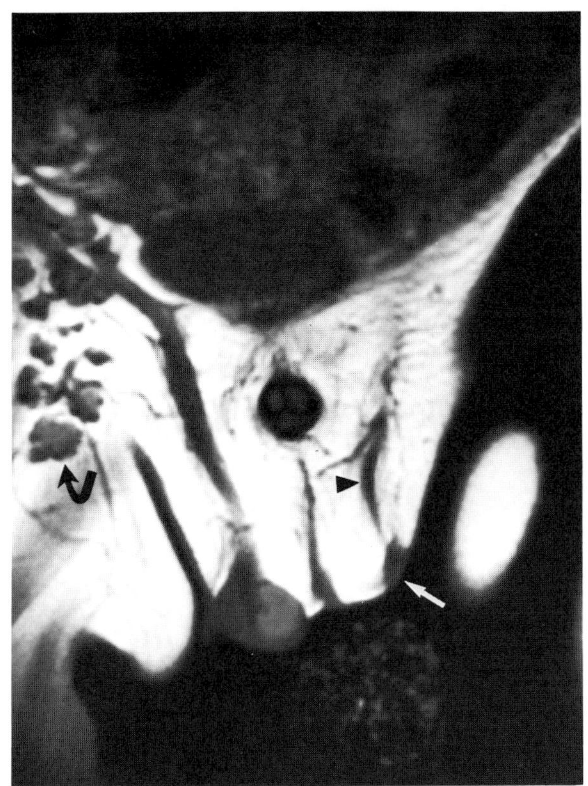

A

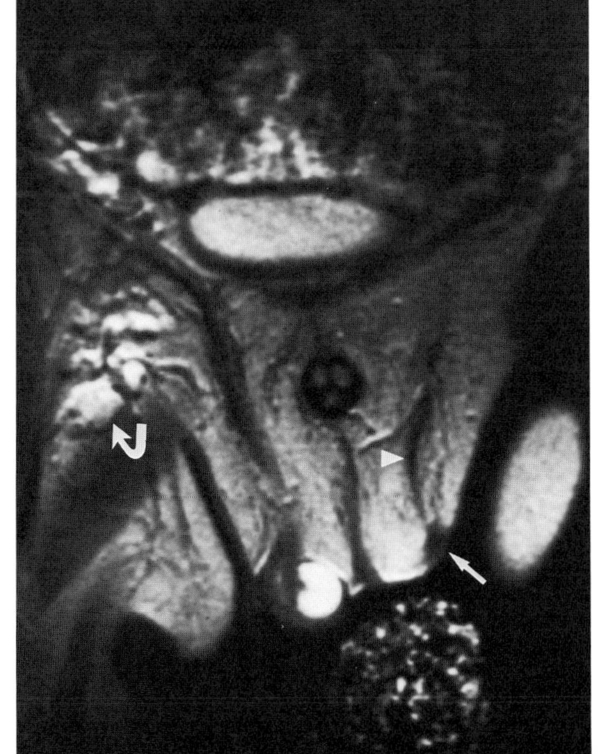

B

of the internal inguinal ring region. The technique described above would allow such assessment. The 5-inch surface coil should be centered over the pubic region and not the scrotum to place the cryptorchid testis at an optimal position in the field.

The undescended testes studied at our institution had a normal ovoid shape with clear demonstration of the tunica albuginea. These testes assumed four positions. They were either in the subcutaneous space anterior to the external inguinal ring, in the spermatic canal (Fig. 12-22), in the inguinal canal (Fig. 12-21), or just lateral to the internal inguinal ring in an intra-abdominal location (Fig. 12-23). Intracanalicular testes were easily differentiated from lymph

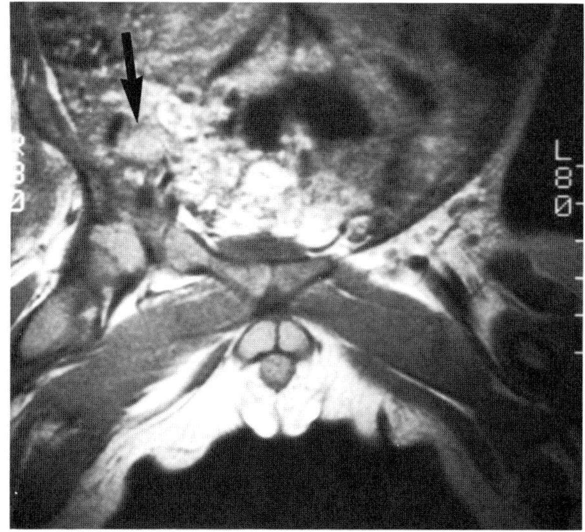

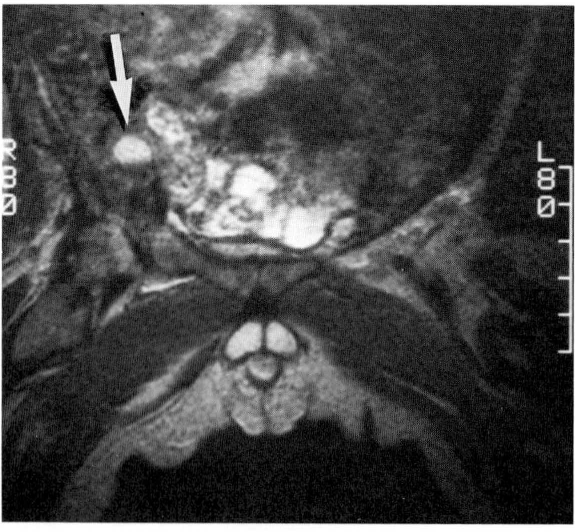

FIG. 12-23. Right intra-abdominal testis (arrow) is seen on (A) hydrogen density-weighted and (B) T_2-weighted images in a typical location in a coronal plane. Note normal testicular signal on both sequences. (From Gylys-Morin et al.,[44] with permission.)

nodes, since their tunica albuginea could be discerned, they were associated with cord structures or epididymis, were surrounded by fluid, and were located in the path of the spermatic cord on axial scans (Fig. 12-21). Lymph nodes, while of similar signal behavior, present different morphology and are lateral to the cord (Figs. 12-21 and 12-22).

Testicular atrophy, most likely related to missed extravaginal torsion, was easily diagnosed. This noninvasive diagnosis, possible with only MRI, has far-reaching clinical implication. This diagnosis must be reserved for those cases with an atrophic cord that reaches the base of the empty scrotum (Fig. 12-22). This finding has been specific for testicular atrophy proven surgically in 9 of 9 cases.[41] Given the reliability of the MRI diagnosis and given the proper clinical setting, the remaining five cases with atrophy diagnosed by MRI are being followed clinically.[41] Surgical resection to eliminate the potential for malignant degeneration is not required in these cases since viable testicular tissue is no longer present. If further clinical experience shows that MRI can indeed diagnose this entity with no false-positive results, surgical exploration in this subset of patients could be eliminated. This ability would have eliminated exploration in 14 of 35 patients in our series (40 percent).

SEMINAL VESICLES

Conditions affecting the seminal vesicles are either malignant, most frequently resulting from prostatic cancer invasion, infectious, most commonly secondary to prostatitis, or congenital. Since the development of the seminal vesicles is closely associated with the development of the vas deferens and ureters, congenital conditions afflicting the seminal vesicles are frequently associated with vas deferens, ureteral, and renal anomalies.[46]

Before the advent of CT, imaging the seminal vesicles was mostly by radiography following the opacification of the urethra, bladder, or rectum or by direct seminal vesiculography. With the advent of CT, vesiculography was gradually abandoned. CT became the primary imaging modality. Transabdominal sonography, while useful, did not replace CT as the primary tool to assess this region, particularly since it was limited in its ability to evaluate the prostate. The use of sonography for the assessment of the seminal vesicles and associated prostatic abnormalities has taken a new role with the increased popularity of transrectal ultrasound. CT and MRI now have to compete with this versatile and powerful modality. Given the higher accuracy of MRI in staging prostate cancer than either CT or sonography, and the frequent involvement of the seminal vesicles with this disease, MRI is commonly called upon to evaluate the integrity of these glands.

Normal Seminal Vesicles

The paired glands lie posterior to the urinary bladder within the perivesical space. Their position is cephalad and posterior to the prostate and anterior to the rectum. The seminal vesicle duct joins with the ipsilateral vas deferens to form the ejaculatory duct. The paired ejaculatory ducts course within the substance of the prostate along its posterior aspect to reach and pierce the verumontanum.

Each gland is approximately 3 cm long and 1.5 cm in diameter.[47] It is made up of convoluted ducts filled with seminal fluid containing nutrients and support for sperm viability. Seminal fluid constitutes the major volume of the ejaculate. Seminal vesicles are asymmetric in size in nearly one-third of patients.[47]

CT appearance of the seminal vesicles is that of soft tissue densities extending cranially and laterally from the prostate just posterior to the bladder. On MRI,

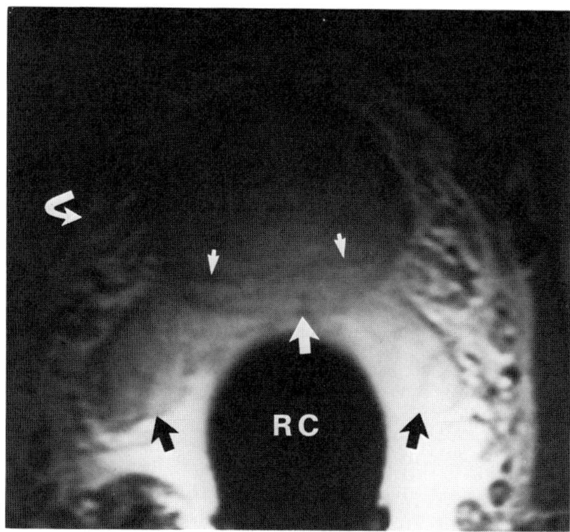

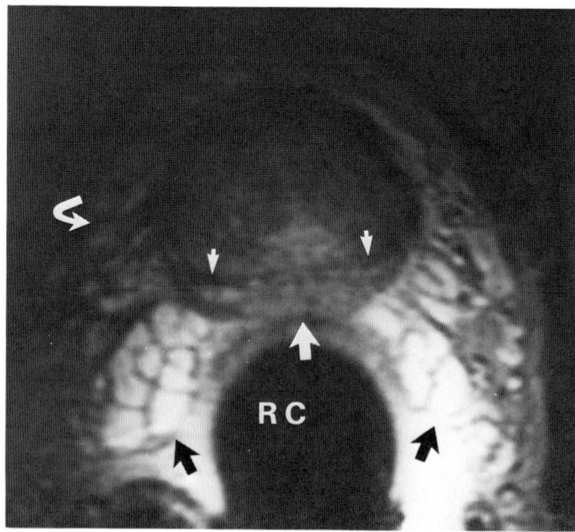

FIG. 12-24. High resolution images of normal seminal vesicles seen on (A) hydrogen density weighting and (B) T₂-weighting. Note the intermediate density of the seminal vesicles (Fig. A, thick black arrows) imaged with an insertable inflatable rectal coil (RC). Note the marked increase in signal of the seminal vesicles relative to fat on T₂-weighting (Fig. B) and the multiple saclike collections of fluid within the glands. Note the hypertrophied central region of the prostate, separated from the peripheral zone by the surgical capsule (white arrows). The dark area between the seminal vesicles (thick white arrow) is the region of the right and left vas deferens where these join the seminal vesicle ducts to form the ejaculatory ducts. Also note the extensive periprostatic vessels (venous plexus) that increase in signal on T₂-weighting (curved arrow).

the predominant signal comes from the seminal fluid. Therefore, the glands are slightly brigher than water on T_1- and hydrogen density-weighted images but are much darker than fat (Fig. 12-24). On T_2-weighted images, the gland becomes brighter than fat (Fig. 12-24). In some patients they can become isointense with fat and indistinguishable from the extensive venous plexus that invests that region. They can also at times be brighter than urine on T_2-weighted images, owing to their shorter T_1 and to urine turbulence within the bladder. In some patients, the seminal vesicles remain darker than fat on T_2-weighted images. The precise reason for this is not clear but seems to be associated with decreased ejaculatory volume (unpublished data).

Tumors

By far the most frequent neoplasm affecting the seminal vesicles is invasive cancer that originates in the prostate (Fig. 12-25), and much less frequently the bladder or the rectum. Primary neoplasm of the seminal vesicles is extremely rare with less than 70 reported cases. There is a high degree of suspicion that some of the early reported cases were prostatic in origin. Primary neoplasia of the seminal vesicles, like that of the prostate, is adenocarcinoma and affects men over 50 years of age. When present, cancer is seen as asymmetric homogeneous[48] or inhomogeneous[46] enlargement of the gland, with normal ap-

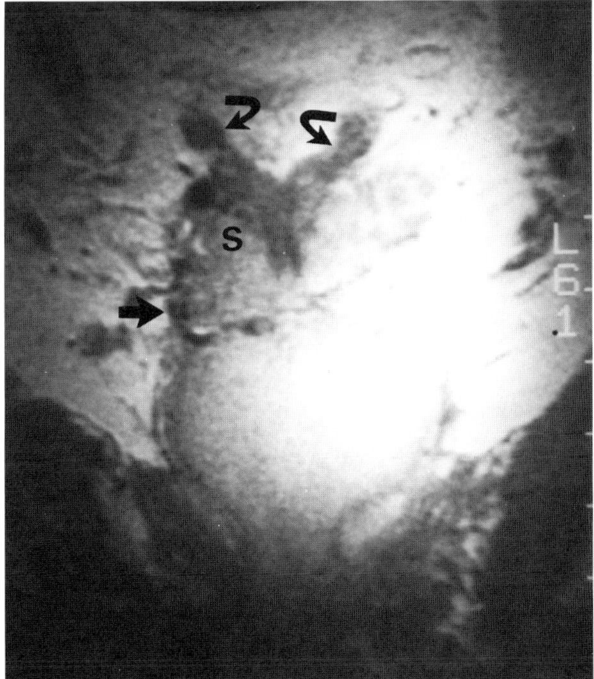

FIG. 12-25.   Prostate cancer (arrow) is seen on a hydrogen density weighted image acquired with the inflatable rectal coil in a coronal plane invading the base of the right seminal vesicle (S) and effacing the prostate seminal vesicle angle. This angle is normal on the left. Note the normal vas deferens (curved arrows).

pearance of the adjacent bladder and prostate.[48] Lesions may obstruct the seminal vesicle duct, causing cystic distention of the gland and presenting as a complex cyst indistinguishable from an abscess.[49]

While no reports of the MRI appearance of primary seminal vesicle neoplasm are available, it would be expected that in addition to affecting the size and shape of the gland, such lesions would darken the normal seminal vesicle signal on T_2-weighted images. This is because lesions replace the high water content of the gland by less-water-containing-tumor tissue as is observed with invasive prostate cancer. However, in cases of obstruction of the ejaculatory duct, it may be difficult to distinguish cancer from a complicated cyst by appearance alone. Cancerous involvement of the seminal vesicles should be suspected when the signal from the right and left glands is asymmetric. Except in cases with hemorrhagic seminal vesicle (Fig. 12-26), the darker gland on T_2-weighting is the abnormal gland.

Infection

Infections of the seminal vesicles go unrecognized in nearly 25 percent of cases with prostatitis.[50] On the other hand, it is estimated that 13 percent of cases suspected of having prostatitis actually have primary seminal vesiculitis.[51] Clinical diagnosis of seminal vesiculitis can be difficult, owing to the complexity of symptoms. While our experience is limited, all reports of seminal vesiculitis are limited to those cases with abscess, hemorrhage, or obstruction of the duct,[52] raising the suspicion that imaging in pure seminal vesiculitis is probably nonspecific.

Seminal vesicle abscesses are rare. Infections of the seminal vesicles leading to abscess formation may be secondary to a hematologic source, or may be due to a predisposing factor such as urinary infection, diabetes, indwelling catheters, instrumentation, and pre-existing anomalies. Several reports have described the CT appearance of seminal vesicle involvement with abscesses,[46,50–53] including tuberculosis.[54] CT may at times have difficulty distinguishing prostatic from seminal vesicle abscesses, since it is limited to the transverse plane. Transrectal sonography is more versatile in demonstrating this relationship.[50] MRI may be equally specific to sonography.[55]

Congenital

Congenital abnormalities of the seminal vesicles most frequently include cyst formation associated with either ipsilateral anomalies of the ureter and kidney or ectopic insertion of the ipsilateral ureter into the cyst. Other events include ectopic insertion or absence of the vas deferens.[55] It is hypothesized that since absence of the vas deferens, which takes its origin from the mesonephric duct, need not be associated with seminal vesicle or ureteral anomalies that take their origin from a slightly more caudal position, abnormal differentiation of

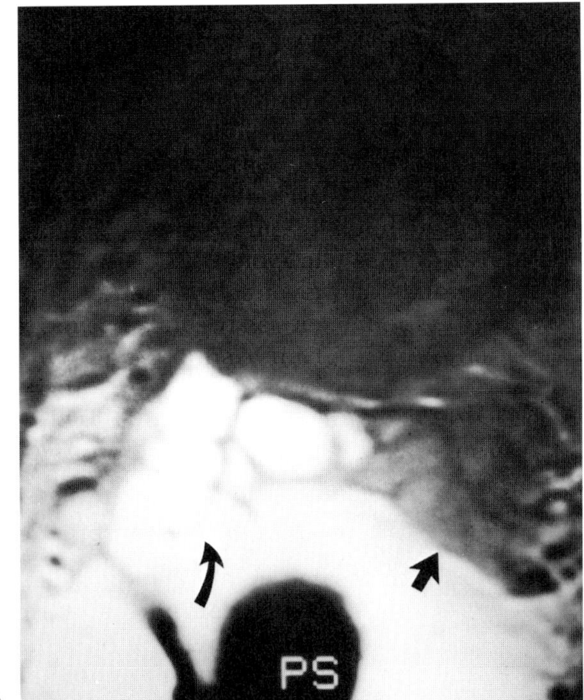

A

FIG. 12-26. Hemorrhagic seminal vesicle secondary to prostate biopsy. Note the normal signal behavior of the left seminal vesicle (black arrow) seen on (A) hydrogen density-weighted and (B) T_2-weighted images. The right seminal vesicle (curved arrow), while normal in shape, assumes a bright signal on both hydrogen density weighting (Fig. A) and T_2-weighting (Fig. B). The right seminal vesicle was bright on a T_2-weighted series (not shown), consistent with blood.

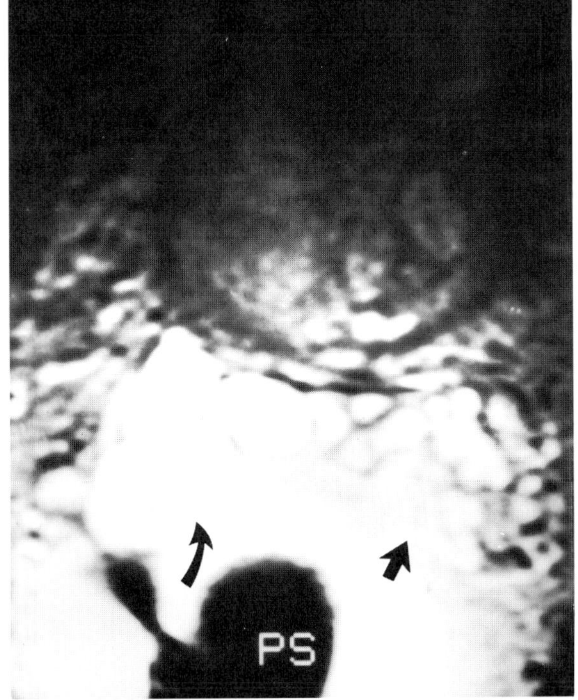

B

the mesonephric duct may be localized.[56] Failures in the ureteral bud, because of failures in the differentiation of the mesonephric duct, will result in failure in the development of the ureter and the ipsilateral kidney leading to renal dysplasia, hypoplasia, or agenesis. The development of the ureteral bud, seminal vesicles, and vas deferens from the mesonephric duct during embryogenesis and the absorption process of some of the associated developmental structures at that location must occur in a precise fashion, or anomalies of the ureter, seminal vesicle, trigone, and kidney may ensue. For instance, should the ureteral bud take origin more cephalad than normal, it results in delayed absorption, placing the ureteral insertion in an ectopic position within the trigone, bladder neck, urethra or any of the structures that result from the mesonephric duct: the ejaculatory duct, seminal vesicle, and vas deferens.[57] Congenital absence of the vas deferens, which was the cause of infertility in 1.2 percent of males, was associated with both seminal vesicles being normal, both hypoplastic, or one hypoplastic in 46, 23, and 31 percent respectively.[56]

Congenital seminal vesicle cysts may be asymptomatic. Patients, should they become symptomatic, develop symptoms at the time of sexual development, when spermatogenesis and seminal fluids form. Stenosis at the level of the ejaculatory duct result in obstruction, accumulation of fluids, and cyst formation. Furthermore, these cysts can become complicated with hemorrhage or infection. Symptoms are vague and may include prostatism, urinary frequency, dysuria, painful ejaculation, and perineal pain or discomfort. Chronic epididymitis may develop secondary to these anomalous conditions, bringing the patient to medical attention.

While these cysts have had varied appearance on CT and are typically cystic on sonography, two recent MRI reports have shown bright signals on both T_1- and T_2-weighted images.[46,55] Congenital cysts contain brownish fluid of complex composition, which includes spermatozoa and other cells. Although the signal suggests old hemorrhage, it may be due to the proteins and other paramagnetic materials not yet characterized.

The differential diagnosis of seminal vesicle cysts includes the prostatic utricle or müllerian duct cyst. These two cysts are easily differentiated from seminal vesicle cysts, since the former are in the midline and the latter are off-center. They may themselves cause obstruction of the ejaculatory duct and produce seminal vesicle cysts. Utricle cysts and müllerian duct cysts have different embryologic development. The prostatic utricle communicates with the urinary tract but may become obstructed from infection or trauma leading to cyst formation. The prostatic utricle, a remnant of the urogenital sinus, is typically found in young patients and is highly associated with hypospadias and abnormal genitalia.[58] On the other hand, müllerian duct cysts present in older men with normal genitalia, do not communicate with the urinary tract, and are due to incomplete resorption of the müllerian duct.[58]

Another entity that needs to be differentiated from congenital cysts, which may be difficult at times, is the acquired cyst of the seminal vesicle.[46] These cysts are due to obstruction of the ejaculatory duct, which could be caused by stones or stenosis resulting from surgery, infection, tumors, or prostatic disease. Acquired cysts are suspected when appropriate predisposing factors are known and there is a normal ipsilateral kidney and vas deferens.

URETHRA

The entire course of the urethra is well visualized by MRI (Figs. 12-11, 12-12, and 12-27). CT is unable to demonstrate the urethra within the substance of the prostate or penis. While the corpora cavernosa can be seen by CT owing to the higher density of the tunica albugenia, sufficient detail of the penis is limited. However, CT is more sensitive than radiography in depicting the calcifications of Pyronnie's disease and may demonstrate early lesions not yet clinically palpable.[59] MRI is able to demonstrate penile anatomy in detail and with sufficient contrast (Figs. 12-11 and 12-27). In one patient in whom a penile prosthesis was removed because of infection, MRI showed the scar in the corpora cavernosa (Fig. 12-28). Indeed, preliminary results in a variety of penile abnormalities demonstrated by MRI, including scarring, trauma, congenital abnormalities, and tumors, were encouraging.[60] Further experience is needed to better establish the role of MRI in the assessment of the penis and urethra.

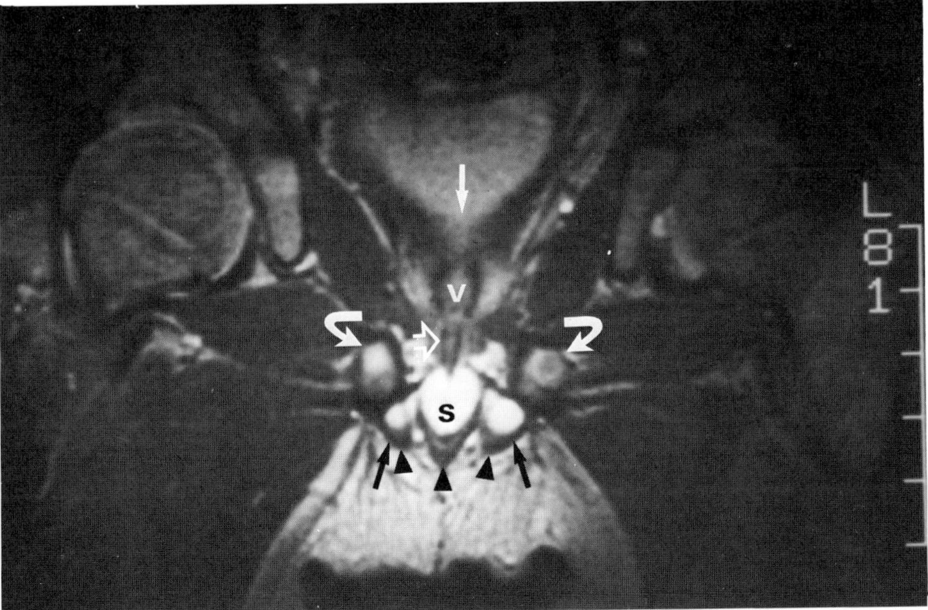

FIG. 12-27.   Five-inch surface coil T$_2$-weighted image obtained at the level of the prostate in a 3-month-old boy. The urethra is seen from the bladder base (white arrow) to the level of the corpora spongiosa (s). The verumontanum (v) and distal prostatic urethra (open arrow) are evident. The corpora spongiosa (s) and cavernous (black arrows) are well seen, accompanied by their respective bulbospongiosus and ischio-cavernosus (arrowheads) muscles. The ischial rami (curved arrows) are seen in close proximity to the corpora cavernosa.

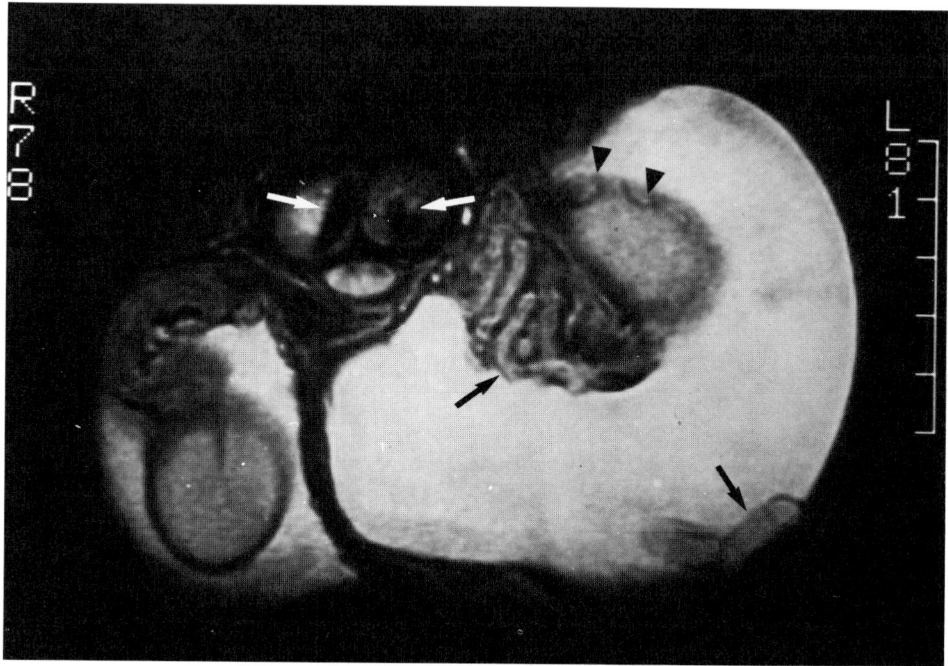

FIG. 12-28.   Scars in the corpora cavernosa from a removed penile implant are seen on a T_2-weighted image as dark signals within each corpora cavernsa (white arrows). There are bilateral large hydroceles outlining the bare area in cross-section. Note the dilated spermatic veins with stagnant blood in the left scrotum (black arrows). Superficial left testicular vessels can also be seen (arrowheads).

Competing techniques include clinical assessment, which is particularly efficacious in the pendulous portion of the penis; endoscopy and urethrography, limited to intraluminal visualization; and sonography, which is capable of displaying anatomic detail of the penis, urethra, and periurethral tissues.[61,62]

CONCLUSION

MRI adds a new dimension to the assessment of scrotal disease. It demonstrates exquisite anatomic detail of the entire scrotum and inguinal region. It allows for the recognition of each intrascrotal structure on the basis of its characteristic appearance and signal rather than strictly its anatomic location. The interpretation of MRI is less subjective and less misleading than ultrasound, particularly when the normal relationship of scrotal contents is disturbed. Being less subjective, it is my belief that MRI is sufficiently specific to permit differentiation of the various pathologic processes, although this hypothesis requires proof. It also appears that MRI may be the most accurate noninvasive tool in localizing and guiding the management of patients with nonpalpable testes. In this setting, it can decrease significantly the number of laparoscopies performed and potentially eliminate the need for surgery in as many as 40 percent of cases.[41]

The ability of MRI to evaluate all conditions affecting the seminal vesicles has not been sufficiently explored. It appears, however, that MRI offers similar findings as CT but, in addition, it offers multiplanar imaging capability and added tissue characterization potential. The competition with MRI is not CT, but rather transrectal sonography. Sonography is versatile, efficacious, inexpensive, and highly accessible to the referring physician. In the assessment of the seminal vesicles, except in prostate cancer staging, I believe that MRI and CT will be the secondary imaging modalities reserved for select cases.

ACKNOWLEDGMENT

The author is the recipient of Career Development Award NCI-KO8-CA01319.

REFERENCES

1. Leopold GR, Woo VL, Scheible FW, et al: High resolution ultrasonography of scrotal pathology. Radiology 131:719, 1979
2. Leopold GR: Superficial organs. p. 123. In Goldberg B (ed): Ultrasound in Cancer. Churchill Livingstone, New York, 1981
3. Hricak H, Filly RA: Sonography of the scrotum. Invest Radiol 18:112, 1983
4. Glazer HS, Lee JKT, Melson GL, McClennan BL: Sonographic detection of occult testicular neoplasms. AJR 138:673, 1982
5. Carroll BA, Gross DM: High frequency scrotal sonography. AJR 140:511, 1983
6. Baker LL, Hajek PC, Burkhard TK, et al: Magnetic resonance imaging of the scrotum: Normal anatomy. Radiology 163:89, 1987
7. Baker LL, Hajek PC, Burkhard TK, et al: Magnetic resonance imaging of the scrotum: Pathologic conditions. Radiology 163:93, 1987
8. Rholl KS, Lee JKT, Ling D, et al: MR imaging of the scrotum with a high resolution surface coil. Radiology 163:99, 1987
9. Seidenwurm D, Smathers RL, Lo RK, et al: Testes and scrotum: MR imaging at 1.5T. Radiology 164:393, 1987
10. Thurnher S, Hricak H, Carroll PR, et al: Imaging the testis: Comparison between MR imaging and US. Radiology 167:631, 1988
11. Johnson JO, Mattrey RF, Philpson J: Differentiation of seminomatous from non-seminomatous testicular tumors by MRI. AJR 154:539, 1990
12. Morse MJ, Whitmore WF: Neoplasms of the testes. p. 1535. In Walsh PC, Gittes RF, Permutter AD, Stamey TA (eds): Campbell's Urology. WB Saunders, Philadelphia, 1986
13. Sokal M, Peckham MJ, Hendry WF: Bilateral germ cell tumours of the testis. Br J Urol 53:158, 1980
14. Schwerk WB, Schwerk WN, Rodeck G: Testicular tumors: Prospective analysis of real-time ultrasound patterns and abdominal staging. Radiology 164:369, 1987
15. Lupetin AR, King W III, Rich P, Lederman RB: Ultrasound diagnosis of testicular leukemia. Radiology 146:171, 1983
16. Bird K, Rosenfield AT: Testicular infarction secondary to acute inflammatory disease: Demonstration by B-scan ultrasound. Radiology 152:785, 1984
17. Gullenwater JY, Grayhack JT, Howards SS, Duckett JW: Adult and Pediatric Urology. Year Book Medical Publishers, Chicago, 1987

18. Finkelstein MS, Rosenberg HK, Snyder HM III, Duckett JW: Ultrasound evaluation of scrotum in pediatrics. Urology 27:1, 1986

19. Hricak H, Jeffrey RB: Sonography of acute scrotal abnormalities. Radiol Clin North Am 21:595, 1983

20. Williamson RCN, Anderson JB: The fate of the human testes following unilateral torsion. Br J Urol 58:698, 1986

21. Ryan PC, Whelan CA, Gaffney EF, Fitzpatrick JM: The effect of unilateral experimental testicular torsion on spermatogenesis and fertility. Br J Urol 62:359, 1988

22. Trambert MO, Mattrey RF, Levine D, Berthoty D: Subacute scrotal pain: Torsion versus epididymitis with MR imaging. Radiology 175:53, 1990

23. Landa HM, Gylys-Morin V, Mattrey RF, et al: Detection of testicular torsion by magnetic resonance imaging in a rat model. J Urol 140:1178, 1988

24. Mueller DL, Amundson GM, Rubin SZ, Wesenberg RL: Acute scrotal abnormalities in children: Diagnosis by combined sonography and scintigraphy. AJR 150:643, 1988

25. Bretan PN, Vigneron DB, Hricak H, et al: Assessment of testicular metabolic integrity with P-31 MR spectroscopy. Radiology 162:867, 1987

26. Fischman AJ, Palmer EL, Scott JA: Radionuclide imaging of sequential torsions of the appendix testis. J Nucl Med 28:119, 1987

27. Ziffer JA, Nelson RC, Chezmar JL, et al: Subclinical varicocele: Detection with MRI (abstract). Presented at SMRI 1989, Los Angeles. Mag Res Imaging 7(suppl):78, 1989

28. Scorer CG, Farrington GH: Congenital Deformities of the Testis and Epididymis. Appleton-Century-Crofts, E. Norwalk, CT, 1972

29. Cour-Palar IJ: Spontaneous descent of the testicle. Lancet 1:403, 1966

30. Hadziselimovic F: Cryptorchidism. Springer-Verlag, Berlin, 1983

31. Batata MA, Whitmore WF Jr, Hilaris BS, et al: Cryptorchidism and testicular cancer. J Urol 124:382, 1980

32. Pinch L, Aceto T Jr, Meyer-Bahlburg HFL: Cryptorchidism. A pediatric review. Urol Clin North Am 1:573, 1974

33. Rajfer J: The testis and epididymis: Cryptorchidism. p. 422. In Kaufman JJ (ed): Current Urologic Therapy. WB Saunders, Philadelphia, 1986

34. Weiss RM, Carter AR, Rosenfield AT: High resolution real-time ultrasonography in the localization of the undescended testis. J Urol 135:936, 1986

35. Wolverson MK, Houttin E, Heiberh E, et al: Comparison of CT with high resolution ultrasound in the localization of the undescended testis. Radiology 146:133, 1983

36. Lee JKT, McClennan BL, Stanley RJ, Sagel SS: Utility of CT in the localization of the undescended testis. Radiology 135:121, 1980

37. Green JR: Computerized axial tomography vs. spermatic venography in localization of the cryptorchid testis. Urology 26:513, 1985

38. Glickman MF, Weiss RM, Itzchak Y: Testicular venography for undescended testes. AJR 129:67, 1977

39. Diamond AB, Meng CH, Kodroff M, Goldman SM: Testicular venography in the non-palpable testis. AJR 129:71, 1977

40. Lowe DH, Brock WA, Kaplan GW: Laparoscopy for localization of the nonpalpable testis. J Urol 131:728, 1984

41. Gylys-Morin VM, Landa HM, Mattrey RF, et al: MRI localization of the undescended testis and its potential impact on surgical management. AJR (submitted)

42. Landa HM, Gylys-Morin V, Mattrey RF, et al: MRI of the cryptorchid testis. Eur J Pediatr 146(suppl):516, 1987

43. Fritsche PJ, Hricak H, Kogan BA, et al: Undescended testis: Value of MRI. Radiology 164:169, 1987

44. Kier R, McCarthy S, Rosenfield AT et al: Nonpalpable testes in young boys: Evaluation with MR imaging. Radiology 169:429, 1988

45. Friedland GW, Chang P: The role of imaging in the management of impalpable undescended testis. AJR 151:1107, 1988

46. King BF, Williamson B, Hattery RR, et al: Seminal vesicle imaging. Radiographics 9:653, 1989

47. Silverman PM, Dunnick NR, Ford KK: Computed tomography of the normal seminal vesicles. Comput Radiol 9:379, 1985

48. Sussman SK, Dunnick NR, Silverman PM, Cohan RH: Carcinoma of the seminal vesicle: CT appearance. J Comput Assist Tomogr 10:519, 1986

49. Kawahara M, Matsushima M, Matsuhashi M, et al: Primary carcinoma of the seminal vesicle. Urology 32:269, 1988

50. Zagoria RJ, Papanicolaou N, Pfister RC, et al: Seminal vesicle abscess after vasectomy: Evaluation by transrectal sonography and CT. AJR 149:137, 1987

51. Patel PS, Wilbur AC: Cystic seminal vesiculitis: CT demonstration. J Comput Assist Tomogr 11:1103, 1987

52. Sue DE, Chicola C, Brant-Zawadski MN, et al: MR imaging in seminal vesiculitis. J Comput Assist Tomogr 13:662, 1989

53. Premkumar A, Newhouse JH: Seminal vesicle tuberculosis: CT appearance. J Comput Assist Tomogr 12:676, 1988

54. Fox CW, Vaccaro JA, Kiesling VJ, Belville WD: Seminal vesicle abscess: The use of CT for diagnosis and therapy. J Urol 139:384, 1988

55. Kneeland JB, Auh YH, McCarron JP, et al: Computed tomography, sonography, vesiculography and MR imaging of a seminal vesicle cyst. J Comput Assist Tomogr 9:964, 1985

56. Goldstein M, Schlossberg S: Men with congenital absence of the vas deferens often have seminal vesicles. J Urol 140:85, 1988

57. Roehrborn CG, Scheider H, Rugendorff EW, Hamann W: Embryological and diagnostic aspects of seminal vesicle cysts associated with upper urinary tract malformation. J Urol 135:1029, 1986

58. Ritchey ML, Benson RC, Kramer SA, Kelalis PP: Management of Müllerian duct remnants in the male patient. J Urol 140:795, 1988

59. Musante F, Zambelli A, Piacentino A: Computerized tomography in Peyronie's disease. Radiol Med 74:308, 1987

60. Hricak H, Marotti M, Gilbert TJ, et al: Normal penile anatomy and abnormal penile conditions: Evaluation with MR imaging. Radiology 169:683, 1988

61. Gluck CD, Bundy AL, Fine C, et al: Sonographic urethrogram: Comparison to roentgenographic techniques in 22 patients. J Urol 140:1404, 1988

62. Merkle W, Wagner W: Sonography of the distal male urethra—a new diagnostic procedure for urethral strictures: Results of a retrospective study. J Urol 140:1409, 1988

63. Mattrey RF, Trambert MA: MR imaging of the scrotum and testis. Ch. 34. In Edelman RR, Hesselink JR (eds): Magnetic Resonance: Clinical Applications/Advanced Techniques. WB Saunders, New York (in press)

64. Berthoty D, Mattrey RF, Twidwell J, et al: High resolution MR imaging of prostate cancer: Preliminary results. Radiology (submitted)

13 CT and MRI of the Transplanted Kidney

JUDITH L. CHEZMAR
BRUCE R. BAUMGARTNER
HARVEY V. STEINBERG
MICHAEL E. BERNARDINO

Renal transplantation has become a widely accepted, effective treatment for end-stage renal disease. Although the introduction of effective immunosuppressive drugs has led to marked improvement in renal transplant survival, significant complications of the procedure still occur frequently. Allograft rejection is common and is difficult to differentiate clinically from other causes of transplant dysfunction including acute tubular necrosis (ATN) and cyclosporin toxicity, which require different forms of treatment. Urologic and vascular complications requiring surgical intervention are not infrequent and include urinary obstruction or extravasation, vascular obstruction, and peritransplant fluid collections. Prompt and correct diagnosis of a complication is essential, as delay in proper treatment may jeopardize both allograft and patient.

A number of imaging modalities have been evaluated for the diagnosis of post-transplant complications. These include ultrasonography, scintigraphy, CT, and MRI. Ultrasound is the usual imaging method of choice in the initial investigation of post-transplant complications because of its wide availability, lack of ionizing radiation, and relatively low cost. Real-time ultrasound allows the detection of urinary obstruction and peritransplant fluid collections, and may be used to guide diagnostic aspiration of these collections. The addition of Doppler ultrasound to real-time scanning (duplex ultrasound) also allows for a diagnosis of acute transplant rejection with reported sensitivity of 75 to 95 percent and specificity of 90 to 96 percent,[1-3] as well as a diagnosis of vascular complications.[4] CT and MRI do, however, continue to play a role in the diagnosis and management of renal transplant complications. This chapter focuses on the application of CT and MRI in the evaluation of renal transplant recipients.

CT

While CT is used less extensively than ultrasound as the initial modality employed for the evaluation of renal transplants, CT is able to provide excellent anatomic information in the pelvis. Hydronephrosis or the presence of peritransplant fluid collections are readily detected, as they are with ultrasound. CT, however, has definite advantages over ultrasound in the evaluation of some complex post-transplant complications that require whole-body assessment. It is particularly indicated for investigation of abscess or hemorrhage that may be extensive or involve multiple organ systems. CT is also indicated when evaluation of the transplant is clinically warranted but the ultrasound examination is suboptimal due to obesity, surrounding bowel gas, or the presence of a wound infection. In addition, CT may be employed in patients in whom the ultrasound evaluation is negative, but there is strong clinical suspicion of a urologic complication.

The often complex nature of transplant complications referred for CT evaluation dictates that the entire abdomen and pelvis be examined. The CT examination is performed following administration of oral and rectal contrast medium for complete bowel opacification. Intravenous (IV) contrast medium is not routinely administered in these patients due to possible compromise of renal function by iodinated contrast material. If indicated for bladder opacification, contrast medium may be instilled into the bladder via a catheter. Occasionally, if additional information regarding the renal collecting system or leakage of urine is needed, IV contrast may be administered.

Peritransplant fluid collections are probably the most common transplant complication evaluated by CT. Fluid collections are detected by sonography in approximately 50 percent of renal transplant recipients.[5] Most of these collections are small and are detected early in the post-transplant period. Most resolve over time and are not associated with symptoms. They are presumed to represent small collections of blood[5] and are without clinical significance. Other peritransplant collections may require further evaluation, which may include diagnostic aspiration, percutaneous drainage, or surgery. The need for such assessment is based on a number of factors, including size, location, presence of obstruction, or clinical symptoms.

Suspicion of a large hematoma may warrant investigation with CT. Although hematomas may have a variable appearance on CT, because of the increased attenuation of acute blood, CT may be useful in differentiating acute hemorrhage from other peritransplant fluid collections,[6] which include lymphocele, urinoma, and abscess (Fig. 13-1). In addition, CT often provides a more accurate assessment of the true extent of a large hematoma than ultrasound.

Lymphoceles are the most commonly documented post-transplant fluid collection.[5,7] Lymphoceles may be detected on a CT scan, as on ultrasound, as fluid collections usually located medial or inferior to the lower pole of the transplant. On CT, lymphoceles are usually rounded or hour-glass shaped with sharp borders and attenuation values of 10 to 20 HU[7] (Fig. 13-2). Lymphoceles may cause obstruction of the ureter, necessitating surgical interven-

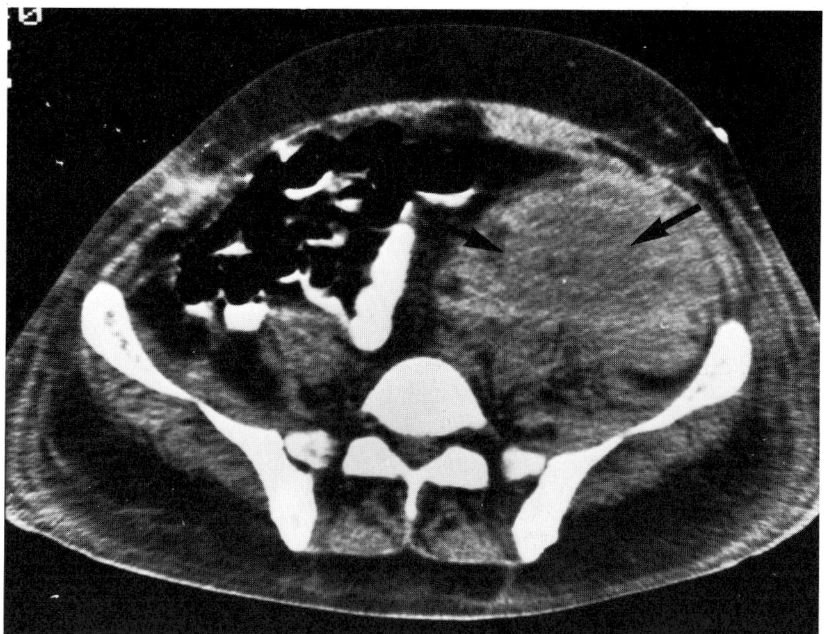

FIG. 13-1.   CT performed with oral contrast demonstrates a high attenuation collection surrounding the renal transplant (arrows) in the pelvis due to acute hemorrhage.

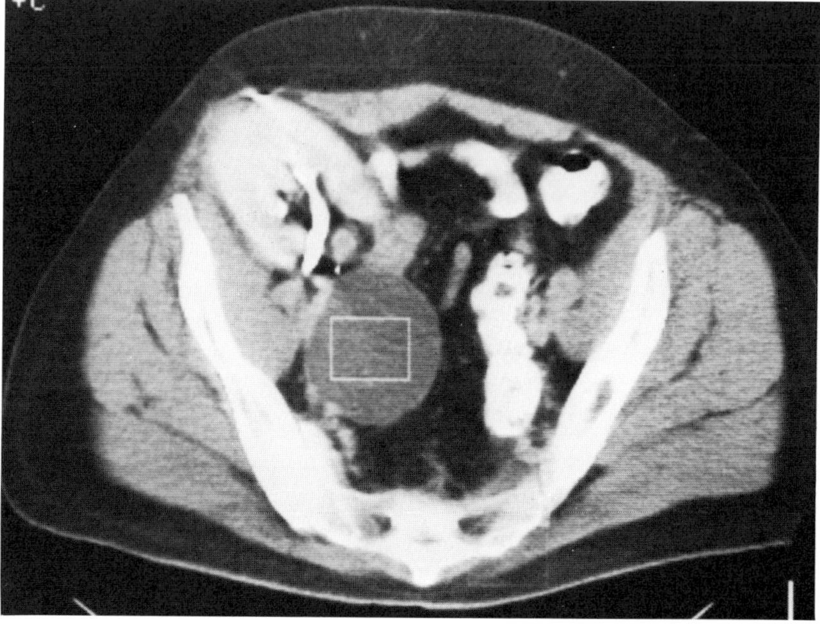

FIG. 13-2.   CT performed after administration of oral and intravenous contrast demonstrates a well circumscribed water density collection medial to the renal transplant. At surgery, this proved to be a lymphocele.

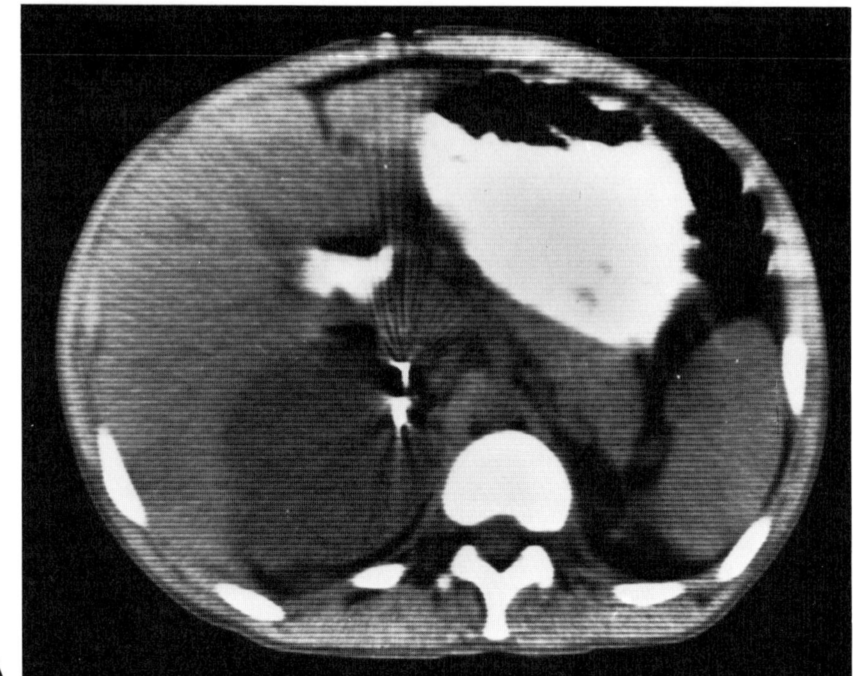

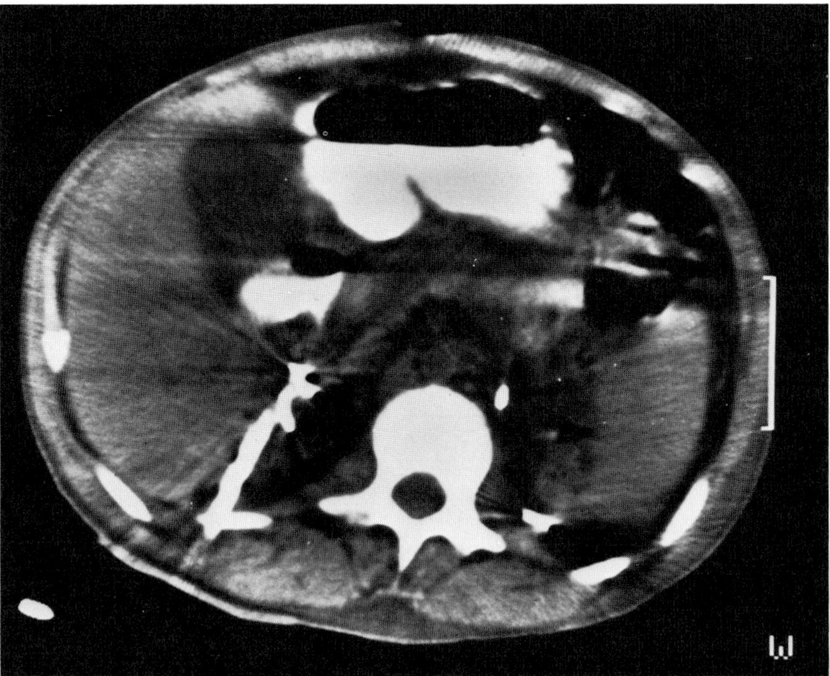

FIG. 13-3.   CT performed with oral contrast in a febrile patient following renal transplantation with removal of native kidneys. (A) A large fluid collection is present in the right renal fossa. CT-guided aspiration of the collection yielded purulent material. (B) The collection was successfully drained percutaneously. A percutaneous drainage catheter is seen in good position. (*Figure continues.*)

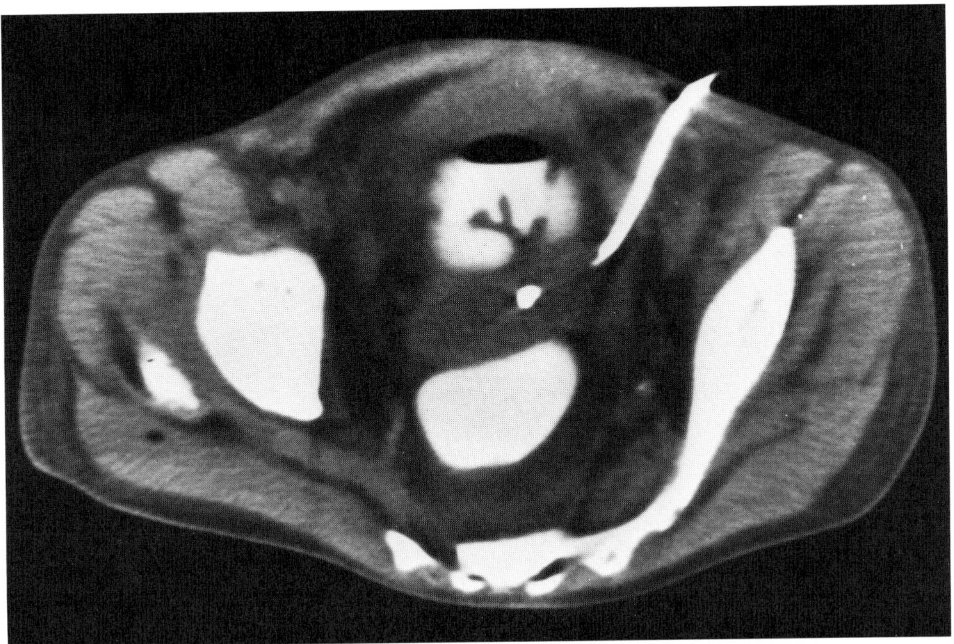

FIG. 13-3 (*Continued*).   (C) a second abscess in the pelvis in the same patient was also percutaneously drained.

tion. The diagnosis may be confirmed by diagnostic aspiration under CT guidance.

Urinomas are also potential peritransplant fluid collections, frequently detected in the early post-transplant period. The appearance of urinomas on CT, a water-density fluid collection, is not specific,[6,7] with the diagnosis often made either by aspiration of the fluid collection or demonstration of accumulation of contrast material in the collection after contrast has been instilled into the bladder or on postcontrast CT.

Abscesses must also be considered a complication of renal transplantation when a fluid collection is seen in a febrile patient. The CT appearance of abscess is variable and may be difficult to differentiate from other fluid collections on the basis of the imaging appearance alone. The presence of gas within a fluid collection, although uncommon, suggests abscess as the etiology of the fluid collection.[7] In a post-transplant patient in whom abscess is suspected, the ability of CT to evaluate the entire abdomen and pelvis rapidly makes CT the imaging study of first choice in this patient group (Fig. 13-3).

Both CT and ultrasound may be used for localization of the renal transplant prior to biopsy. CT may be reserved for those patients in whom sonographic identification of the kidney is difficult, particularly obese patients. Both modalities may also be used to guide diagnostic aspiration of peritransplant fluid collections.

Percutaneous catheter drainage of peritransplant fluid collections may also be performed under ultrasound or CT guidance. We prefer to use ultrasound guidance when the collection is large and superficial, reserving CT for small or deep collections and lesions in critical anatomic areas such as near the renal transplant hilus or adjacent to bowel.[8]

Although the value of CT following renal transplant rests largely in the diagnosis and therapy of urologic complications, the value of dynamic CT in evaluating the physiologic status of renal transplants has been investigated.[9] This technique has little application because of the possible compromise of renal function by injection of iodinated contrast, a problem not shared by other techniques that are able to aid in the diagnosis of transplant rejection, including Doppler ultrasound,[1-3] scintigraphy,[10] or MRI.[11-13]

Transplant recipients are at increased risk of the development of malignancy in their native kidneys. Another indication for CT in the transplant recipient is in the diagnosis of post-transplant neoplasms, particularly lymphoma.[14]

MRI

Several investigators have studied the potential of MRI for evaluation of renal transplants.[11-13] The MRI features of a normal renal transplant have been well described (Fig. 13–4). Because a distinct corticomedullary junction is best seen on relatively T_1-weighted images, MRI scans of a renal transplant are usually obtained using a spin-echo sequence with a repetition time (TR) of 200 to 500 ms and an echo time (TE) of 20 to 30 ms. At our institution, both axial and coronal T_1-weighted images are obtained using a surface coil. The superficial location of renal transplants in the pelvis make it ideal for surface coil MRI evaluation.[12]

MRI, as well as CT, provide excellent anatomic information in the pelvis. This facilitates recognition of hydronephrosis, as well as identification of peritransplant fluid collections (Fig. 13-4). Hricak et al.[12] reported the value of MRI in characterization of some peritransplant fluid collections. Postoperative seromas, lymphoceles, and urinomas had uniformly low signal intensity on T_1-weighted spin-echo images. Abscesses were described as more heterogeneous, with higher signal intensity than seromas, lymphoceles, or urinomas, regardless of the MRI sequence used. Adjacent inflammatory changes in the transplanted kidney, causing heterogeneity of signal intensity and loss of sharpness in the renal outline, have also been described by these investigators. The MRI appearance of hematomas varied with age, with acute hemorrhage appearing more homogeneous and of intermediate signal intensity and older hemorrhage more heterogeneous. Because ultrasound is able to identify most peritransplant fluid collections and is less expensive and more widely available, ultrasound remains a procedure of choice for screening the transplant patient for urologic complications. However, Hricak et al. suggest that MRI may be helpful when multiple fluid collections are present, possibly permitting intervention in one specifically targeted area.

Early hopes were that MRI would be the noninvasive modality best able to

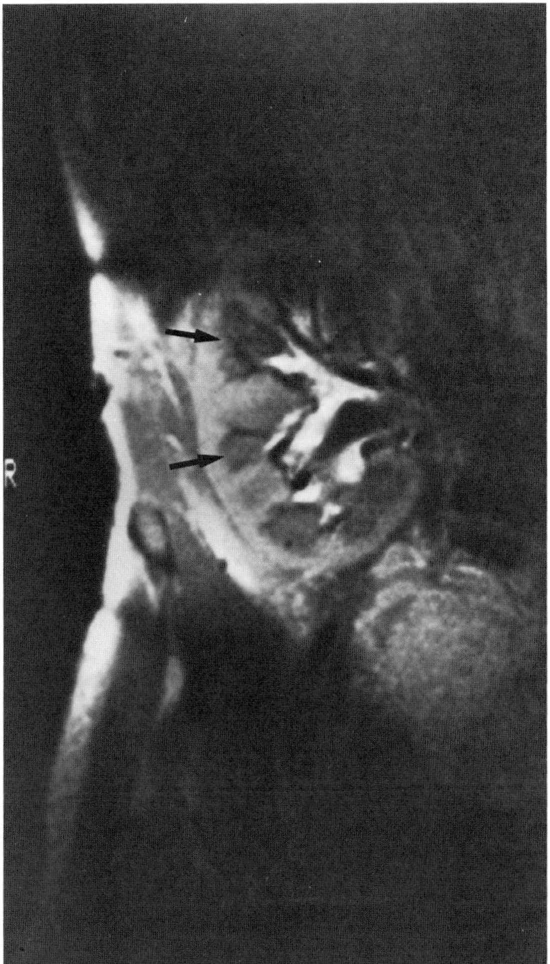

FIG. 13-4.   Normal renal transplant. Coronal surface coil spin-echo (30/500 ms) image clearly demonstrates normal corticomedullary differentiation (arrows). (From Baumgartner et al.,[13] with permission.)

aid in the differential diagnosis of renal transplant rejection from ATN and cyclosporin toxicity. These hopes were based on the observation that the corticomedullary differentiation seen in normal kidneys and normally functioning renal transplants was lost in kidneys undergoing rejection[11–14] (Figs. 13-5 and 13-6). In normal kidneys, the longer T_1 relaxation time of renal medulla allows for clear distinction between the higher signal intensity renal cortex and the lower signal intensity renal medulla on T_1-weighted spin-echo images. Loss of corticomedullary distinction on MRI was not found to be specific for rejection, however, having been reported in a number of other conditions including hydronephrosis, renal artery and renal vein thrombosis, glomerulonephritis, diabetes, drug abuse, acquired immune deficiency syndrome (AIDS), hypertension, and following contrast agent administration.[15] ATN may variably affect corticomedullary differentiation on MRI with normal,

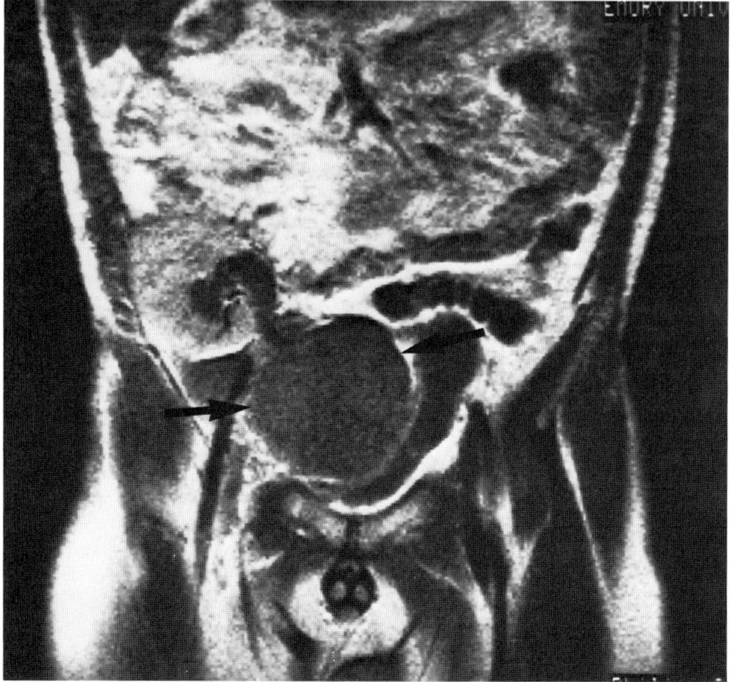

FIG. 13-5.   Coronal spin-echo image (30/700 ms) reveals a large perinephric fluid collection (arrows) displacing bladder to the left and causing mild hydronephrosis. The collection is of homogeneous low signal intensity on this sequence. A smaller collection is located adjacent to the lower pole. Note loss of corticomedullary differentiation in the transplant, which may be seen with obstruction in the absence of rejection. (From Baumgartner et al.,[13] with permission.)

slightly decreased, or absent corticomedullary differentiation having been reported.[11–13] In the limited number of patients with cyclosporin toxicity so far reported in the literature, five have maintained normal corticomedullary differentiation,[12] while two cases with loss of corticomedullary differentiation have been published.[3,16] Thus, MRI of renal transplants has been shown to be less sensitive and specific in the diagnosis of renal transplant rejection than originally hoped for, with one prospective study[13] showing Doppler ultrasound to be more sensitive (95 percent vs. 70 percent) and specific (95 percent vs. 75 percent) in the detection of transplant rejection than MRI.

It is hoped that higher sensitivity and specificity of MRI in the diagnosis of transplant rejection will be possible with the implementation of MRI spectroscopic techniques. If metabolic changes identifiable by spectroscopy could be recognized early in the course of graft rejection, treatment could be instituted even before rejection becomes clinically evident or detectable by current imaging techniques. Ongoing research is focused on this potential application.

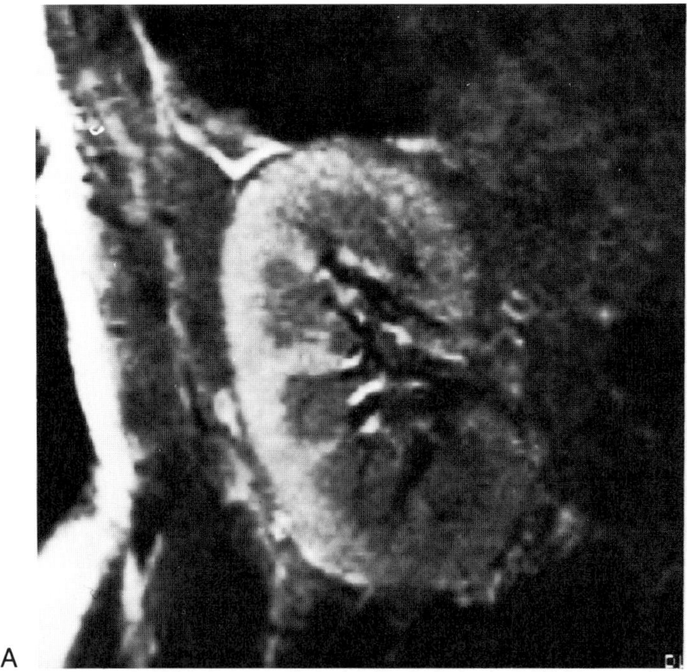

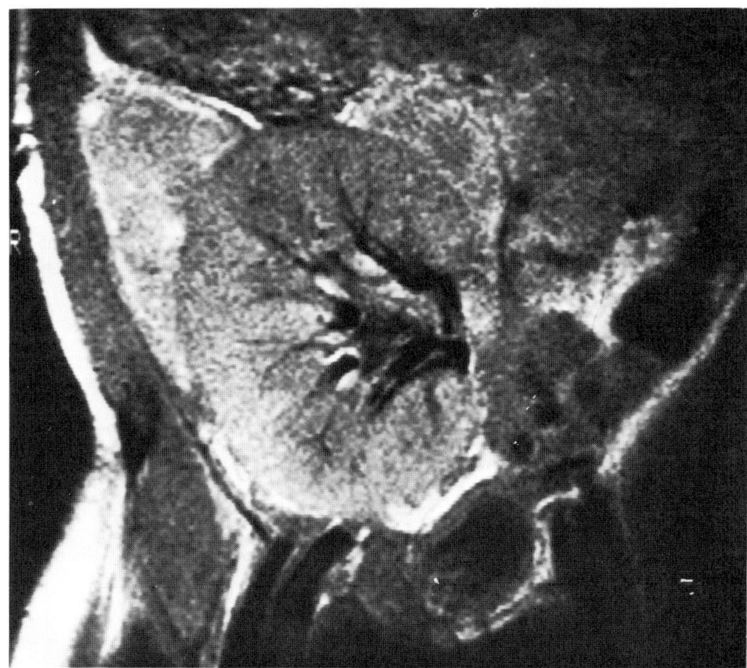

FIG. 13-6.   Coronal spin-echo (30/500 ms) images. (A) Normal corticomedullary differentiation 1 day following renal transplant. (B) Two weeks later, the transplant is larger and more globular, with absent corticomedullary differentiation associated with acute rejection. (From Baumgartner et al.,[13] with permission.)

REFERENCES

1. Berland LL, Lawson TL, Adams MB, et al: Evaluation of renal transplants with pulsed Doppler duplex sonography. J Ultrasound Med 1:215, 1982
2. Rigsby CM, Taylor KJW, Weltin G, et al: Renal allografts in acute rejection: Evaluation using duplex sonography. Radiology 158:375, 1986
3. Steinberg HV, Nelson RC, Murphy FB, et al: Renal allograft rejection: Evaluation by Doppler ultrasound and MR imaging. Radiology 162:337, 1987
4. Taylor KJW, Morse SS, Rigsby CM, et al: Vascular complications in renal allografts: Detection with duplex Doppler US. Radiology 162:31, 1987
5. Silver TM, Campbell D, Wicks JD, et al: Peritransplant fluid collections: Ultrasound evaluation and clinical significance. Radiology 138:145, 1981
6. Novick AC, Irish C, Steinmuller D, et al: The role of computerized tomography in renal transplant patients. J Urol 125:15, 1981
7. Nakstad P, Kolmannskog F, Kolbenstvedt A, Sodal G: Computed tomography in surgical complications following renal transplantation. J Comput Assist Tomogr 6:286, 1982
8. Bernardino ME, Baumgartner BR: Abscess drainage in the genitourinary tract. Radiol Clin North Am 24:539, 1986
9. Fuld IL, Matalon TA, Vogelzang RL, et al: Dynamic CT in the evaluation of physiologic status of renal transplants. AJR 142:1157, 1984
10. Delmonico FL, McKusick KA, Cosimi AB, Russell PS: Differentiation between renal allograft rejection and acute tubular necrosis by renal scan. AJR 128:625, 1977
11. Geisinger MA, Risus B, Jordan ML, et al: Magnetic resonance imaging of renal transplants. AJR 143:1229, 1984
12. Hricak H, Terrier F, Demas BE: Renal allografts: Evaluation by MR imaging. Radiology 159:435, 1986
13. Baumgartner BR, Nelson RC, Ball TI, et al: MR imaging of renal transplants. AJR 147:949, 1986
14. Tubman DE, Frick MP, Hanto DW: Lymphoma after organ transplantation: Radiologic manifestations in the central nervous system, thorax and abdomen. Radiology 149:625, 1983
15. Newhouse JH, Nickloff EL, Rogers JK: Loss of corticomedullary distinction in MR imaging of native kidneys: Specificity, etiology, and optimization of pulse sequences. Presented at the Seventy-third Scientific Assembly and Annual Meeting of the Radiological Society of North America, Chicago, November 1987
16. Lund G, Letourneau JG, Day DL, Crass JR: MRI in organ transplantation. Radiol Clin North Am 25:281, 1987

CASE NO. 1   Elliot K. Fishman

HEMATURIA AND PNEUMATURIA

A 50-year-old woman presented with a history of recent hematuria and pneumaturia. The patient had known Crohn's disease. A CT scan was done with select images shown in Figure 1A–C.

DISCUSSION

CT has been shown to be important in the evaluation of the complications of Crohn's disease.[1–4] Although barium studies are often satisfactory for the detection of fistulas, their extent as well as associated organ involvement often cannot be accurately defined on barium studies. CT has the advantage not only of being able to visualize the presence of a fistulous tract but to define its extension into adjacent muscle, bone, or viscera. This difference can be clearly shown in the evaluation of suspected enterovesical fistulas. Prior to CT scanning, the success rate for the detection of enterovesical fistulas was less than 50 percent regardless of the imaging modality used.

Standard radiographic techniques have proved of little value in the detection of enterovesical fistulas. Plain films show gas in the bladder in less than 30 percent of cases. On intravenous pyelography (IVP), a fistula is demonstrated in less than 18 percent of cases. Cystography will demonstrate only 35 percent of fistulas and barium enema 20 to 40 percent of cases. Proctosigmoidoscopy and cystoscopy will only visualize the fistulas in 20 to 50

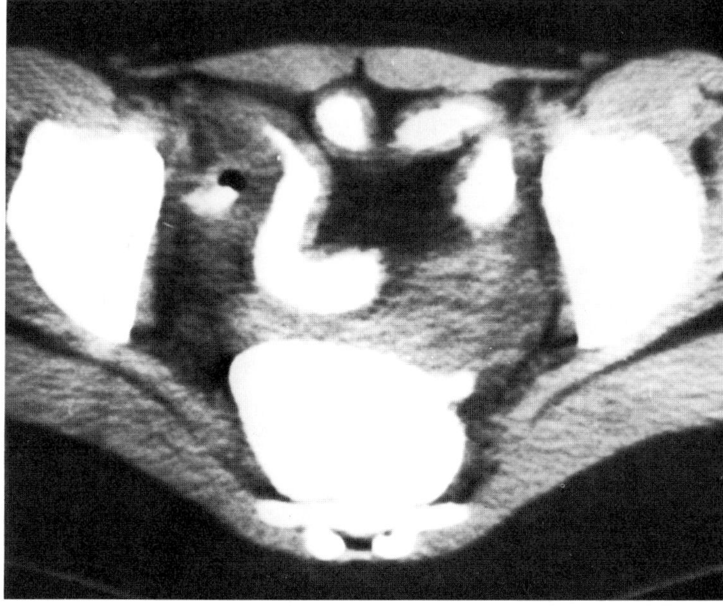

A

FIGURE 1   (A) CT scan demonstrating multiple thickened and inflamed small bowel loops. (*Figure continues.*)

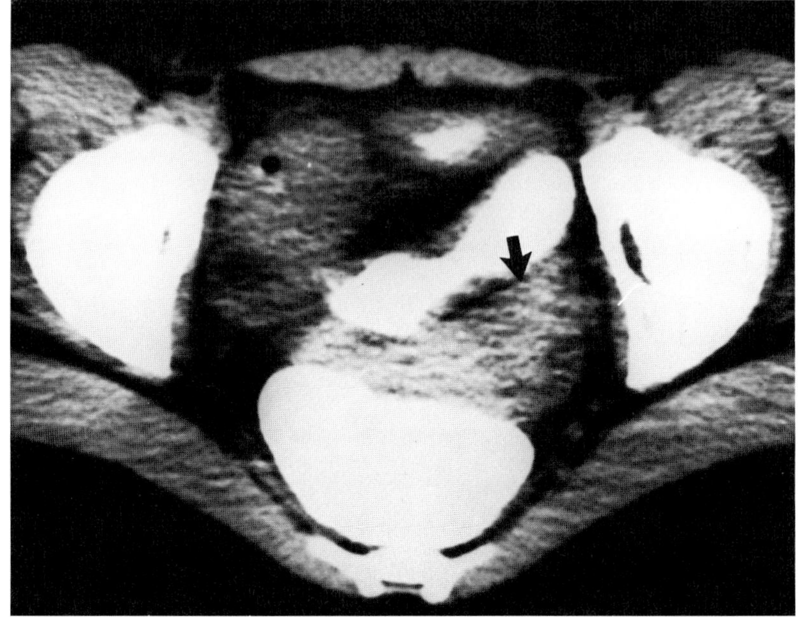

FIG. 1 (*Continued*). (B) Soft tissue mass with fistulous tract seen extending down into pelvic region (arrow). (C) Thickening of right bladder was noted as well as air in the bladder.

percent of cases. Using a carefully performed CT study, we have been able to detect the presence of an enterovesical fistula in more than 90 percent of cases.

The following CT criteria are used to diagnose the presence and nature of a colovesical fistula:

1. Air in the bladder in the absence of recent catheterization or infection
2. Demonstration of contrast material in the bladder without antecedent administration of intravenous contrast material
3. Fistulous tract between bowel and bladder
4. Focal bladder wall thickening usually adjacent to focal small or large bowel thickening
5. The presence of an abscess intervening between bowel and bladder wall
6. Direct adherence of inflamed bowel to bladder

Genitourinary complications of Crohn's disease include nephrolithiasis, hydroureteronephrosis, renal amyloidosis, cystitis, and ileoureteral fistula. These occur in 5 to 20 percent of patients with Crohn's disease. In a prior review of 275 consecutive patients with symptomatic Crohn's disease, we found 14 patients with bladder involvement. These included 10 patients with an enterovesical fistula.

In the present case, multiple thickened and inflamed small bowel loops were seen consistent with Crohn's disease. On following the downward sequence of images thickening of the anterior right bladder wall as well as air in the bladder is seen. This fistulous communication is seen anteriorly.

DIAGNOSIS:

Enterovesical fistulas in a patient with Crohn's colitis

REFERENCES

1. Merine DS, Fishman EK, Kuhlman JE, et al: Bladder involvement in Crohns disease: Role of CT in detection and evaluation. J Comput Assist Tomogr 13:90, 1989
2. Goldman SM, Fishman EK, Gatewood OMB, et al: CT in the diagnosis of enterovesicle fistulae. AJR 144:1229, 1985
3. Fishman EK, Wolf EJ, Jones B, et al: CT evaluation of Crohns disease: Effect of patient management. AJR 148:537, 1987
4. Goldman SM, Fishman EK, Gatewood OMB, et al: CT demonstration of colovesical fistulae secondary to diverticulitis. J Comput Assist Tomogr 8:462, 1984

CASE NO. 2   William J. Marasco

HYPERTENSION AND LEFT FLANK PAIN

A 68-year-old white man with medically treated hypertension presented with a 1-month history of intermittent left flank pain, radiating to his left lower quadrant. A diagnosis of diverticulitis was made clinically and the patient was started on Keflex. The patient's clinical symptoms failed to improve, and further workup revealed an elevated creatinine level. The patient was then referred for an intravenous pyelogram (IVP) (Fig. 1). A CT scan of the abdomen was then requested (Fig. 2).

DISCUSSION

The patient presented with a history of chronic abdominal pain without systemic signs. Coupled with the rising creatinine, primary or secondary renal disease was suspected. The IVP (Fig. 1) demonstrates obstruction of the left kidney with delayed function. Delayed films showed opacification of the left collecting system and medial deviation of the left ureter. Some of the common causes of renal obstruction are nephrolithiasis, ureteral compression due to intrinsic or extrinsic masses, and ureteral stricture. However, no obvious source of obstruction was found. Therefore, a CT scan was done for further evaluation of the left renal obstruction.

The CT scan revealed the upper aorta to be extensively calcified to the level of the mid-kidneys, where an associated soft tissue mass was seen involving the wall of the aorta (Fig.

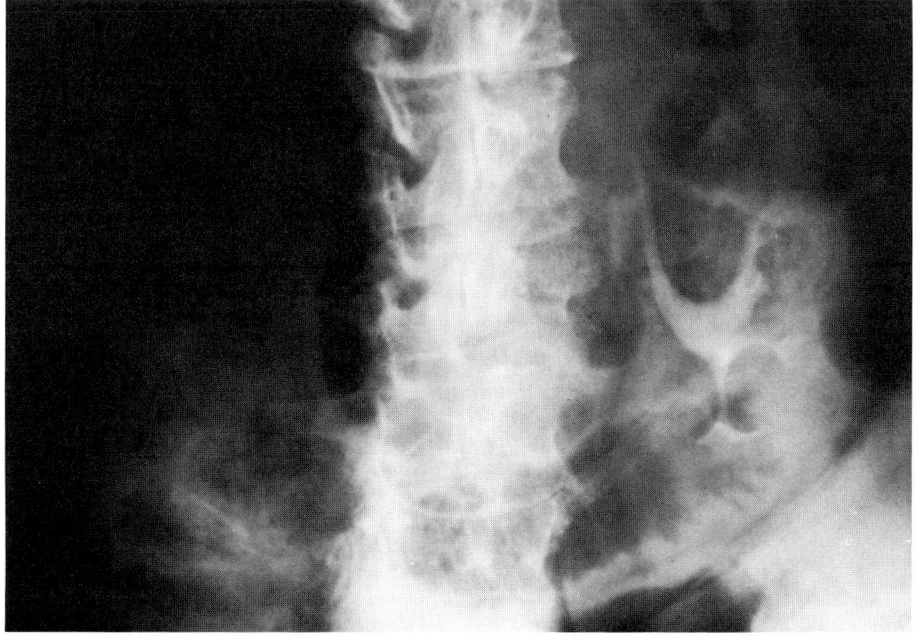

FIGURE 1   IVP demonstrates delayed function of the left kidney.

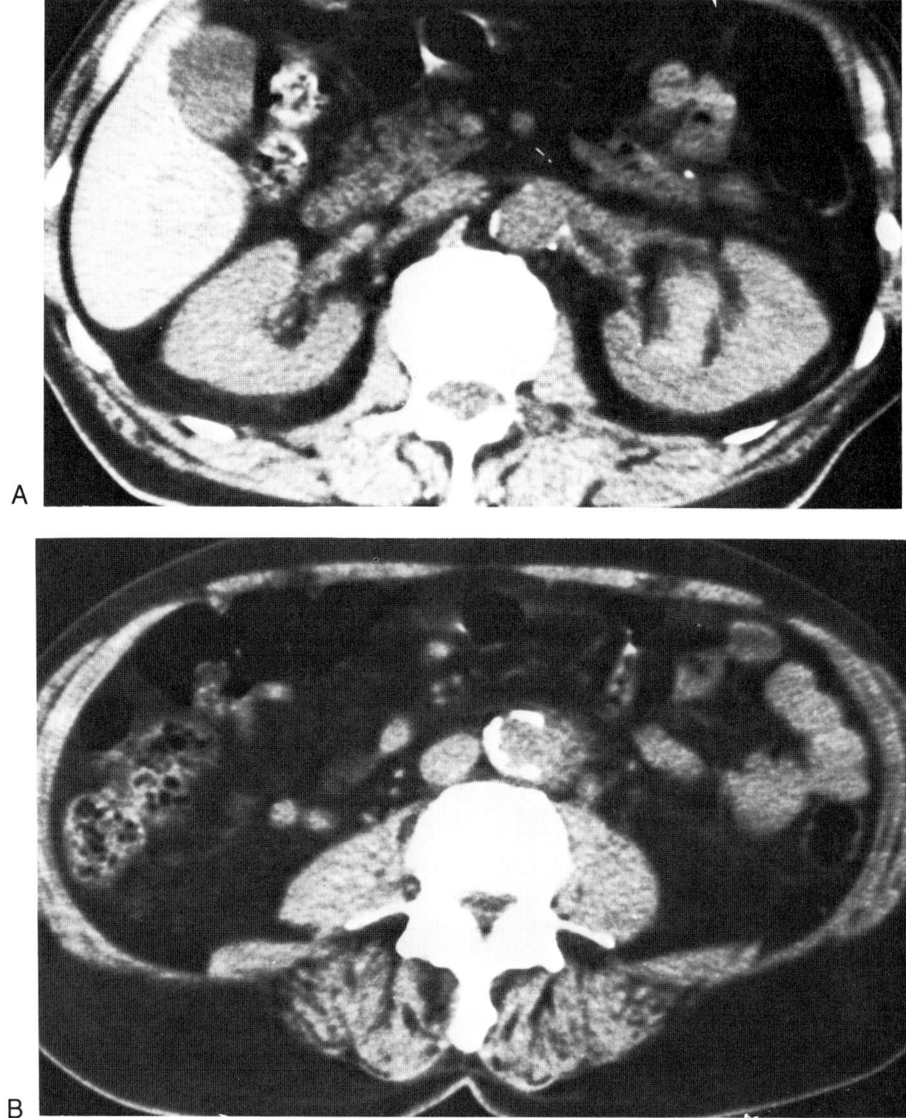

FIGURE 2   (A) Scan at level of left renal hilum demonstrates left hydronephrosis. (B) Scan at approximately L4 level demonstrates a soft tissue mass on left side of aorta. Note the break in the aortic calcification of the left side.

2). Hydronephrosis of the left kidney was also seen. Processes that can cause this appearance are retroperitoneal fibrosis (RPF), perianeurysmal inflammation, leaking or uncomplicated abdominal aneurysms, urinomas, prior radiation or malignant adenopathy.[1-3] The aorta was diffusely calcified, except for an area of the left side of the aorta, where an associated soft tissue mass was seen. Based on the clinical and radiographic findings, a diagnosis of retroperitoneal fibrosis with perianeurysmal fibrosis was made. The patient subsequently underwent surgery for repair of his abdominal aortic aneurysm.

Retroperitoneal fibrosis is a fibrotic process that most frequently involves the inferior aspect of the retroperitoneum. On histologic examination, RPF is composed of densely packed collagen fibers surrounded by inflammatory cells. The etiology is varied. The causes include methylsergide (Sansert) ingestion, irradiation, abdominal aortic aneurysms, metastases, desmoplastic reactions from primary neoplasms, extravasation from the urinary tract, retroperitoneal hemorrhage, previous surgery, diverticulitis, appendicitis, tuberculosis, brucellosis, syphilis, histoplasmosis, and trauma.[4] However, up to 70 percent of cases are categorized as idiopathic since no identified source can be found.[5]

Patients with RPF are mostly men, 40 to 70 years of age. The symptomatology is usually abdominal, pelvic, back, or flank pain. The diagnosis is often suggested by excretory urography by the characteristic medial deviation of the midureter and mild hydronephrosis.[4] CT scanning is a noninvasive method for diagnosing RPF. The CT findings include hydronephrosis, loss of clear delineation between the aorta and vena cava, and a soft tissue mass located in the midline anterior to the aorta and vena cava that can encircle either structure. The mass can envelop the ureter beginning medially and posteriorly but usually spares the anterolateral aspect of the involved ureter. Other causes for these retroperitoneal findings, such as lymphomas, primary retroperitoneal tumors, hematomas, and leaking abdominal aneurysms, can usually be excluded by the characteristic CT findings of these individual entities.[6]

Diagnosis:

Perianeurysmal retroperitoneal fibrosis

REFERENCES

1. Osmond JK: Bilateral ureteral obstruction due to envelopment and compression by an inflammatory retroperitoneal process. J Urol 59:1072, 1948
2. Kaude J: Retroperitoneal fibrosis. Acta Radiol [Diagn] (Stockh) 4:331, 1966
3. Stephens DH, Williamson B, Sheedy PF, et al: Computed tomography of the retroperitoneal space. Radiol Clin North Am 15:377, 1977
4. Lepor H, Walsh PC: Idiopathic retroperitoneal fibrosis. J Urol 1:1, 1979
5. Fagan CJ, Larrieu AJ, Amparo EG: Retroperitoneal fibrosis: Ultrasound and CT features. AJR 133:239, 1979
6. Feinstein RS, Olga M, Gatewood B, et al: Computerized tomography in the diagnosis of retroperitoneal fibrosis. J Urol 126:255, 1981

CASE NO. 3   Timothy J. Miller

INTERMITTENT ABDOMINAL PAIN

An 18-month-old white boy presented with a 7-week history of intermittent crampy abdominal pain associated with constipation and a 1-week history of poor urinary stream. A palpable mass was present in the lower abdomen. Ultrasound showed a large solid polypoid

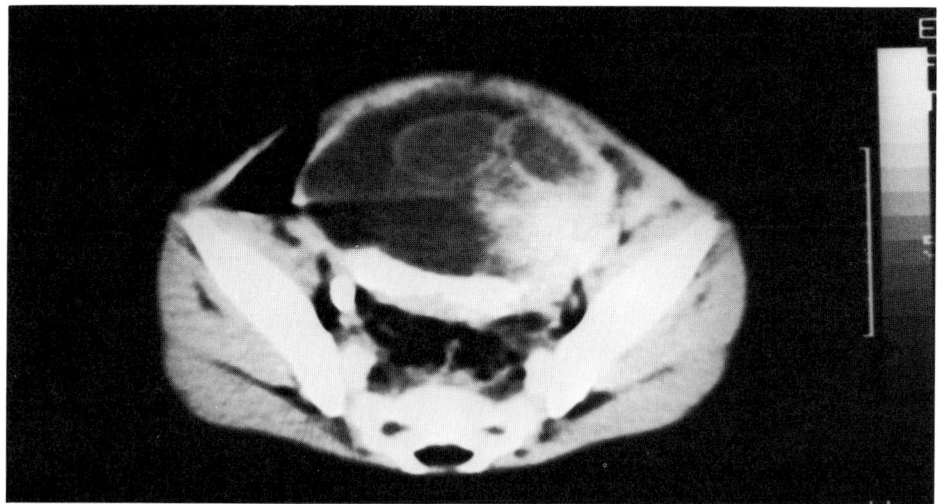

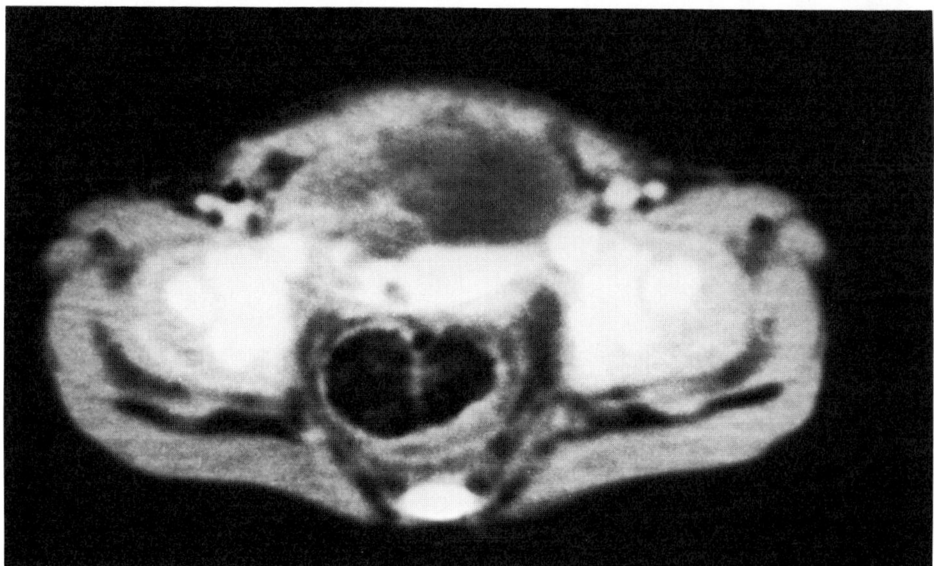

FIGURE 1 (A & B)   CT scans demonstrate lobulated mass arising from left wall of bladder. Also noted is associated bladder wall thickening.

bladder mass and bilateral hydronephrosis. A CT scan was done (Fig. 1). Tissue diagnosis was made by cystoscopy and biopsy.

DISCUSSION

Although rare, rhabdomyosarcoma is the commonest neoplasm of the lower urinary tract in children. Because of its polypoid, lobulated appearance, it is also called sarcoma botryoides (bunch of grapes). The tumor most often affects children between 2 and 5 years of age. It orginates in the vagina or bladder in girls or in the prostate, bladder, or urethra in boys. Rhabdomyosarcoma tends to metastasize early by direct invasion and via hematogenous and lymphatic spread.[1-3]

Usual clinical manifestions of rhabdomyosarcoma include hematuria, urinary retention, or other symptoms of urinary tract obstruction. The neoplasm may have an insidious onset and present with a large palpable mass.[2,3]

When a mass is discovered by physical examination or on another imaging study, such as excretory urogram, voiding cystourethrogram, or barium enema, an ultrasound can be the first choice for evaluation because it does not involve ionizing radiation. When ultrasound is equivocal or suggests a malignancy, CT is necessary to determine the extent of disease.[1,4-6]

The CT findings of rhabdomyosarcoma of the bladder include an intrinsic polypoid soft tissue mass with density readings similar to muscle usually originating in the inferior wall of the bladder. Large tumors may show central areas of necrosis. Calcifications are occasionally seen, and variable enhancement is present after administration of intravenous contrast. Direct invasion of adjacent structures, pelvic adenopathy, hydronephrosis, or distant metastatses to lung or liver may be seen on CT. Although less common, bladder tumors with an appearance similar to rhabdomyosarcoma include pheochromocytoma, neurofibroma, hemangioma, bladder wall invasion by leukemia or lymphoma, leioymosarcoma, or transitional cell carcinoma.[1,2,5,6]

Following surgical resection of at least part of the tumor, radiotherapy, and chemotherapy, the survival rate is 60 to 70 percent. Prognosis is worse when the tumor occurs in the first year of life.[2]

Diagnosis:

Rhabdomyosarcoma of bladder

REFERENCES

1. Lee JK, Sagel SS, Stanley RJ: Computed Body Tomography with MRI Correlation. Raven Press, New York, 1989
2. Silverman FN: Caffey's Pediatric X-ray Diagnosis. Year Book Medical Publishers, Chicago, 1985
3. McDougal WS, Persky L: Rhabdomyosarcoma of the bladder and prostate in children. J Urol 124:882, 1980
4. Eklof O, Brun B, Claessom I, et al: Tumours of the lower urinary tract in children. Acta Radiol [Diagn] (Stockh) 19:171, 1978
5. Siegel MJ, Glasier CM, Sagel SS: CT of pelvic disorders in children. AJR 137:1139, 1981
6. Carter B, Kahn P, Wolpert S, et al: Unusual pelvic masses: A comparison of computed tomographic and ultrasound. Radiology 121:383, 1976

CASE NO. 4   Steven H. Millmond

RIGHT FLANK MASS

A 46-year-old woman presented with hematuria. A right flank mass was appreciated on physical examination. An enhanced CT scan was performed (Fig. 1), revealing a large unilateral mass replacing the majority of the right kidney.

DISCUSSION

The CT scan revealed a large, unilateral multilocular mass composed of multiple cysts of variable size and attenuation values, separated from one another by thick-walled septae. Right nephrectomy specimen demonstrated the mass to be surrounded by a thick capsule, which when bisected, yielded cysts containing clear, turbid yellow, or bloody fluid. Pathologically, this was a *Multilocular Cystic Nephroma*.

Multilocular cystic nephroma (MLCN) is an uncommon renal neoplasm that is characterized by a large well-circumscribed mass that contains multiple noncommunicating fluid-filled locules.[1-4] The mass is usually solitary but rarely can be multiple. It predominantly affects male children and adult females. The lesion can present as a palpable mass, as new-onset hematuria, or as an incidental finding. MLCN is widely thought to represent either a benign tumor of the kidney, probably derived from metanephrogenic blastema, or a focal multicystic dysplasia.

Excretory urography with nephrotomography occasionally can reveal evidence of the septae with displaced collecting structures, accompanied by focal absence of the urographic nephrogram. Cysts can herniate into the pelvis, creating a smooth, round filling defect,

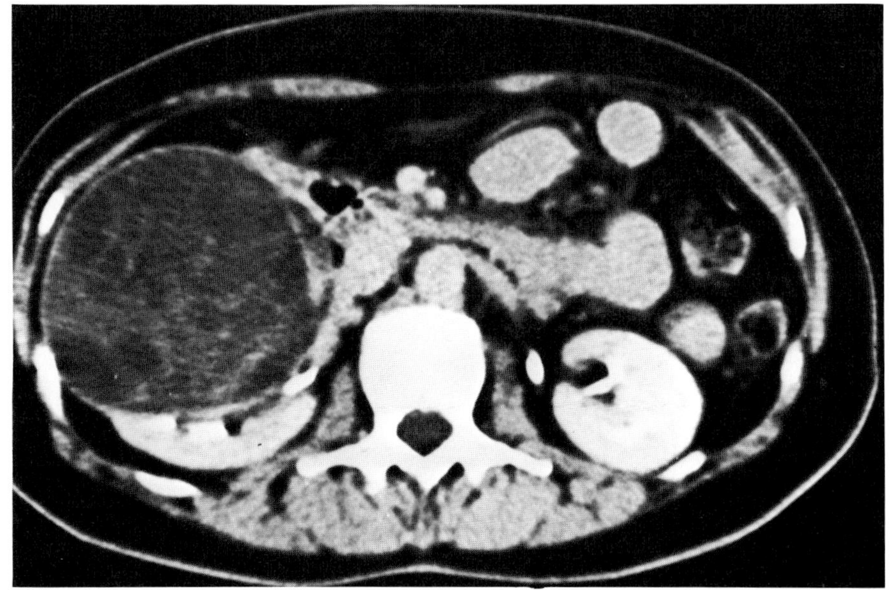

FIGURE 1   CT scan revealing a large unilateral mass replacing most of the right kidney.

sometimes causing obstruction. CT demonstrates a well-marginated mass, with an appearance as described in the case example above. The cysts have an attenuation value near water and varying upwards. Ultrasound reveals a sharply defined often septated mass containing components of anechoic and hyperechoic texture. Angiography reveals displacement of normal vessels by a mass of variable vascularity. The septae may occasionally be seen on the angiographic nephrogram. The differential diagnosis includes Wilms' tumor in children, renal cell carcinoma in adults (M>F), and *Echinococcus* cysts.

Diagnosis:

Multilocular cystic nephroma

REFERENCES

1. Madewell JE, Goldman SM, Davis CJ Jr, et al: Multilocular cystic nephroma: A radiographic-pathologic correlation of 58 patients. Radiology 146:309, 1986
2. Davidson AJ: Radiology of the Kidney, WB Saunders, Philadelphia, 1985, pp 383–386
3. Parienty RA, Pradel J, Imbert M-C, et al: Computed tomography of multilocular cystic nephroma. Radiology 140:135, 1981
4. Hartman DS, Davidson AJ: Renal cystic disease. AFIP Atlas of Radiologic-Pathologic Correlation, fascicle I. WB Saunders, Philadelphia, 1989

CASE NO. 5   Michael Hallowell

MASS IN A CYSTIC KIDNEY

A middle-aged man with a history of renal failure secondary to chronic glomerulonephritis presented with left flank pain. An unenhanced and enhanced CT of the abdomen was performed.

DISCUSSION

Cystic degeneration of the kidneys is a known complication in patients suffering from chronic renal failure.[1] The development of this entity, known as acquired renal cystic disease (ARCD), is related to the duration of chronic renal failure, and especially to the length of time the patient has been maintained on hemodialysis. Up to 79 percent of patients undergoing hemodialysis for more than 3 years may develop ARCD.[2] Similar findings have been observed in patients undergoing chronic peritoneal dialysis.[3]

Major complications of ARCD are hemorrhage and the development of renal tumors. Both benign and malignant tumors are known to occur in patients with ARCD; the reported incidence of renal cell carcinoma is 5.8 percent.[4] The size and CT appearance of these hypernephromas are quite variable. Detection and diagnosis of small lesions may be complicated by hemorrhage or distortion of the renal architecture caused by the presence of multiple cysts. It is now generally recommended that patients with end stage renal failure being maintained on dialysis have a baseline CT or ultrasound evaluation of the kidneys with periodic follow-up examinations.

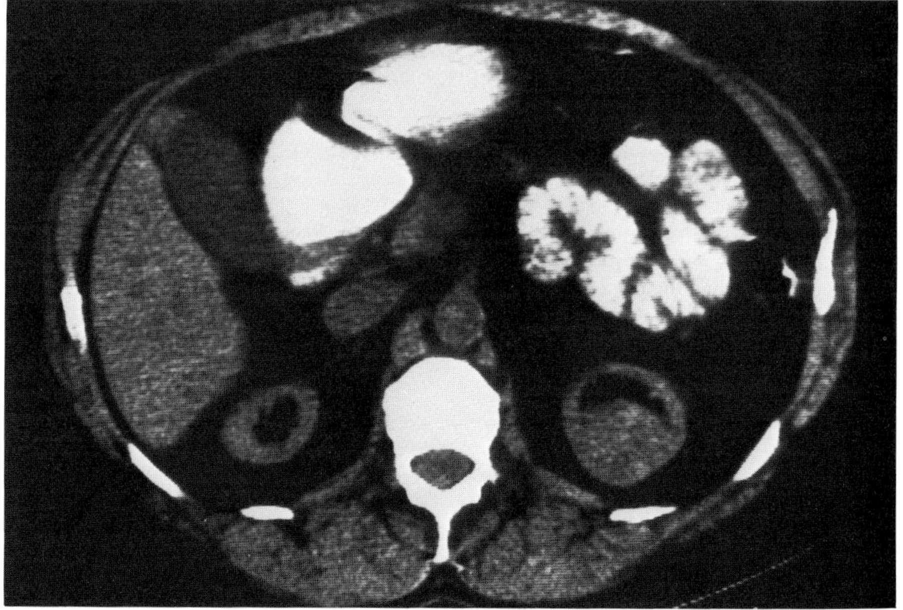

FIGURE 1   Unenhanced CT through the levels of the upper poles of the kidneys.

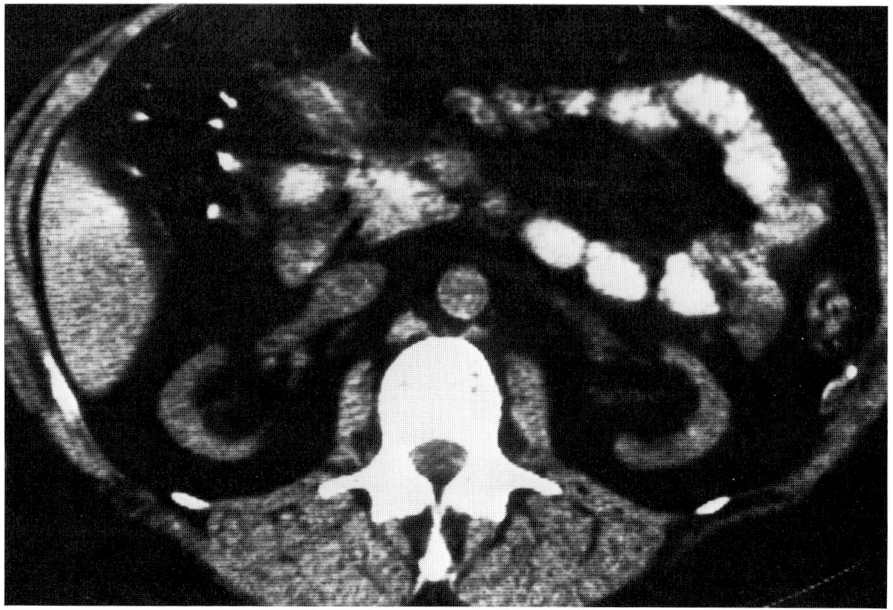

FIGURE 2   Contrast-enhanced CT at the level of the renal hila.

In the case presented here, CT shows a 4-cm mass arising from the upper pole of the left kidney. A radical nephrectomy was performed and a hypernephroma was diagnosed by pathologic examination.

Diagnosis:

Hypernephroma in acquired renal cystic disease

REFERENCES

1. Dunnill MS, Millared PR, Oliver D: Acquired cystic disease of the kidneys: A hazard of long-term intermittent haemodialysis. J Clin Pathol 30:868, 1977
2. Ishikawa I: Uremic acquired cystic disease of the kidney. Urology 26:101, 1985
3. Jabour BA, Ralls PW, Tang WW, et al: Acquired cystic disease of the kidneys computed tomography and ultrasonography appraisal in patients on peritoneal and hemodialysis. Invest Radiol 9:728, 1987
4. Hughson MD, Buchwald D, Fox M: Renal neoplasia and acquired cystic disease in patients receiving long term dialysis. Arch Pathol Lab Med 110:592, 1986

CASE NO. 6   Ron Khazan

ABNORMAL URINALYSIS IN TWO PATIENTS
WITH THE SAME ABNORMALITY

A 23-year-old man presented with progressive renal failure. Renal biopsy revealed membranous nephropathy (Fig. 1).

A 57-year-old woman presented with flank pain, hematuria, and proteinuria (Fig. 2).

DISCUSSION

Figures 1 and 2 demonstrate that the renal veins can be well visualized on transaxial CT and MRI scans. In addition, these modalities yield high contrast between thrombus and flowing blood, making them suitable direct noninvasive modalities for evaluation of possible renal vein thrombosis (RVT).

RVT is a relatively common complication of the nephrotic syndrome. In their prospective study, Lloch et al. noted a 22 percent incidence of RVT in nephrotic patients.[1] Most patients with RVT were asymptomatic and unable to recall any discrete episode of abdominal or flank pain.[2,3]

Anticoagulation[4] and even thrombolytic therapy[5–7] have been advocated in the treatment of RVT. Many modalities have been used to confirm this diagnosis in the past. Selective renal venography remains the most definitive examination[8] but, like renal arteriography, it is invasive and not suitable as a screening study. Intravenous urograms have been reported

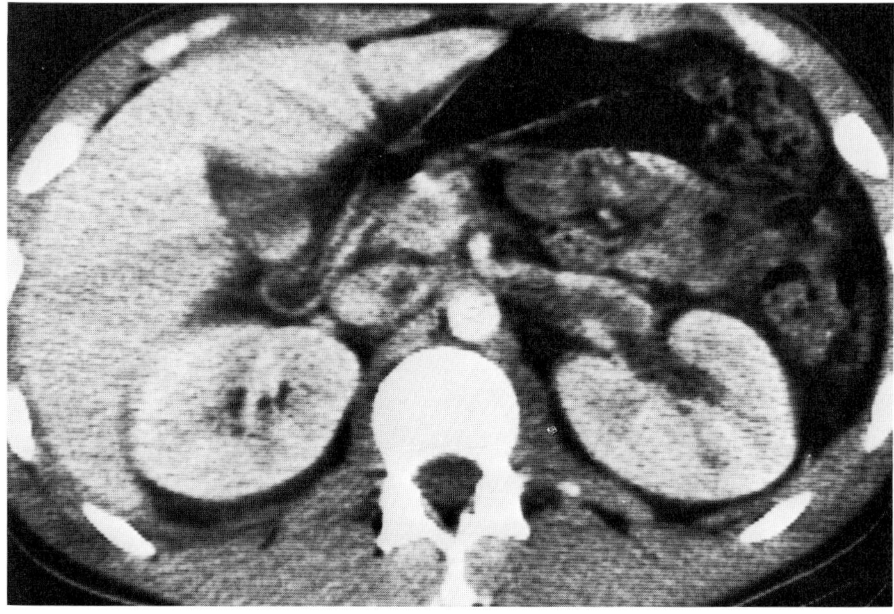

FIGURE 1   Contrast-enhanced CT scan through the level of the renal hila.

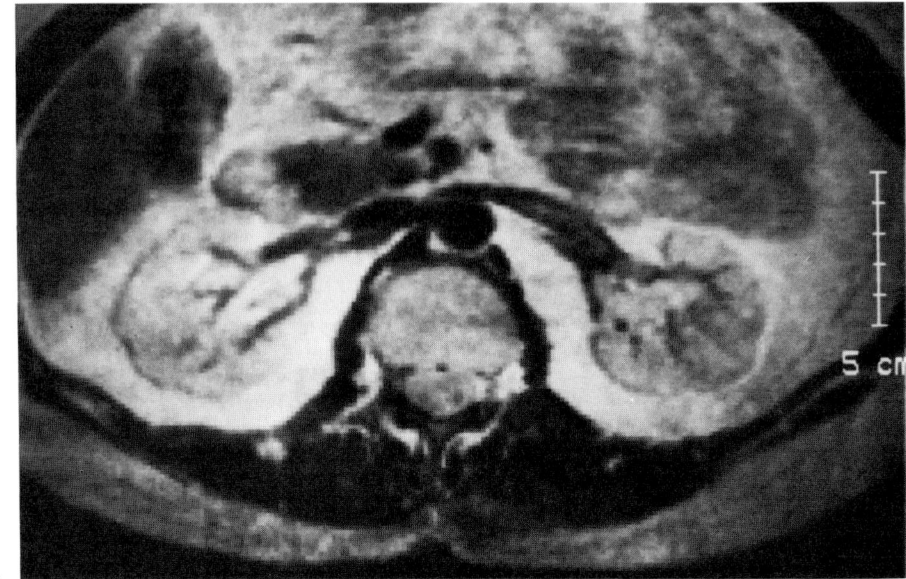

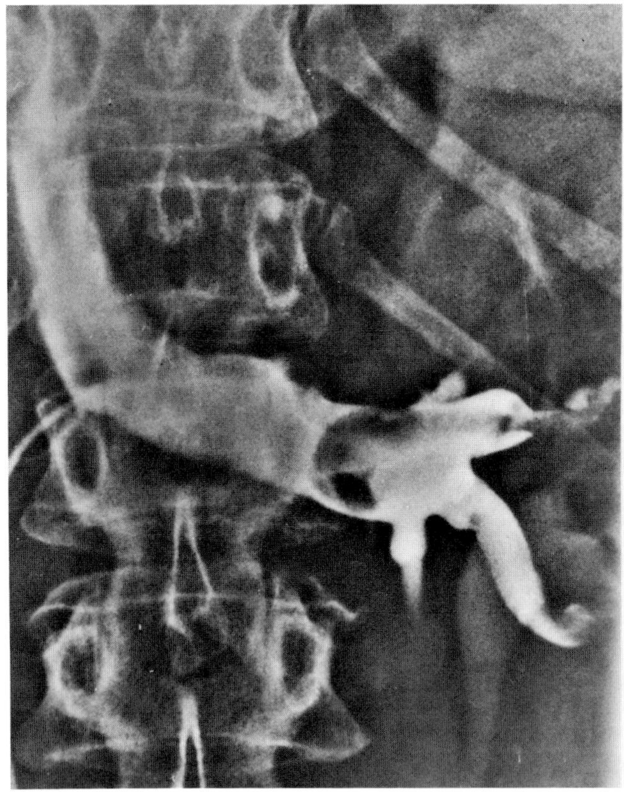

FIGURE 2 (A) Axial MRI scan through renal hila. (B) Renal venography confirming the abnormal finding on the MRI scan.

as negative in a large number of patients with RVT and are only suggestive or nonspecific in many others.[3,8,9]

Recently, CT has been used to visualize the thrombus within the renal veins as well as the frequently associated IVC thrombus.[10] MRI has also successfully detected RVT, as shown in the example presented here, as well as other case reports.[11] With the availability of multiplane imaging, as well as newer flow-sensitive imaging techniques, MRI may prove the most appropriate modality for noninvasive direct imaging of possible RVT.

REFERENCES

1. Llach F, Papper S, Massry SG: The clinical spectrum of renal vein thrombosis: Acute and chronic. Am J Med 69:819, 1980
2. McCarthy LJ, Titus JL, Daugherty GW: Bilateral renal-vein thrombosis and the nephrotic syndrome in adults. Ann Intern Med 58:837, 1963
3. Llach F, Koeffler A, Finch E, Massry SG: On the incidence of renal vein thrombosis in the nephrotic syndrome. Arch Intern Med 137:333, 1977
4. Balabanian MB, Schnetzler DE, Kaloyanides GJ: Nephrotic syndrome, renal vein thrombosis and renal failure: Report of a case with recovery of renal function, loss of proteinuria and dissolution of thrombus after anticoagulant therapy. Am J Med 54:768, 1973
5. Burrow CR, Walker WG, Bell WR, Gatewood OMB: Streptokinase salvage of renal function after renal vein thrombosis. Ann Intern Med 100:237, 1984
6. DiMarco PL, Sheinfeld J, Gutierrez OH, Cockett ATK: Direct fibrinolytic therapy for renal vein thrombosis: Radiographic follow-up. J Urol 132:966, 1984
7. Robinson JM, Cockrell CH, Tisnado J, et al: Selective low-dose streptokinase infusion in the treatment of acute transplant renal vein thrombosis. Cardiovasc Intervent Radiol 9:86, 1986
8. Clark RA, Colley DP: Radiological evaluation of renal vein thrombosis. CRC Crit Rev Diagn Imaging 13:337, 1980
9. Mulhern CB, Arger PH, Miller WT, Chait A: The specificity of renal vein thrombosis. AJR 125:291, 1975
10. Glazer GM, Francis RK, Gross BH, Amendola MA: Computed tomography of renal vein thrombosis. J Comput Assist Tomogr 8:288, 1984
11. Honda H, Yuh WTC, Lu CC: Magnetic resonance imaging of renal vein and inferior vena cava thrombosis in a patient with glomerulonephritis: A case report. Comput Tomogr 12:147, 1988

Index

Page numbers followed by f refer to figures; those followed by t indicate tables.